# ORAL ONCOLOGY



edited by I. VAN DER WAAL
G. B. SNOW

1984
MARTINUS NIJHOFF PUBLISHING
A MEMBER OF THE KLUWER ACADEMIC PUBLISHERS GROUP
BOSTON/THE HAGUE/DORDRECHT/LANCASTER

Softcover reprint of the hardcover 1st edition 1984



Distributors:

for North America

Kluwer Academic Publishers
190 Old Derby Street
Hingham, MA 02043

for all other countries

Kluwer Academic Publishers Group
Distribution Centre
P.O. Box 322
3300 AH Dordrecht
The Netherlands

**Library of Congress Cataloging in Publication Data**
Main entry under title:

Oral oncology.

(Developments in oncology)
Includes index.
1. Mouth—Cancer. I. Waal, I. van der. II. Snow,
G. B. III. Series. [DNLM: 1. Mouth neoplasms—Pathology.
2. Mouth neoplasms—Therapy. 3. Mouth rehabilitation.
4. Precancerous conditions. WU 280 0656]
RC280.M60748 1984 616.99'431 84-1524

ISBN-13: 978-1-4612-9796-3 e-ISBN-13: 978-1-4613-2845-2
DOI: 10.1007/978-1-4613-2845-2

# ORAL ONCOLOGY

# DEVELOPMENTS IN ONCOLOGY

F.J. Cleton and J.W.I.M. Simons, eds. Genetic Origins of Tumour Cells. 90-247-2272-1

J. Aisner and P. Chang, eds. Cancer Treatment Research. 90-247-2358-2

B.W. Ongerboer de Visser, D.A. Bosch and W.M.H. van Woerkom-Eykenboom, eds. Neuro-oncology: Clinical and Experimental Aspects. 90-247-2421-X

K. Hellman, P. Hilgard and S. Eccles, eds. Metastasis: Clinical and Experimental Aspects. 90-247-2424-4

H.F. Seigler, ed. Clinical Management of Melanoma. 90-247-2584-4

P. Correa and W. Haenszel, eds. Epidemiology of Cancer of the Digestive Tract. 90-247-2601-8

L.A. Liotta and I.R. Hart, eds. Tumour Invasion and Metastasis. 90-247-2611-5

J. Bánóczy, ed. Oral Leukoplakia. 90-247-2655-7

C. Tijssen, M. Halprin and L. Endtz, eds. Familial Brain Tumours. 90-247-2691-3

F.M. Muggia, C.W. Young and S.K. Carter, eds. Anthracycline Antibiotics in Cancer. 90-247-2711-1

B.W. Hancock, ed. Assessment of Tumour Response. 90-247-2712-X

D.E. Peterson and S.T. Sonis, eds. Oral Complications of Cancer Chemotherapy. 0-89838-563-6

R. Mastrangelo, D.G. Poplack and R. Riccardi, eds. Central Nervous System Leukemia. Prevention and Treatment. 0-89838-570-9

A. Polliack, ed. Human Leukemias. Cytochemical and Ultrastructural Techniques in Diagnosis and Research. 0-89838-585-7

W. Davis, C. Maltoni and S. Tanneberger, eds. The Control of Tumor Growth and its Biological Bases. 0-89838-603-9

A.P.M. Heintz, C.Th. Griffiths and J.B. Trimbos, eds. Surgery in Gynecological Oncology. 0-89838-604-7

M.P. Hacker, E.B. Douple and I. Krakoff, eds. Platinum Coordination Complexes in Cancer Chemotherapy. 0-89838-619-5

M.J. van Zwieten. The Rat as Animal Model in Breast Cancer Research: A Histopathological Study of Radiation- and Hormone-Induced Rat Mammary Tumor. 0-89838-624-1

B. Löwenberg and A. Hagenbeek, eds. Minimal Residual Disease in Acute Leukemia. 0-89838-630-6

## CONTENTS

## CONTRIBUTING AUTHORS

Mario Altini
Senior Lecturer
Department of Oral Pathology
School of Pathology
University of the Witwatersrand and South
African Institute for Medical Research
Johannesburg, SOUTH AFRICA

Jolan Bánóczy
Department of Conservative Dentistry
Faculty of Dentistry
Semmelweis Medical University
Mikszath Kalman ter 5
H-1088 Budapest, HUNGARY

Joseph R. Bertino
American Cancer Society Professor of Medicine
and Pharmacology
Yale University School of Medicine
333 Cedar Street
New Haven, Connecticut 06510, USA

J. Conley
2111 Central Park West
New York, NY 10024, USA

B. J. Cummings
The Princess Margaret Hospital
500 Sherbourne Street
Toronto, Ontario M4X 1K9, CANADA

S. E. W. Engels
Associate Professor and Head
Department of Maxillofacial Prosthodontics
Free University Hospital
1117 de Boelelaan
1007 MB Amsterdam, THE NETHERLANDS

R. B. Lucas
Emeritus Professor of Oral Pathology
University of London
Leicester Square
London, WC2H 7LJ, UNITED KINGDOM

J. J. Pindborg
Professor and Head
The Royal Dental College Copenhagen
Dept. of Oral Pathology
3C Blegdamsvej
DK-2200 Copenhagen, DENMARK

Susan W. Pitman
Assistant Professor of Medicine
Yale University School of Medicine
333 Cedar Street
New Haven, Connecticut 06510, USA

Mervyn Shear
Professor and Head
Department of Oral Pathology
University of the Witwatersrand and South African Institute for Medical Research
Johannesburg, SOUTH AFRICA

G. B. Snow
Professor and Head
Department of Otolaryngology
Free University Hospital
1117 de Boelelaan
1007 MB Amsterdam, THE NETHERLANDS

A. C. Thackray
Emeritus Professor of Morbid Histology
University of London
Leicester Square
London, WC2H 7LJ, UNITED KINGDOM

R. M. Tiwari
Associate Professor
Department of Otolaryngology
Free University Hospital
1117 de Boelelaan
1007 MB Amsterdam, THE NETHERLANDS

I. van der Waal
Professor and Head
Department of Oral Pathology
Free University Hospital
1117 de Boelelaan
1007 MB Amsterdam, THE NETHERLANDS

## PREFACE

A multidisciplinary approach to the problems related to the diagnosis, treatment, and rehabilitation of patients with oral cancer and precancer is reflected in the various specialties of the authors who contributed to this book. Today, patients with tumors of the oral cavity are dealt with preferably by a team of specialists who have been properly trained in the field of oncology, who have learned to appreciate each other's knowledge and experience, and who are able to operate as an integrated team.

This book is intended for use by every physician and dentist involved in the diagnosis and management of oral cancer. It is presented in such a way as to be useful for both the physician in training as well as the specialist in the field of head and neck oncology. The text concentrates on the common as well as the unusual aspects. For those who look for more detailed information, an extensive list of references is provided at the end of each chapter.

It should be emphasized that treatment policies may vary not only in different parts of the world, but also from institution to institution, depending on the expertise of the members of the oncologic team and the available facilities.

I. VAN DER WAAL AND G. B. SNOW, editors.

# I. DIAGNOSIS

The four chapters in part I discuss the clinical and histological aspects of tumors of the oral mucosa, jaws, and the salivary glands. They are all written by scientists who have a high repute for valuable and original contributions in their fields

Tumors of oral mucosa, jaws, and salivary glands are areas characterized by a vivid scientific activity in recent years both with regard to clinical aspects and histopathological features. This fact is documented by the extensive bibliographies accompanying the chapters.

All six authors have succeeded in giving a comprehensive but still succinct and readable state-of-the-art in their respective fields.

When one compares just 25 years ago with the content of these four chapters, one is astonished to see how much progress has been made. The progress has led to an improvement in our diagnostic capabilities and thereby to a better service to our patients.

JENS J. PINDBORG

# 1. CLINICAL AND HISTOPATHOLOGICAL ASPECTS OF PREMALIGNANT LESIONS

JOLÁN BÁNÓCZY

## 1. INTRODUCTION

Carcinoma of the oral cavity may be associated with or preceded by lesions that carry a serious risk of malignant changes. These so-called precancerous lesions may precede the development of carcinoma by months or by years. The WHO has defined a precancerous *lesion* as "a morphologically altered tissue in which cancer is more likely to occur than in its apparently normal counterpart," whereas a premalignant *condition* is defined as "a generalized state associated with a significantly increased risk of cancer" [1]. According to the present viewpoints, the following pathological lesions and conditions are considered premalignant: leukoplakia, erythroplakia, and submucous fibrosis.

Although the removal of oral pigmented nevi has often been recommended because of possible malignant transformation, insufficient data are available to substantiate that recommendation [2,3]. Therefore, no further attention will be paid to pigmented nevi in this chapter.

## 2. LEUKOPLAKIA

Leukoplakia is considered to be the most frequent precancerous change of the mouth. The lesion was first described in the second half of the last century by

A more detailed treatise on the subject of oral leukoplakia has been published by the author of this chapter in 1982 [107].

*I. van der Waal and G.B. Snow (eds), ORAL ONCOLOGY.* 

the Hungarian dermatologist Schwimmer [4]. The concept of oral leukoplakia has been subject to many variations in the course of time, with different authors employing the term either in a clinical or histological sense. Recently, the WHO recommended that the term *leukoplakia* should carry no histologic connotation and should be used in a clinical descriptive sense only [5], meaning a white patch on the oral mucosa that cannot be removed by rubbing and that cannot be classified clinically or pathologically as any other diagnosable disease (lichen planus, candidiasis, white sponge nevus, migratory glossitis, discoid lupus erythematosus, morsicatio buccarum). The use of this term is unrelated to the absence or presence of histological dysplasia.

Although leukoplakia has been known for more than a hundred years, interest has been focused on this premalignant lesion mainly in the last 20 to 30 years.

## 2.1. Epidemiology

The incidence and prevalence of oral leukoplakia has been investigated in rather few countries [6,7,8]. The first epidemiological investigations in Europe were performed by Bruszt [9], who reported data from 5,613 persons over 14 years of age living in seven villages of Hungary and found leukoplakia in 3.6% of the inhabitants. The data of Axéll [10], with 3.2% in city inhabitants, are very similar to these numbers. Rough epidemiological data of unselected populations (table 1–1) show a frequency that varies between 0.4 and 11.7%, of which the higher values were found in New Guinea and India.

The onset of leukoplakia is generally after the 40th year. However, the peak incidence of leukoplakia lies above the age of 50 years [24,25]. The development of carcinoma from leukoplakia has been observed in somewhat older age groups, with a peak incidence over 60 years. This observation points to the fact that leukoplakia is a chronic lesion. Its malignant transformation takes a rather long time from the clinical diagnosis to the development of carcinoma, which emphasizes the importance of early diagnosis.

The sex distribution generally shows a higher involvement of the male sex. In most studies a male-female ratio of about 3 to 1 or 2 to 1 has been demonstrated, findings that may be correlated with a higher occurrence of etiologic factors, especially that of smoking in men.

## 2.2. Etiologic factors

In the etiology of oral leukoplakia, the following factors have been reported to play a role: smoking, mechanical irritants, alcohol, electrical potential differences, Candida albicans infection, and chronic alterations of the oral mucosa due to syphilis, anaemia (sideropenic dysphagia), and submucous fibrosis. In this respect syphilis, sideropenic dysphagia, and submucous fibrosis are considered to be precancerous conditions.

The etiological role of smoking in connection with oral leukoplakia has been considered from two different viewpoints: (1) the effect of tobacco on the oral

**Table 1–1.** Epidemiological data on the prevalence of leukoplakia

| Author | Year | Country | Number of examined persons | Examined population | Occurrence of leuko-plakia in percentage |
|---|---|---|---|---|---|
| Gerry et al. [11] | 1952 | Guatemala | 2,004 | rural | 0.4 |
| Mehta et al. [12] | 1961 | India | 4,734 | urban | 3.5 |
| Bruszt [9] | 1962 | Hungary | 5,613 | rural | 3.6 |
| Atkinson et al. [6] | 1964 | New Guinea | 3,996 | rural | 8.1 |
| Pindborg et al. [13,14,15] | 1965 a,b 1966 | India | 30,000 | urban | 1.5–3.3 |
| Zachariah et al. [16] | 1966 | India | 10,000 | urban | 2.4 |
| Pindborg, Barmes, Roed-Petersen [17] | 1968 | New Guinea | 1,266 | rural | 4.6 |
| Bánóczy, Radnai, Reményi [18] | 1969 | Hungary | 16,332 | rural | 0.57 |
| Wahi, Mital [9] | 1970 | India | 7,286 | rural | 5.2 |
| Mehta et al. [19] | 1969 | India | 50,915 | rural | 0.2–4.9 |
| Gangadarhan, Paymaster [20] | 1971 | India | 203,249 | urban | 0.7 |
| Sonkodi, Tóth [21] | 1973 | Hungary | 1,071 | urban | 1.21 |
| Axéll [10] | 1975 | Sweden | 8,696 | urban | 3.2 |
| Silverman et al. [22] | 1976 | India | 57,518 | urban | 11.7 |
| Wilsch et al. [23] | 1978 | Germany | 4,000 | urban | 2.2 |

mucosa in causing leukoplakia and (2) the effect related to the malignisation of leukoplakia, which will be discussed separately [1,8]. Investigators have supported the etiological role of smoking, with the majority having performed clinical longitudinal studies on large populations of patients [7,26,27]. Clinical, cytological, and histological investigations have proven the hyperkeratosis-inducing effect of smoking on the oral mucosa. The development and location of the lesion seemed to be related to the category of smoking habit and to the quantity of tobacco consumed [28]. The ratio of smokers in oral leukoplakia patients was significantly higher than in control groups and related to the amount of cigarettes consumed and to the duration of smoking [23,27]. Roed-Petersen et al. [29] observed that sex differences in the distribution of oral leukoplakia were correlated with smoking habits. Following the cessation of smoking, many leukoplakias showed regression.

In India special correlation has been found between tobacco habits and occurrence and site of leukoplakia. "Bidi" smoking causes lesions, particularly in the commissures and on the buccal mucosa; different tobacco habits cause various characteristics of lesions [12,19,30]. Leukoplakia of the lower lip in man is commonly related to pipe smoking; Pindborg, Roed-Petersen, and

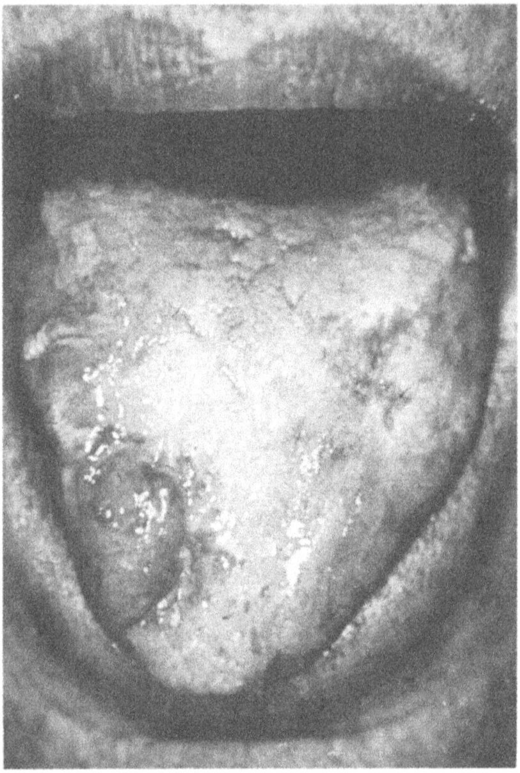

**Figure 1–1.** Carcinoma developed on the tongue of a 50-year-old, heavy smoker and alcoholic man, who has been aware of his leukoplakia for 20 years.

Renstrup [31] reported the association of leukoplakia of the floor of the mouth with cheroot smoking.

*Chronic mechanical irritation* by carious, broken teeth and/or ill-fitted bridges or dentures had been believed to cause oral leukoplakia. Indeed, a high incidence of mechanical factors could be demonstrated, especially in those cases having undergone malignant transformation [27].

*Alcohol consumption* in itself is not believed to cause leukoplakia, but by causing and sustaining chronic inflammation of the oral mucosa, it may act as a predisposing factor (figure 1–1).

*Electrogalvanism* as an etiologic factor in oral leukoplakia has been described as early as in 1932 by Lain [32] and Ullmann [33]. Although not very frequently noted, the presence of electrical potential differences should not be neglected, even today, with special regard to their role in the process of malignisation. Electrogalvanism has been found to occur rather often in carcinoma cases developed from oral leukoplakia [27]. In a Hungarian-Danish collabora-

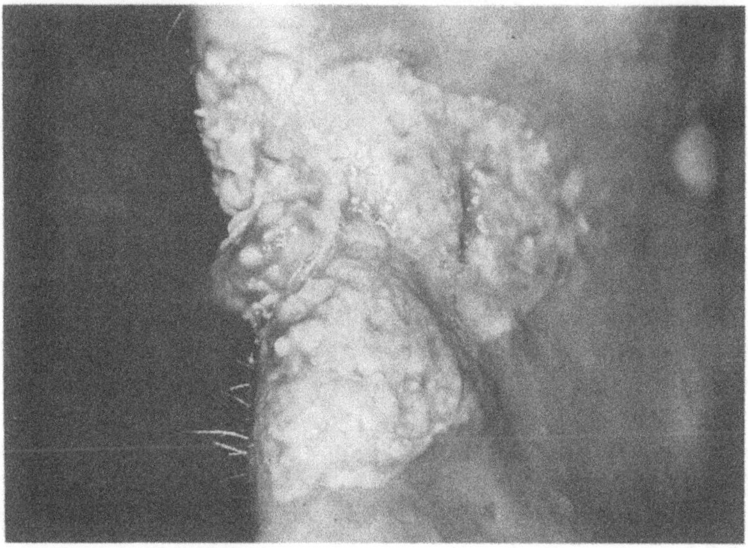

**Figure 1–2.** Nodular leukoplakia with Candida albicans infection in the commissure.

tive study, the data of 1,128 leukoplakia patients were analyzed; among them were found 16 patients whose lesions could be attributed to electrogalvanism. Malignant transformation developed in 4 of these 16 cases, a rather high ratio that is indicative of the importance of electrogalvanism as a cofactor [34].

The possibility of a relationship between *Candida infection* and oral leukoplakia was shown by Jepsen and Winther [35] in 1965, who found Candida hyphae in 39% of their leukoplakia patients. Since then several studies have supported this concept, with findings of Candida albicans in 6.8 to 31% of their leukoplakia patients [27,36,37,38,39]; a high occurrence of epithelial dysplasia in Candida-leukoplakias was also reported. The suspicion of Candida infection arises in cases of erosive or speckled leukoplakia, with a typical clinical appearance (figure 1–2). Candida cultures and histology by PAS staining, with Candida hyphae in the epithelium, are conclusive evidence. The frequent association of Candida infection with aforementioned clinical types was observed by Renstrup [37], who found Candida in 61% of erosive leukoplakias.

Antimycotic treatment often leads to total or partial disappearance of the lesions. Regression of "high-risk" leukoplakias has been observed by several investigators after antimycotic treatment: the speckled type of leukoplakia changed to homogeneous [35], and the erosive leukoplakia transformed into the simplex type [40].

Some decades ago *syphilis* was considered the most important etiologic agent in leukoplakia. In this respect the syphilitic glossitis was brought into connection with the development of oral leukoplakia, when the chronic inflammatory state of the tongue might have acted as predisposing factor. Recent data, however, do not support the importance of the etiologic role of syphilis, although in some cases it might act as a cofactor.

Mucosal changes associated with *anaemia* are not infrequent. Hunter-glossitis often accompanies the pernicious type of anaemia. Well known are the atrophic inflammatory changes of the tongue and oral mucosa in sideropenic dysphagia, which constitute a part of the so-called *Plummer-Vinson* or *Paterson-Kelly* syndrome. Concerning the latter, in Scandinavian countries a positive correlation has been demonstrated with the development of oral leukoplakia caused by other local irritants.

The oral mucosal changes of *submucous fibrosis*, experienced mainly in India, might act also in favor of the development of oral leukoplakia. This condition will be discussed later in this chapter.

The above-mentioned factors may all contribute as predisposing or inducing cofactors to the development of oral leukoplakia, but today the important etiological agents are considered to be smoking and Candida albicans infection.

**2.3. Site of leukoplakia in the oral cavity**

Leukoplakia may develop anywhere in the oral cavity. The most frequent locations are the commissures and the buccal mucosa. There are, however, geographical differences related to habits (smoking and chewing habits) and other possible etiological factors.

For the systemic and standardized recording of the different sites, a topographical scheme by Roed-Petersen and Renstrup [42] has been proposed which facilitates the exact classification and makes comparisons possible between different reports. This classification is also used in the *WHO Oral Mucosa Manual* [43] (see figure 2–18). Studies using this topographical classification scheme found a prevalence of leukoplakia in 62.8% of the cases in the commissures and buccal mucosa [27] (table 1–2). In these locations leukoplakia occurs often on both sides in a symmetrical form (figures 1–2, 1–3, 1–4). Other frequent locations are the tongue (figures 1–1, 1–5), hard palate, lips (figure 1–6), and floor of the mouth. A leukoplakia is not very often located on the alveolar ridge and soft palate and very rarely affects the gingiva.

The distribution of leukoplakia shows differences according to sex and habits. Leukoplakia of the lip, especially of the lower lip, has been found more often in men, whereas leukoplakia of the tongue is seen more frequently in women. These differences might be explained by etiological factors. Studies from India [44] have shown that most of the labial mucosa leukoplakias are associated with the habit of hookli smoking; the short stem of the hookli may be responsible for the lesion. In Europe the leukoplakia of the lower lip in pipe smokers is well known, as is the development of labial leukoplakia on the basis

**Table 1–2.** Distribution of leukoplakia and carcinoma developed from leukoplakia according to site

| Location | Percentage of leukoplakia (670 cases) | Percentage of carcinoma (40 cases) |
|---|---|---|
| Commissures | 37.5 | 7.5 |
| Buccal mucosa | 25.3 | 12.5 |
| Lips | 6.8 | 15.0 |
| Tongue | 8.2 | 37.5 |
| Hard palate | 8.5 | 5.0 |
| Soft palate | 1.3 | 2.5 |
| Floor of mouth | 5.7 | 12.5 |
| Alveolar ridge | 6.7 | 7.5 |
| Total | 100.0 | 100.0 |

From reference 27.

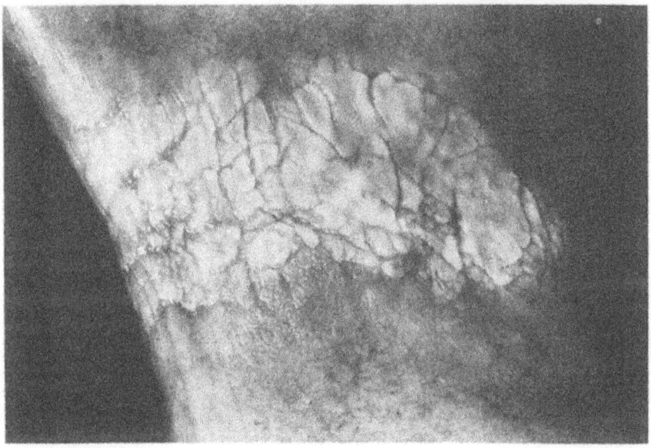

**Figure 1–3.** Leukoplakia simplex located in the commissure of the mouth: the oral mucosa is thickened, whitish.

of an actinic cheilitis in outdoor workers. In India studies found that leukoplakias associated with bidi smoking show a preference for the commissures and those associated with chewing habits are more likely to occur on the buccal mucosa. Leukoplakias of the hard palate are generallly reported in India to be associated with the habit of reverse smoking, while in Europe that are found especially in patients with ill-fitting dentures. Floor of the mouth leukoplakia is exceptional in India, but occurs frequently in Western countries. The higher prevalence of the tongue site in women might be related to the frequent occurrence of precancerous conditions such as anaemia and sideropenic dysphagia in some countries, which favor the development of leukoplakia.

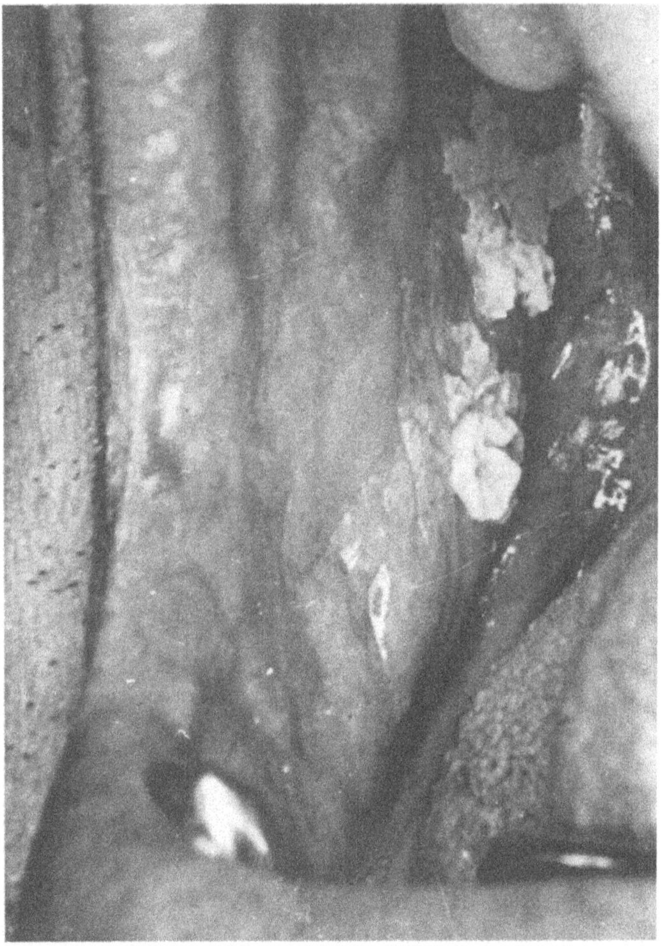

**Figure 1-4.** Verrucous leukoplakia: strongly elevated proliferations on the buccal mucosa caused by mechanical irritation of bad dentures.

### 2.4. Clinical aspects

Several classifications have been recommended to differentiate clinical types within the "white patch" symptom of the oral mucosa. The etiological-nosological classification of Hornstein [45,46] divides leukoplakias into two groups: leukoplakias in the broad sense (so-called hereditary and endogenous-irritative leukoplakias) and leukoplakias in the narrow sense (so-called exogenous-irritative and precancerous leukoplakias). Other classifications consider histopathological characteristics. However, based on the clinical appearance of leukoplakia, two classifications are generally accepted and used.

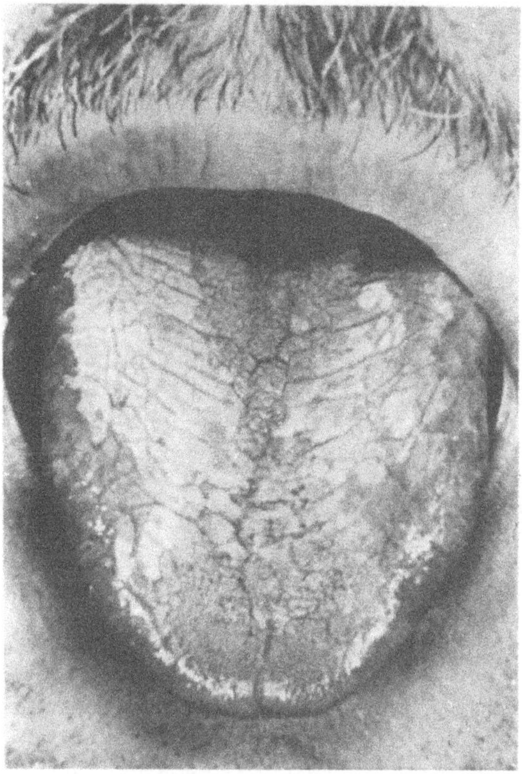

**Figure 1–5.** Simplex and verrucous leukoplakia on the dorsal surface of the tongue: homogeneous, thickened, elevated white areas with wrinkled surface; the patient was a heavy cigarette smoker.

Sugár and Bánóczy [47,48] distinguished three clinical types of oral leukoplakia:

Type I: *Leukoplakia simplex*: white, homogeneous keratinized lesion, slightly elevated from the surface of the oral mucosa (figures 1–3, 1–6).
Type II: *Leukoplakia verrucosa*: white, verrucous proliferations with wrinkled surface (figures 1–4, 1–5).
Type III: *Leukoplakia erosiva*: white lesions with erythematous areas, erosions, fissures (figure 1–2).

Pindborg et al. [49] differentiate two main groups according to the clinical appearance:

1. *Homogeneous* type of leukoplakia—a white patch with variable appearance:

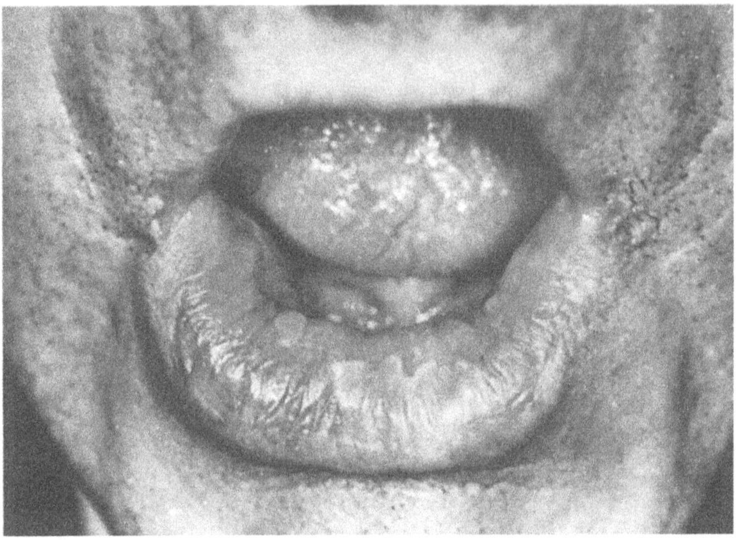

**Figure 1–6.** Leukoplakia simplex of the lower lip: white, slightly elevated patches on the vermillion border.

the surface may be smooth or wrinkled; smooth-surfaced lesions may be traversed by small cracks or fissures (figures 1–3 to 1–6).

2. *Speckled* or *nodular* type of leukoplakia—on an erythematous base characteristic white patches giving a "speckled" appearance, or nodular white excrescences are to be seen [5] (figure 1–2).

The two aforementioned clinical classifications are in good agreement with each other, as far as the "simplex" and "verrucous" types might fit into the "homogeneous" group, and the erosive type might be considered identical to the "speckled" type [45].

Clinical follow-up studies showed definite correlations between clinical types and rate of malignant transformation, as will be discussed later. Transitions or changes among the different clinical types of oral leukoplakia have been observed. Bánóczy and Sugár [40], in longitudinal studies, found a change in the clinical type in 12.7% of the leukoplakias, of which 9.0% showed a regressive and 3.7% a progressive tendency. Thus, leukoplakia must not be considered a stationary condition, but rather a dynamic one, which in the course of time might show gradual changes in the clinical type pattern.

### 2.5. Diagnostic procedures

Although characteristic clinical symptoms of oral leukoplakia might already awake the suspicion of malignancy, the nature of leukoplakia must be assured by histopathological investigation [50]. The clinical appearance of leukoplakia may already cover histopathological changes as dysplasia, carcinoma in situ, or invasive carcinoma. Therefore, a biopsy is necessary or even obligatory in certain cases. However, several additional diagnostic procedures may be performed earlier or in connection with a biopsy and might serve as valuable help in the diagnosis of malignisation.

Additional diagnostic procedures other than a biopsy are performed in order to support the clinical diagnosis without surgical intervention. These additional procedures are stomatoscopy, toluidine blue staining, and exfoliative cytology.

*2.5.1. Stomatoscopy*

Stomatoscopy is called the method of direct observation of the oral mucosa. With the aid of a special optical system, under intense light and with an enlarged view, the distinction of certain characteristic morphological details is possible. The system has been adopted from the gynecology by Fasske et al. [51] in 1958, who attributed great value to this procedure in the diagnosis of neoplastic conditions. Their results, completed with cytology and control biopsies, were confirmed later by others [52], accentuating that this auxiliary method might serve as a valuable means in the early diagnosis of cancer. However, this method did not gain a widespread use.

*2.5.2. Toluidine blue staining*

The toluidine blue test is based on the principle that malignant cells contain quantitatively more DNA and RNA, and to these nucleic acids the toluidine blue dye has an affinity. The staining solution applied in vivo on the oral mucosa reacts metachromatically with malignant epithelial cells and thus delineates the region of malignancy of the epithelial mucosa. The method has been used with good results with parallel performed cytological and histopathological controls. Its greatest value is considered to be its ability to indicate and delineate the adequate site of biopsy in order to obtain the most representative tissue of the lesion [53].

*2.5.3. Exfoliative cytology*

Exfoliative cytology examines the morphological characteristics of exfoliated or scraped off superficial cells of the oral mucosa. The exfoliated cells are stained, usually according to the method of Papanicolaou and Traut [54]. From the cytological smears the type and intensity of keratinization might be assessed. However, the main scientific and practical value of cytology lies in the diagnosis of malignancy.

The use of exfoliative cytology in diagnosing malignant transformation in leukoplakias is controversial. One group of investigators found that the keratinized layer in oral leukoplakia did not interfere with the good results of cytodiagnosis. Another group of investigators, consisting of a significantly larger number, considers the efficacy of oral exfoliative cytology in oral leukoplakia to be low, since the superficial cornified layer impedes the emergence of deeper dyskeratotic cells [53]. False negative cytologic results in hyperkeratotic leukoplakias were observed in 63.9% [56] and in 62% [57] of the cases. However, none of these investigators took the clinical type of leukoplakia into consideration. Recently, comparative cytologic and histologic studies in oral leukoplakia in correlation with clinical type of lesion [58] showed an agreement between cytologic and histologic results of 201 oral leukoplakias in 76.7% of all cases, with a higher efficacy of cytology in detecting malignancy in the erosive leukoplakia group. This finding is in accordance with results of previous investigations [59] concerning the expectations of the cytologic method in cases of ulcerated leukoplakias. Considering the experience that in erosive leukoplakia a higher rate of malignant transformation occurs, the importance of exfoliative cytology seems to be accentuated. Numerous reports substantiate the fact that the use of exfoliative cytology has accelerated the taking of a biopsy in lesions that looked clinically rather harmless. According to Silverman and Galante [60], an immediate biopsy of every lesion is impractical and not indicated. Therefore, a simple, reliable, and acceptable technique like exfoliative cytology might be of great use in the diagnosis of early malignancy. However, it must be accentuated that cytology is an adjunct and not a substitute for biopsy.

### *2.5.4. The biopsy: Indications and techniques*

The indication when to perform a biopsy in oral leukoplakia varies considerably. Some authors believe a biopsy is obligatory at the patient's first visit, when the clinical diagnosis of leukoplakia has been established, regardless of its clinical appearance. Others perform a biopsy not necessarily at the first visit of the leukoplakia patient but either when the lesion is clinically suspected of being malignant (in the "high risk" groups: erosive or speckled types) or when the leukoplakia, although clinically not suspicious, has been treated previously and does not show signs of regression after a certain period of treatment.

The biopsy might be performed technically by use of a punch of 2 to 5 mm diameter or with a scalpel. Punch biopsies are done with the direct aim of histopathological investigations of the lesion and therefore must be taken from the most suspicious area. Generally, the leukoplakic lesion is more extended than the area of the planned punch biopsy. Therefore, its exact place has to be determined by thorough clinical examination and/or additional diagnostic procedures already mentioned. When the lesion is not too extended, a surgical in toto excision is recommended by use of a scalpel, which also serves therapeutic purposes. In these cases, when the biopsy is done in association with the surgical elimination of the lesion, the histopathological examination by serial sections of the whole specimen is indicated. Special attention must be paid to the clinically suspected areas and to the transitional border between normal and pathological areas of the specimen. The fixation and staining procedures vary according to the aim of the investigation.

**2.6. Histopathological aspects**

The histopathological aspects of oral leukoplakia can be studied by the light microscope, and on an ultrastructural level by the electron microscope. For practical purposes the histopathological diagnosis with light microscopy is of decisive importance.

As previously mentioned, the up-to-date definition of leukoplakia does not carry histologic connotation in itself [5]. Although the histological characteristics of oral leukoplakia have been abundantly studied [61,62] and an agreement on epithelial dysplasia and carcinoma in situ has been established [5], no uniform histological criteria for the clinical concept of leukoplakia are available. However, some definitions of the individual histological characteristics are used, which might facilitate the histological description of oral leukoplakia but *not* show epithelial dysplasia or carcinoma in situ. Of these the most commonly used and accepted are the following terms:

Changes in the epithelium (figures 1–7 and 1–8):

*Orthokeratosis:* The uppermost cell layers of the epithelium are almost homogeneous, eosinophile, without nuclei, with a stratum granulosum always present.

*Hyperorthokeratosis:* The thickness of the orthokeratotic layer exceeds the thickness that is considered normal for the area.

*Parakeratosis:* The outer cell layers of the epithelium are acidophilic and flattened, containing pyknotic nuclei. A stratum granulosum may or may not be present.

*Hyperparakeratosis:* The thickness of the parakeratotic layer is increased.

*Dyskeratosis:* Keratinization of cells in the prickle cell layer. It is not identical with epithelial atypia, but considered as a component of it.

*Intraepithelial edema:* Intra- and intercellular edema of epithelium.

*Hyperplasia:* Proliferation of all layers of the epithelium causing the thickening of epithelium in that area.

*Atrophy:* Reduction in the normal thickness of the epithelium due to a decrease in the number of cells.

Changes in the connective tissue:

*Inflammation:* In the subepithelial connective tissue, cell elements in various groupings and characteristic of chronic inflammation are to be found. In some studies the inflammatory changes have been included in the histologic classification of leukoplakia [63].

*Hyaline degeneration:* The interspaces of the subepithelial connective tissue are permeated with some hyaline material and thereby become homogeneous and stain eosinophilic.

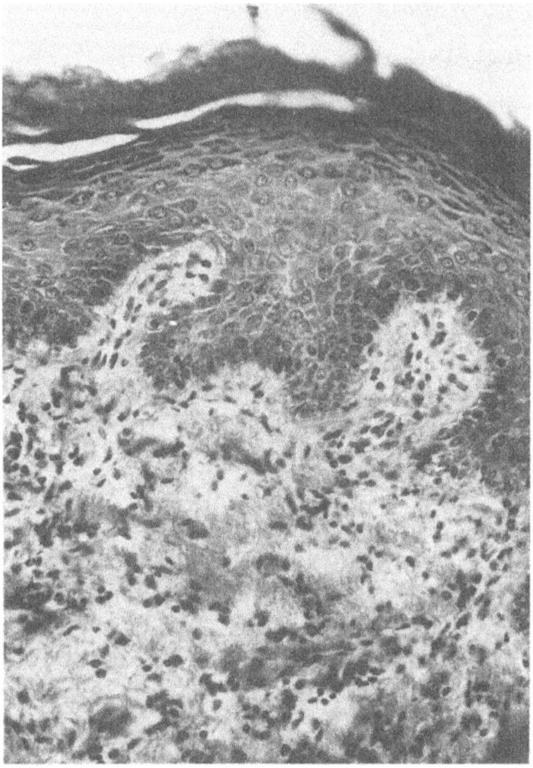

**Figure 1–7.** Histopathological picture of leukoplakia simplex: epithelial hyperplasia, acanthosis, hyperorthokeratosis, strongly expressed granular layer, mild infiltration in the connective tissue. HE Magn. 250 ×.

Recently, attempts have been made to define by computer-aided studies the most frequently occurring histological characteristics in oral leukoplakia [64, 65] and those occurring in leukoplakias that developed later carcinoma [66,67, 68]. Correlations have been established among the clinical type of leukoplakia and histopathological characteristics. Burkhardt [39] differentiated three microscopic forms in oral leukoplakia—(1) the plain form, which corresponds clinically to the leukoplakia simplex, (2) the papillary-endophytic form, and (3) the papillomatous exophytic form—with the latter two forms corresponding to the verrucous and erosive clinical forms of leukoplakia. Dysplasias occurred most frequently in the papillary-endophytic forms. In the high-risk group (speckled or erosive type) leukoplakias, parakeratosis, hyperparakeratosis, hyperplasia, and connective tissue inflammation were present with an increased occurrence of epithelial dysplasia (figure 1–8). In simplex or

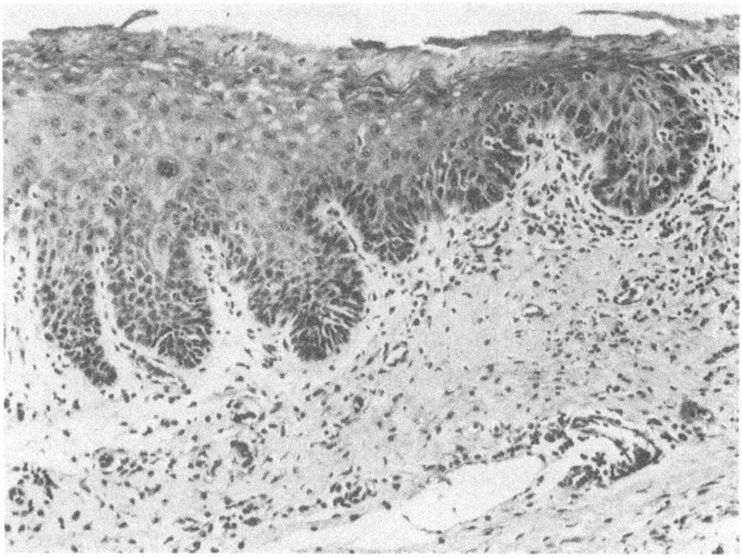

**Figure 1–8.** Histopathological picture of leukoplakia erosiva: epithelial hyperplasia, parakeratosis, signs of moderate epithelial dysplasia, mild infiltration of the connective tissue with inflammatory cells. HE Magn. 200 ×.

homogeneous leukoplakia, epithelial hyperpasia and hyperorthokeratosis are generally characteristic (figure 1–7) [49,38,69].

*Epithelial dysplasia* and carcinoma in situ denote changes of the epithelium and point toward a possible and definite, respectively, subsequent development of malignancy.

*Epithelial dysplasia* connotates a general disturbance in the epithelium, where the individual cell changes are referred to as atypia (figure 1–8).

The following are some of the changes that may occur in epithelial dysplasia [5]:

1. Loss of polarity of the basal cells.
2. Hyperplasia of the basal layer.
3. Increased nuclear-cytoplasmic ratio.
4. Drop-shaped rete-processes.
5. Irregular epithelial stratification.
6. Increased number of mitotic figures (a few abnormal mitoses may be present).
7. The presence of mitotic figures in the superficial half of the epithelium.
8. Cellular pleomorphism.
9. Nuclear hyperchromatism.

10. Enlarged nucleoli.
11. Loss or reduction of intercellular adherence.
12. Keratinization of single cells or cell groups in the prickle cell layer.

Necessarily, not all of these changes might be seen in the epithelium. The histological diagnosis of dysplasia is generally established when two or more of the dysplastic changes are present. According to the number/ratio of changes, the dysplasia might be classified as mild, moderate, or severe.

Severe grades of epithelial dysplasia are not completely separable from the lesion customarily designated as *carcinoma in situ*, in which the whole or almost the whole thickness of the epithelium is involved, but the epithelium–connective-tissue borderline remains intact. "However, whether the histologic convention of distinguishing between severe dysplasia and carcinoma in situ is of practical value in the case of the oral mucosa, remains to be seen" [5]. In invasive carcinoma the epithelial–connective-tissue borderline is not any more intact and the connective tissue is invaded by the malignant epithelial cells (figure 1–9).

From the viewpoint of early diagnosis of potentially malignant leukoplakias, the histopathological diagnosis of dysplasia seems to be decisive. Leukoplakias showing histologically epithelial dysplasia are considered to have a greater disposition for malignant transformation. The ratio of epithelial dysplasia has been found between 3.7 and 28.8% in a large histological sample of oral leukoplakias [70]. Regarding the grade of dysplasia, Waldron and Shafer [62] found mild and moderate dysplasia in 12.2%, and severe dysplasia and carcinoma in situ in 4.5% of their histological sample from 3,256 leukoplakias. Burkhardt and Seifert [38], who analysed the histology of 656 oral leukoplakias, observed in 17% moderate dysplasia and in 6% severe dysplasia. Dysplasia showed a strong correlation with the speckled-erosive clinical type of leukoplakia. In 68% and 51%, respectively, of this clinical group, dysplasia was present [49,70]. On the other hand, a correlation between histological dysplasia and Candida albicans infection of oral leukoplakia was found [38]. An increased ratio of severe dysplasias has been found in the lip and tongue leukoplakias, when compared with other sites [38,39,62,70]. Taking into account the possibility of malignisation, complete removal of all lesions showing more than slight degrees of dysplasia seems advisable.

Electron microscopic investigations to study the histopathological changes in oral leukoplakia on an ultrastructural level have been performed abundantly both by transmission and scanning electron microscopy. By the former method histologically nonmalignant leukoplakias showed differences in keratinization [71], alterations of tonofibrils, and keratohyalin granules [72]. In histologically dysplastic, precancerous leukoplakias, characteristic alterations of the basement membrane and of structures connected with the basement membrane were described [73–76]. Clinically erosive and histologically dysplastic leukoplakias showed ultrastructural alterations characteristic of oral

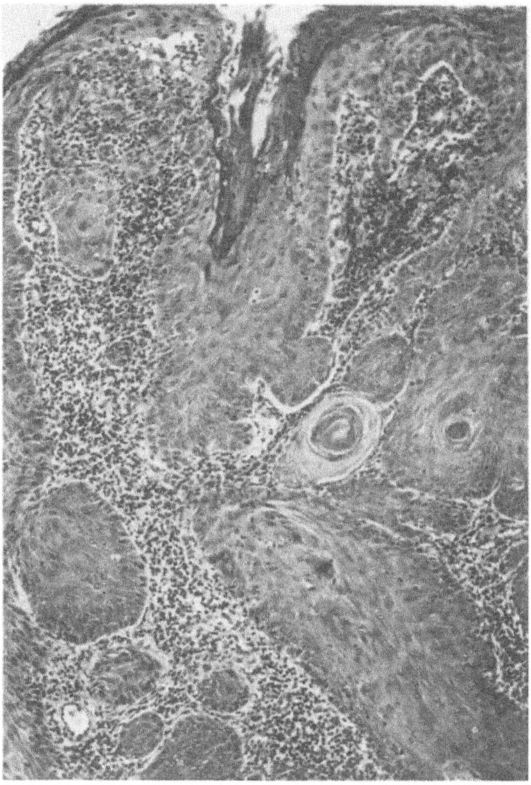

**Figure 1–9.** Histopathological picture of well-differentiated squamous cell carcinoma, developed on the basis of long-standing leukoplakia with invasion of the connective tissue.

carcinomas [77]. By the scanning electronmicroscopical method, the cytoplasmic projections of superficial epithelial cells in leukoplakia, dysplasia, and carcinoma appeared irregular and rough when compared with cells of the normal oral mucosa [76,78,79,80]. The appearance of the superficial leukoplakia cells varied with the clinical type. In leukoplakia simplex and leukoplakia verrucosa, the epithelial cells appeared keratinized, with little alterations of the superficial network pattern in the latter type (figure 1–10), in leukoplakia erosiva the epithelial surface was discontinuous and the cytoplasmic protrusions on the cell surface showed alterations characteristic of dysplasia and carcinoma [81] (figure 1–11).

### 2.7. Differential diagnosis

Through recent knowledge of the so-called "white-lesions" of the oral mucosa, several clinicopathological entities can be separated from oral leukoplakia. These, as already mentioned at the definition of leukoplakia, are lichen

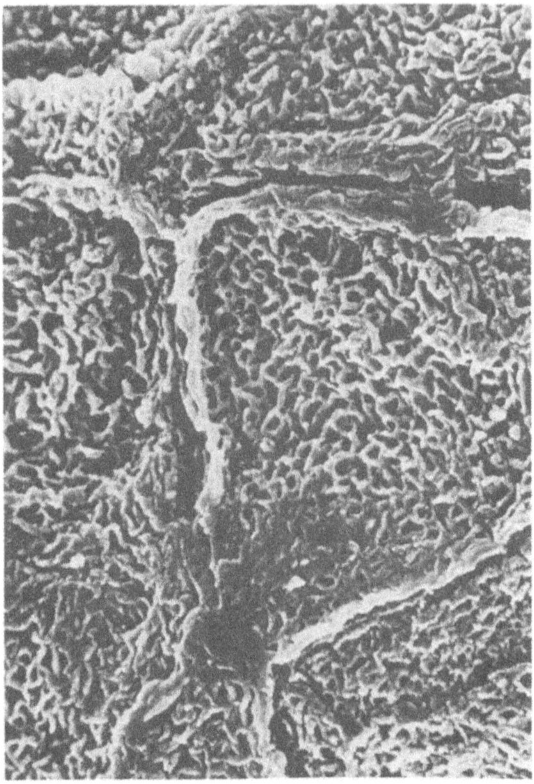

**Figure 1–10.** Scanning electron microscopy of leukoplakia simplex: the neighbouring cells are connected; the superficial structure of the cells is regular.

planus, candidiasis, white sponge nevus, migratory glossitis, discoid lupus erythematosus, and morsicatio buccarum.

*Lichen planus* is a disease that might affect the skin or oral mucosa, or both. Oral mucosal lesions may persist without skin lesions for a long time. The etiology is unknown. Smoking, in contrast to the etiology of leukoplakia, seems to occur rather infrequently. Electrical potential differences [34,82], as well as diabetes and psychic stress, seem to play a role in the development of the lesions [83]. The lesions are clinically characteristic: little white papules, grouped in different ways, give the clinical aspect of the reticular (figure 1–12) papular, plaque type of lichen. The presence of the so-called Wickham striae (white lines irradiating from the center of the lesion) is of differential diagnostic importance in that type, as well as in the bullous, atrophic, and erosive type. The latter three types occur mostly in cases of chronic, long-standing lichen. The histopathology of lichen is characteristic: corresponding to the clinically visible papules, the epithelium is thickened, shows signs of acan-

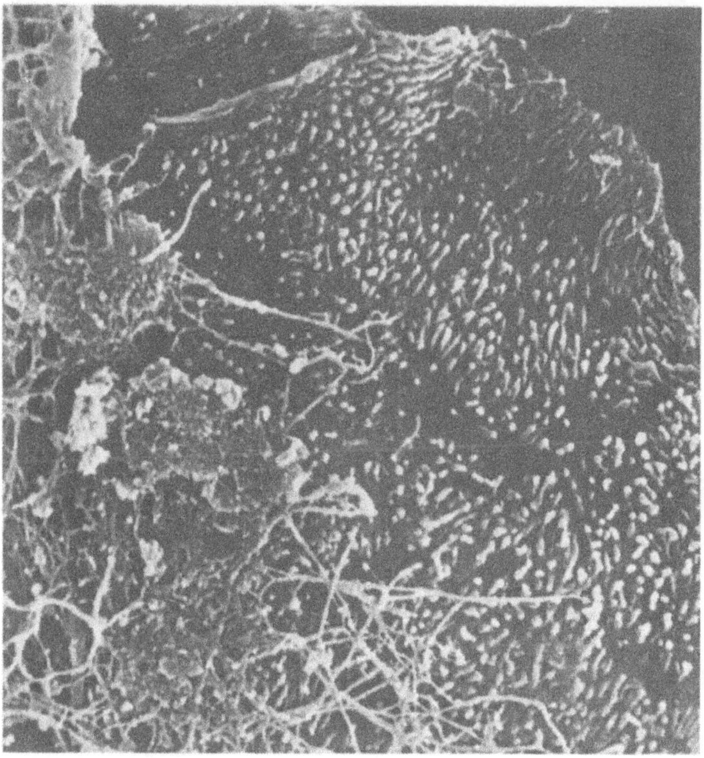

**Figure 1–11.** Scanning electron microscopy of leukoplakia erosiva: the intercellular connections were loosened; the microrugae are irregular, scattered.

thosis and hyper/para/keratosis, with liquefaction degeneration of the basal layer, and a well-defined inflammatory zone in the connective tissue. In long-standing cases the oral epithelium shows the histopathologic signs of atrophy.

The precancerous character of oral lichen has been a subject of discussion for a long time. Carcinomas arising from oral lichen have been reported several times. Some investigations estimated its frequency to be between 0 and 10% [84]. It is not yet fully established whether the common occurrence of lichen and carcinoma is only a coincidence or a consequence of irritations on the atrophic, eroded oral mucosa in cases of long-standing chronic lichen. Regardless, caution and constant supervision are advisable, especially in the atrophic and eroded cases of oral lichen in order to prevent the development of malignancies.

*Candidiasis* is a chronic disease of the oral mucosa caused by Candida albicans, which may occur secondarily as a superimposed infection on already existing oral lesions (leukoplakia, lichen) or primarily when, as a consequence of some disturbances in the host/microorganism relation, Candida albicans

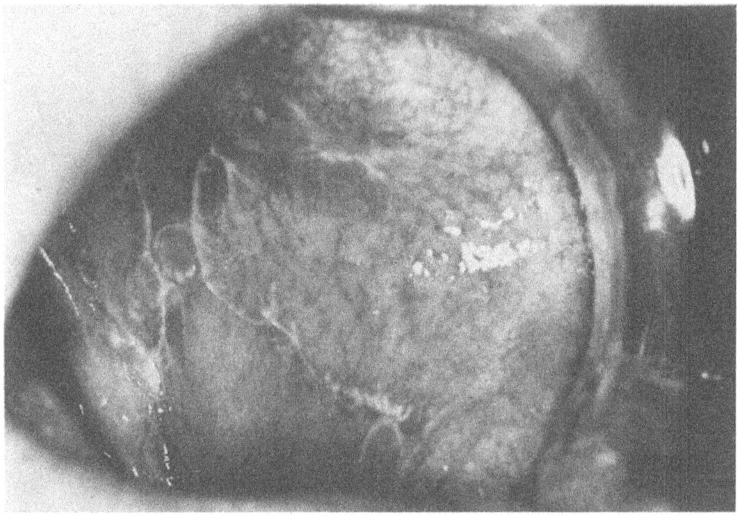

**Figure 1–12.** Reticular type of lichen of the buccal mucosa: the papules are coalescent, forming characteristic patterns, Wickham striae.

prevails and causes pathological symptoms. The latter forms are seen as generalized candidiasis in malnourished, cachectic patients, or after long-lasting antibiotic treatment. In denture-wearing patients localized forms in connection with the dentures may develop.

The clinical picture of oral candidiasis, especially in the chronic forms, is characterized by thick, white patches of different size, which may coalesce. The white plaques are removable by strong rubbing and leave a reddened, erythematous, and sometimes bleeding surface underneath (figure 1–2). Histopathologically, the epithelium is thickened, shows hyperplasia, parakeratosis, and infiltration of polymorph nuclear leukocytes. The Candida hyphae can be demonstrated by PAS staining in the superficial layers of the epithelium. Dysplastic changes may occur, especially in connection with oral leukoplakias.

*White sponge nevus* (leukoedema exfoliativum mucosae oris) is an autosomal, dominant hereditary dyskeratotic hyperplasia of the oral mucosa, which might also affect other mucosal sites. The lesions appear at early infancy or childhood and become less pronounced by advancing age.

The clinical appearance shows grayish-whitish, continuously thickened, folded or desquamating oral mucosa, extended generally on all those sites that have an underlying submucosa. The lesions might be rubbed off, but reappear after a certain lapse of time. White sponge nevus does not cause complaints, but, because of the thickened, desquamating mucosa, is sometimes associated with cheek biting. Histopathological investigation shows epithelial hyperplasia with characteristic spongiosis of the spinous layer and hyperparakeratosis, which, according to ultrastructural investigations, might be related to the faulty desquamation of the superficial cell layers [85]. Generally, the connective tissue has no inflammation. The condition is considered completely benign, and follow-up studies of large patient populations failed to show any evidence of a possible malignisation [86].

*Migratory glossitis*, called "exfoliatio areata linguae" or "geographic tongue" is a chronic inflammatory condition of the tongue mucosa manifested clinically by the appearance of red patches devoid of papillae, which are surrounded by collarlike white elevations consisting of filiform papillae. The lesions change their clinical appearance rather quickly, may manifest in early childhood, and show a preference for the female sex. Similar lesions might be present on the buccal and labial mucosal sites, occasionally referred to as "ectopic geographic tongue." A familial occurrence and the importance of psychic stress in the etiology have been noted. Histopathologically, focal inflammatory changes in the epithelium with the formation of microabcesses and inflammatory infiltrate of the connective tissue are characteristic. No evidence of malignant changes has ever been reported.

*Discoid lupus erythematosus* is a skin disease of general involvement and may present oral signs similar to leukoplakia. The oral lesions are circumscribed: little elevated white patches on an erythematous background, erosions on the clinically atrophic, inflammatory mucosa may develop. Histopathologically characteristic are the atrophic epithelium with hyperorthokeratosis, liquefaction degeneration of the basal layer, a subepithelial acidophilic band (consisting of PAS positive, diastase-resistant material), and a bandlike infiltration of lymphocytes in the connective tissue [5]. Epithelial dysplasia may occur, but there is no direct evidence on the malignisation of these lesions.

*Morsicatio buccarum* (habitual cheek biting, pathomimia) is a chronic disease with a well-defined etiology: the patients are aware of their habits. After stopping the cheek, lip, or tongue biting, the lesions show regression. The clinical picture shows lesions on the sites corresponding to the biting habits: generally, in the occlusal line of the buccal mucosa, on the margins of the tongue and on the lips, which vary from white, slight elevations to thick, desquamating lesions to erosions. Histopathologically, the hyperplastic epithelium shows acanthosis, hyperparakeratosis with a slight bacterial layer on the epithelial surface, and inflammatory changes in the connective tissue. The lesion is not considered potentially malignant.

### 2.8. Rate of malignant transformation

The first clinical follow-up studies to yield information about the rate of malignant transformation were initiated by Sugár and Bánóczy [47] in 1957. Since then several investigators have carried out follow-up examinations in

**Table 1–3.** Clinical follow-up studies on the rate of malignant transformation in oral leukoplakia

| Authors | Country, year | Observation period in years | Number of leukoplakia patients followed up | Percentage of malignisation |
|---|---|---|---|---|
| Sugár, Bánóczy [47] | Hungary, 1957 | 1–11 | 86 | 5.8 |
| Skach, Svoboda, Kubát [87] | Czechoslovakia, 1960 | 3–6 | 71 | 1.4 |
| Mela, Mongini [26] | Italy, 1966 | 3–11 | 141 | 3.5 |
| Einhorn, Wersäll [88] | Sweden, 1967 | 10–20 | 782 | 4.0 |
| Pindborg et al. [7] | Denmark, 1968 | 1–9 | 248 | 4.4 |
| Silverman, Rozen [24] | USA, 1968 | 1–11 | 117 | 6.0 |
| Roed-Petersen [25] | Denmark, 1971 | 12 | 331 | 3.6 |
| Pindborg, Mehta, Daftary [89] | India, 1975 | 7 | 170 | 3.5 |
| Bánóczy [27] | Hungary, 1977 | 1–30 | 670 | 6.0 |

various countries. As is shown in table 1–3, the frequency of carcinomatous changes in oral leukoplakia varies between 1.4 and 6% during an observation period of 1 to 30 years.

The rate of malignant transformation in oral leukoplakia seems to correspond with the percentage of oral carcinomas and malignancies in other organs. The occurrence of oral carcinoma in Europe varies between 1 and 5% [90]: in Denmark 1.5%, in Switzerland 2%, in Italy 3%, in France 4%, and in Hungary, 5% of all neoplasms located in the mouth, which corresponds well with the high percentage of malignisation of oral leukoplakia found in the latter country.

Concerning the clinical course of oral leukoplakia, the natural history might be influenced strongly if certain treatment methods are employed. However, Mehta and Pindborg [91], in their control study of Bombay policemen found some spontaneous regression, in spite of continued smoking habits. Experiences gained on 670 patients [27] in the longitudinal course of treated oral leukoplakias are summarized in table 1–4.

The age and sex distributions seem to be rather characteristic factors associated with carcinoma developing from leukoplakia. The increased percentage of females with carcinomas developed from leukoplakia suggests that although men show a higher occurrence, women undergo a greater risk for malignisation of oral leukoplakia [20]. Roed-Petersen [25] observed a malignisation rate in leukoplakias of 5.8% in women and 2.1% in men. Bánóczy [27] made similar observations: 8.8% of females and 5.1% of males with leukoplakia developed later carcinoma.

Sugár and Bánóczy [47,48] found more carcinoma cases developed from the erosive type of leukoplakia. Similarly Pindborg et al. [49] considered the

**Table 1–4.** Results of follow-up examinations of patients with leukoplakia

| Result | No. of cases with leukoplakia | Percentage |
|---|---|---|
| Cured | 208 | 31.0 |
| Improved | 199 | 29.7 |
| Unchanged | 173 | 25.8 |
| Spread | 50 | 7.5 |
| Cancer | 40 | 6.0 |
| Total | 670 | 100.0 |

From reference 27.

speckled type of leukoplakia as bearing a greater risk for malignisation. In the material of Bánóczy [27] of 670 leukoplakia patients followed up over a period of 30 years, 25.9% of the erosive leukoplakia cases showed signs of malignant transformation, and of the verrucous leukoplakia cases only 5.5%. In the leukoplakia simplex group, no malignisation has been observed. Maerker and Burkhardt [92] found a malignisation rate of 38% in erosive leukoplakias. [7] The follow-up observations of Pindborg et al. on 248 leukoplakia patients support the concept that the speckled (nodular) type of leukoplakia is associated more often with epithelial atypia than the homogeneous type and is therefore more likely to become malignant. Roed-Petersen's [25] data based on the clinical follow-up of 331 leukoplakia patients with a 12-year observation period showed a malignisation rate of 9.1% in the speckled-nodular type and only of 1.3% in the homogeneous group. These observations emphasize the importance of the clinical type with regard to the possibility of malignant transformation. Leukoplakias that show clinically an erythematous base, or erosions, with white patches of verrucous, speckled, or nodular appearance should arouse the suspicion for histological dysplasia or carcinoma. In this way the correct clinical diagnosis might be established in an early phase, which is of great importance in the prevention of malignisation (figures 1–1, 1–2, and 1–7).

The rate of malignisation also differs according to the site of leukoplakia. Malignisation occurs most often when the leukoplakia is located on the tongue (figure 1–1), lips, and floor of the mouth. In a study dealing with 670 leukoplakia patients [27], malignisation has been observed in 27.2% of tongue leukoplakias, mostly occurring in women. The rate of malignisation of lip leukoplakias has been 14.7% and observed mostly in men. These findings are supported by the data of other investigators [25,38,93]. Recent studies on floor of the mouth leukoplakias showed a malignisation rate of 24.1%, on the basis of which some investigators recommend separating this form, called sublingual keratosis, from the other forms of oral leukoplakia [94,95].

Analysing the role of smoking in the malignisation of leukoplakia, comparative studies hitherto have failed to give conclusive evidence. Bánóczy [27] found that 83% of patients with leukoplakia—but only 77% of patients with carcinoma developed from leukoplakia—were smokers. Histological investigations found no differences in the occurrence of epithelial dysplasia between smoker and nonsmoker leukoplakia groups [96]. These data agree with the findings of other investigators [25,88], leading to the conclusion that the etiological role of smoking in leukoplakia is to be accepted, but its role in promoting the malignisation of leukoplakia is not proved yet [97].

In conclusion it can be stated that the natural course of oral leukoplakia might be strongly modified by different treatment methods. Spontaneous regression may occur. However, spreading and malignant transformation of the lesion may also take place in spite of treatment and continuous observation.

### 3. ERYTHROPLAKIA

The term *erythroplakia* originates from the description of Queyrat [98] in 1911, who used the term *erythroplasia* to define a sharply demarcated, bright red, velvety lesion occurring on the glans penis and regarded as precancerous. The ocurrence of erythroplasia in the oral cavity with clinical and histological features similar to the penile lesions has been recognized in the last decades by many authors [99]. In these studies, analogous to the word *leukoplakia,* the term of *erythroplakia* has been used. An identity with Bowen's disease of the skin has also arisen because of similarities in the histologic appearance of the two lesions. However, according to the majority of descriptions, clinical differences between the two conditions were reported.

According to the WHO definition [5], the term *erythroplakia* is used analogous to leukoplakia to designate lesions of the oral mucosa that present as bright red, velvety plaques that cannot be characterised clinically or pathologically as being due to any other condition. In this sense red patches of the oral mucosa caused by dermatoses and inflammatory conditions, as Candidiasis, tuberculosis, and other conditions, are excluded from the denomination of erythroplakia.

Classifications based on the clinical appearance of erythroplakia by Shear [100] differentiated three forms: homogeneous erythroplakia, erythroplakia interspersed with patches of leukoplakia, and granular or speckled erythroplakia. The two latter forms are not easily differentiated from the corresponding forms of oral leukoplakia. Studies on the homogeneous form of erythroplakia considering the clinical aspects revealed no apparent sex predilection; a relatively late age onset during the sixth and seventh decades; and as the most common sites of occurrence, the mandibular alveolar mucosa, gingiva, and sulcus in females and floor of the mouth in males [99]. Mashberg [101] considers erythroplakia as the earliest sign of asymptomatic oral cancer.

Microscopically, erythroplakia is associated with marked epithelial atrophy and a variable degree of epithelial dysplasia, which may amount to carcinoma in situ in the majority of cases. In a series of 58 investigated cases of homogeneous erythroplakia, 91% of the specimens showed either invasive carcinoma in situ or severe epithelial dysplasia and carcinomas were found 17 times more frequently in erythroplakia than in leukoplakic lesions [99,101]. Therefore, every erythroplakia should be biopsied, treated, and kept under control according to the procedure followed in cases of other oral malignancies and precancerous lesions [102].

**4. SUBMUCOUS FIBROSIS**

Submucous fibrosis, first described in 1953, is a slowly progressing chronic disease of the oral mucosa. The disease, which occasionally extends on the mucosa of the pharynx and esophagus, almost exclusively occurs in Indians, Pakistanis, and Burmese, but has been also observed sporadically in individuals from other countries [103]. Epidemiologic surveys conducted in rural and urban districts of India and South Africa report a frequency between 0.03 and 1.2% [104].

Clinically, the disease is sometimes preceded by and/or associated with vesicle formation, is focal in character, and shows pallor or whitish coloration, wrinkling of the mucosa, and minimal induration. By this time the lesions become more diffuse, white, extensive, and indurated, involving one or more anatomical sites, most frequently the buccal mucosa, tongue, and palatal mucosa. Later stages present with stiffness of the oral mucosa and symptoms due to restricted mobility, trismus, stretching at angles of the mouth, inability to protrude the tongue, and altered pronunciation. Firm submucosal bands can be palpated, and the surface may be fissured or ulcerated [104]. Considering the etiology of the disease, hypersensitivity to chili, betel nut chewing, use of tobacco, or vitamin deficiencies have been suggested [104]. According to pathogenetic theories the disease begins in the connective tissue, which leads to secondary changes in the epithelium [1].

Microscopically, submucous fibrosis is characterized by juxtoepithelial inflammatory reaction, which is followed by fibrosis, fibroelastic change in the lamina propria, and changes in the overlying epithelium, which are usually atrophic in nature. In some cases areas of hyperplasia may be seen. The frequency of epithelial dysplasia is rather high: 13 to 14% [1].

The precancerous nature of the disease has been pointed out first in 1956 by Paymaster [106], who described the development of squamous cell carcinoma in one-third of his submucous fibrous patients in Bombay. An increased association with oral leukoplakia has been reported in submucous fibrosis by several observers [104].

On the basis of the high occurrence of epithelial dysplasia, the association with superimposed leukoplakia and/or carcinoma, and the extensive nature of the lesions, submucous fibrosis is considered a precancerous condition [1] of slowly progressing character.

## REFERENCES


1. Pindborg JJ. Oral Cancer and Precancer. Bristol: Wright & Sons, 1980.
2. Buchner A, Hansen LS. Pigmented nevi of the oral mucosa: A clinicopathologic study of 32 new cases and review of 75 cases from the literature. Part 1. Oral Surg (48): 131–142, 1979.
3. Buchner A, Hansen LS. Pigmented nevi of the oral mucosa: A clinicopathologic study of 32 new cases and review of 75 cases from the literature. Part 2. Oral Surg (49): 55–62, 1980.
4. Schwimmer E. A szájüreg és nyelv nyálkahártya némely ritka kóralakjáról. Orv Egyesület Evkönyve, 1877, 48 sz.
5. WHO Collaborating Centre for Oral Precancerous Lesions. Definition of leukoplakia and related lesions: An aid to studies on oral precancer. Oral Surg (46): 518–539, 1978.
6. Atkinson L, Chester IC, Smith FG, Ten Seldam REJ. Oral cancer in New Guinea. A study in demography and etiology. Cancer (17): 1289–1298, 1964.
7. Pindborg JJ, Jolst O, Renstrup G, Roed-Petersen B. Studies in oral leukoplakia: A preliminary report on the prevalence of malignant transformation in leukoplakia based on a follow-up study of 248 patients. J Amer Dent Ass (76): 767–771, 1968.
8. Wahi PN, Mital VP. Epidemiological study of precancerous lesions of the oral cavity: A preliminary report. Indian J Med Res (58): 1361–1391, 1970.
9. Bruszt P. Stomato-onkologische Reihenuntersuchungen in sieben Gemeinden Südungarns. Schw Mschr Zahnheilk (72): 758–766, 1962.
10. Axéll T. A preliminary report on prevalence of oral mucosal lesions in a Swedish population. *Community Dent Oral Epidemiol* (3): 143–145, 1975.
11. Gerry RG, Smith ST, Calton ML. The oral characteristics of Guamanians including the effects of betel chewing on the oral tissues. Oral Surg (5): 762–781, 1952.
12. Mehta F, Sanjana MK, Shroff BC, Doctor RHC. Incidence of leukoplakia among "pan" (betal leaf) chewers and "bidi" smokers: A study of a sample survey. Indian J Med Res (49): 393–398, 1961.
13. Pindborg JJ, Kalapessi HK, Kale SA, Singh B, Talverkhan B. Frequency of oral leukoplakias and related conditions among 10,000 Bombayites. J All India Dent Ass (37): 1–2, 1965.
14. Pindborg JJ, Chawla TN, Misra RK, Nagpaul RK, Gupta P. Frequency of oral carcinoma, leukoplakia, leukoedema, leukokeratosis, submucous fibrosis and lichen planus in 10,000 Indians in Lucknow, Uttar Pradesh, India. J Dent Res (44): 615–618, 1965.
15. Pindborg JJ, Rhatt M, Devanath KR, Narayana HR, Ramachandra S. Frequency of oral white lesions among 10,000 individuals in Bangalore, South India. Indian J Med Sci (20): 349–352, 1966.
16. Zachariah J, Matthew B, Varma NAR, Iqbal AM, Pindborg JJ. Frequency of oral mucosal lesions among 5,000 individuals in Trivandrum, South India. J All India Dent Ass (38): 290–294, 1966.
17. Pindborg JJ, Barmes OD, Roed-Petersen B. Epidemiology and leukoedema among Papuans and New Guineans. Cancer (22): 379–384, 1968.
18. Bánóczy J, Radnai T, Reményi I. Módszertani tapasztalataink Dunakeszi és Felsógöd lakosságán végzett stomato-onkológiai szürővizsgálatok alapján. Fogorv Szle (62): 118–122, 1969.
19. Mehta F, Pindborg JJ, Gupta PC, Daftary DK. Epidemiologic and histologic study of oral cancer and leukoplakia among 50,915 villagers in India. Cancer (24): 832–849, 1969.
20. Gangadarhan P, Paymaster JC. Leukoplakia, an epidemiologic study of 1504 cases observed at the Tata Memorial Hospital, Bombay, India. Brit J Cancer (25): 657–668, 1971.
21. Sonkodi I, Tóth K. Szegedi textilipari munkások stomato–onkológiai vizsgálata. Fogorv Szle (67): 165–169, 1974.
22. Silverman S, Bhargava K, Mani N, Smith LW, Malaowalla MA. Malignant transformation and natural history of oral leukoplakia in 57,518 industrial workers of Gujaret, India. Cancer (38): 1790–1795, 1976.
23. Wilsch L, Hornstein OP, Brüning H, Schwipper V, Lösel F, Schönberger A, Gunselmann W, Prestele H. Orale Leukoplakien II. Ergebnisse einer 1 jährigen poliklinischen Pilotstudie. Dtsch zahnärztl Zschr (33): 132–142, 1978.
24. Silverman S, Rozen RD. Observations on the clinical characteristics and natural history of oral leukoplakia. J Amer Dent Ass (76): 772–776, 1968.
25. Roed-Petersen B. Cancer development in oral leukoplakia. Follow-up of 331 patients. J Dent Res (50): 711–716, 1971.

26. Mela F, Mongini F. La terapie della lesioni leucoplasiche del cavo orale (In base di resultati di uno studio su 141 casi controllati a distanza dall' intervento). Minerva Stomat (15): 804–811, 1966.
27. Bánóczy J: Follow-up studies in oral leukoplakia. J. Max.-Fac. Surg. (5): 69–75, 1977.
28. Baric JM, Alman JE, Feldman RS, Chauncey HH. Influence of cigarette, pipe, and cigar smoking, removable partial dentures, and age on oral leukoplakia. Oral Surg (54): 424–429, 1982.
29. Roed-Petersen B, Gupta PC, Pindborg JJ, Singh B. Association between oral leukoplakia and sex, age and tobacco habits. Bull Wld Hlth Org (47): 13–19, 1972.
30. Mehta S, Daftary DK, Shroff BC, Sanghvi LD. Clinical and histologic study of oral leukoplakia in relation to habits. A five-year follow-up. Oral Surg (28): 372–388, 1969.
31. Pindborg JJ, Roed-Petersen B, Renstrup G. Role of smoking in floor of the mouth leukoplakias. J. Oral Path (1): 22–29, 1972.
32. Lain E. Electrogalvanic lesions of the oral cavity produced by metallic dentures. J Amer Dent Ass (100): 717–723, 1933.
33. Ullmann K. Leukoplakia caused by electrogalvanic current generated on the oral cavity. Wien klin Wschr (45): 840–852, 1932.
34. Bánóczy J, Roed-Petersen B, Pindborg JJ, Inovay J. Clinical and histologic studies on electrogalvanically induced oral white lesions. Oral Surg (48): 319–323, 1979.
35. Jepsen A, Winther JE. Mycotic infection in oral leukoplakia. Acta Odont Scand (23): 239–256, 1965.
36. Daftary DK, Mehta FS, Gupta PC, Pindborg JJ. The prevalence of Candida in 723 oral leukoplakias among Indian villagers. Scand J Dent Res (80): 75–79, 1972.
37. Restrup G. Occurrence of Candida in oral leukoplakias. Acta Path Microbiol Scand B (78): 421–424, 1970.
38. Burkhardt A, Seifert G. Morphologische Klassifikation der oralen Leukoplakien. Dtsch Med Wschr (102): 223–229, 1977.
39. Burkhardt A. Der Mundhöhlenkrebs und seine Vorstadien, G. Fischer. New York: Stuttgart, 1980.
40. Bánóczy J, Sugár L. Progressive and regressive changes in Hungarian oral leukoplakias in the course of longitudinal studies. Community Dent Oral Epidemiol (3): 194–197, 1975.
41. Clemmesen J. Statistical Studies in the Etiology of Malignant Neoplasms. København: Munksgaard, 1965.
42. Roed-Petersen B, Renstrup G. A topographical classification of the oral mucosa suitable for electronic data processing (its application to 560 leukoplakias). Acta Odont Scand (27): 681–695, 1969.
43. World Health Organization. Oral Mucosa Manual, Geneva, 1980.
44. Mehta FS, Pindborg JJ, Hamner JE. Oral Cancer and Precancerous Conditions in India. København: Munksgaard, 1971.
45. Hornstein OP. Leukoplakien der Mundschleimhaut. Zlbl Haut u Geschlechtskrank. (139): 1–18, 1977.
46. Hornstein OP. Orale Leukoplakien I. Klassifikation, Differentialdiagnose, Atiologische Bedingungen der Kanzerisierung, Prognose. Dtsch zahnärztl Z (32): 497–505, 1977/b.
47. Sugár L, Bánóczy J. Vizsgálatok a szájnyálkahártya praecancerosisairól. Fogorv Szle (50): 347–353, 1957.
48. Sugár L, Bánóczy J. Untersuchungen bei Präkanzerose der Mundschleimhaut. Dtsch. Zahn-, Mund-Kieferheilk (30): 132–140, 1959.
49. Pindborg JJ, Renstrup G, Poulsen HE, Silverman S. Studies in oral leukoplakias: V. Clinical and histological signs of malignancy. Acta Odont Scand (21): 407–414, 1963.
50. Fischman SL, Ulmansky M, Sela J, Bab I, Gazit D. Correlative clinico-pathological evaluation of oral premalignancy. J Oral Pathol (11): 283–289, 1982.
51. Fasske E, Hahn W, Morgenroth K, Themann H. Die Leukoplakie der menschlichen Mundschleimhaut. Mitteilungsdienst (2): 7–24, 1958.
52. Popescu V, Sturza M. Stomatoscopy in the early diagnosis of buccal cancer. Int Dent J (18): 694–707, 1968.
53. Sigurdson A. Metodundersökninger vid oral slemmhimmediagnostik. Thesis, Stockholm, 1977.
54. Papanicolaou G, Traut W. Diagnosis of urterine cancer by the vaginal smear. New York, Commonwealth Fund, 1943.

55. Bánóczy J. Exfoliative cytologic examinations in the early diagnosis of oral cancer. Int Dent J (26): 398–404, 1976.
56. Mehta FS, Daftary DK, Sahiar BE. A correlative histocytological study of epithelial atypia in leukoplakia and submucous fibrosis lesions amongst Indian villagers in a mass screening programme. Indian J Cancer (7): 18–25, 1970.
57. Dabelsteen E, Roed-Petersen B, Smith J, Pindborg JJ. The limitation of exfoliative cytology for the detection of epithelial atypia in oral leukoplakias. Brit J Cancer (25): 21–24, 1971.
58. Bánóczy J, Rigó O. Comparative cytologic and histologic studies in oral leukoplakia. Acta Cytol (20): 308–312, 1976.
59. Bánóczy J. Exfoliative cytological changes in oral leukoplakias. J Dent Res (48): 17–21, 1969.
60. Silverman J, Galante M. Oral Cancer. San Francisco: University of California, 1972.
61. Shafer WG, Waldron CA. A clinical and histopathological study of oral leukoplakia. Surg/ Gynecol Obstetr (112): 411–420, 1961.
62. Waldron CA, Shafer WG. Leukoplakia revisited. A clinicopathologic study 3256 oral leukoplakias. Cancer (36): 1386–1392, 1975.
63. Grässel-Pietrusky R, Hornstein OP. Histologische Klassifikation oraler Präkanzerosen. Dtsch A Mund-Kiefer-Gesichts-Chir (6): 343–351, 1982.
64. Kramer IRH, Lucas RB, El-Labban N, Lister L. A computer-aided study on the tissue changes in oral keratoses and lichen planus, and an analysis of cases grouping by subjective and objective criteria. Brit J Cancer (24): 407–426, 1970.
65. Kramer IRH, Lucas RB, El-Labban N, Lister L. The use of discriminant analysis for examining the histological features of oral keratoses and lichen planus. Brit J Cancer (24): 673–686, 1970.
66. Kramer IRH. Precancerous conditions of the oral mucosa. Annals R Coll Surg England (45): 3–19, 1969.
67. El-Labban N, Lucas RB, Kramer IRH. The mitotic values for the epithelium in oral keratoses and lichen planus. Brit J Cancer (25): 411–416, 1971.
68. Kramer IRH, El-Labban N, Sonkodi S. Further studies on lesions of the oral mucosa using computer-aided analyses of histological features. Brit J Cancer (29): 223–231, 1974.
69. Bánóczy J, Csiba A. Comparative study of the clinical picture and histopathologic structure of oral leukoplakia. Cancer (29): 1230–1234, 1972.
70. Bánóczy J, Csiba A. Occurrence of epithelial dysplasia in oral leukoplakia. Oral Surg (42): 766–774, 1976.
71. Haim G. Elektronenmikroskopische Untersuchungen pathologischer Verhornungsvorgänge im Epithel der Schleimhaut. Stoma (17): 292–308, 1964.
72. Silverman J. Ultrastructure studies of oral mucosa. I. Comparison of normal and hyperkeratotic human buccal epithelium. J Dent Res (46): 1433–1443, 1967.
73. Frithiof L. Ultrastructure of the basement membrane in normal and hyperplastic human oral epithelium compared with that in preinvasive and invasive carcinoma. Acta Path et Microb Skand (200): 1–63, 1969.
74. Frithiof L. Ultrastructural changes in the plasma membrane in human oral epithelium. J Ultrastruct Res (32): 1–17, 1970.
75. Frithiof L. Electron microscopic observations on structures related to the epithelial basement membranes in squamous cell carcinoma. Acta Otolaryng (73): 323–334, 1971.
76. Schenk P. Die ultrastrukturelle Morphologie normalen und pathologischen oralen Epithelien unter besonderer Berücksichtigung von dysplastischen und dyskeratotischen Veränderungen, Carcinoma in situ und invasivem Carcinoma. Thesis, Stockholm, 1975.
77. Bánóczy J, Juhász J, Albrecht M. Ultrastructure of different clinical forms of oral leukoplakia. J Oral Pathol (9): 41–53, 1980.
78. Morgenroth K, Morgenroth Kjr. Untersuchungen von Mundschleimhautveränderungen mit dem Rasterelektronenmikroskop. Acta meditechn (18): 18–23, 1970.
79. Morganroth K, Morgenroth Kjr. Vergleichende stomatoskopische und rasterelektronenmikroskopische Untersuchungen von Mundschleimhautveränderungen. Dtsch Zahnärztl Zschr (25): 199–207, 1970.
80. Matsumoto Y, Uchida T, Maruya M, Tokita M, Seto K, Watanabe Y. Scanning electron microscopic study of the human oral mucosa. J Dent Res (55): D. 176, 28, 1976.
81. Bánóczy J, Lapis K, Albrecht M. Scanning electron microscopic study of oral leukoplakia. J Oral Pathol (9): 145–154, 1980.

82. Frykholm O, Frithiof L, Fernström B, Moberger G, Blom S, Björn E. Allergy to copper derived from dental alloys as a possible cause of oral lesions of lichen planus. Acta derm venereol (49): 268–281, 1969.
83. Kövesi G, Bánóczy J. Follow-up studies in oral lichen planus. Int J Oral Surg (2): 13–19, 1973.
84. Lauffer J, Kuffer R. Le Lichen Plan Buccal. Paris: Masson et Cie, 1970.
85. Frithiof L, Bánóczy J. Ultrastructural observations in leukoedema exfoliativum mucosae oris (white sponge nevus). Oral Surg (41): 607–622, 1976.
86. Bánóczy J, Sugár L, Frithiof L. White sponge nevus: Leukoedema exfoliativum mucosae oris. Swed Dent J (66): 481–493, 1973.
87. Skach M, Svoboda O, Kubát K. Prisperich k problému leukoplakia. Acta Univ Carol Sect Med Suppl (10): 363–371, 1960.
88. Einhorn J, Wersäll J. Incidence of oral carcinoma in patients with leukoplakia of the oral mucosa. Cancer (20): 2189–2193, 1967.
89. Pindborg JJ, Mehta FS, Daftary DK. Incidence of oral cancer among 30,000 villagers in India in a 7-year follow-up study of oral precancerous lesions. Community Dent Oral Epidemiol (3): 86–88, 1975.
90. Pindborg JJ. Oral Cancer from an international point of view. J Canad Dent Ass (31): 219–226, 1965.
91. Mehta FS, Pindborg JJ. Spontaneous regression of oral leukoplakias among Indian villagers in a 5-year follow-up study. Community Dent Oral Epidemiol (2): 80–84, 1974.
92. Maerker R, Burkhardt A. Klinik oraler Leukoplakien und Präkanzerosen. Retrospektive Studie an 200 Patienten. Dtsch Z Mund-Kiefer-Gesichts-Chir (2): 206–220, 1978.
93. Pindborg JJ. Epidemiological studies of oral cancer. Intern Dent J (27): 172–178, 1977.
94. Roed-Petersen B, Renstrup G, Pinborg JJ. Candida in oral leukoplakia. Scand J Dent Res (78): 323–328, 1970.
95. Kramer IRH, El-Labban NG, Lee KW. The clinical features and risk of malignant transformation in sublingual keratosis. Brit Dent J (144): 171–180, 1978.
96. Roed-Petersen B, Bánóczy J, Pindborg JJ: Smoking habits and histological characteristics of oral leukoplakias in Denmark and Hungary. Brit J Cancer (28): 575–579, 1973.
97. Cawson RA. Premalignant lesions in the mouth. Brit Med Bull (31): 164–168, 1975.
98. Queyrat L. Erythroplasie du gland. Bull Soc Fr Dermatol Syphiligr (22): 378–382, 1911.
99. Shafer WG, Waldron CA. Erythroplakia of the oral cavity. Cancer (36): 1021–1028, 1975.
100. Shear M. Erythroplakia of the mouth. Int Dent J (22): 460–473, 1972.
101. Mashberg A. Erythroplasia—Earliest sign of asymptomatic oral cancer. J Am Dent Ass (96): 615–620, 1978.
102. Shafer WG. Oral carcinoma in situ. Oral Surg (39): 227–238, 1975.
103. Laskaris G, Bovopoulou O, Nicolis G. Oral submucous fibrosis in a Greek female. Br J Oral Surg (19): 197–201, 1981.
104. Pindborg JJ. Is submucous fibrosis a precancerous condition on the oral cavity? Intern Dent J (22): 474–480, 1972.
105. Wahi PN, Kapur NL, Luthra KU, Srivastava MC. Submucous fibrosis of the oral cavity: 1. Clinical features. Bull Wld Hlth Org (35): 789–792, 1966.
106. Paymaster JC. Cancer of the buccal mucosa; a clinical study of 650 cases in Indian patients. Cancer (37): 431–435, 1956.
107. Bánóczy J. Oral Leukoplakia. The Hague: Martinus Nijhoff, 1982.

# 2. SQUAMOUS CELL CARCINOMA: CLINICAL AND HISTOPATHOLOGICAL ASPECTS

I. VAN DER WAAL

## 1. INTRODUCTION

About 3% of all malignancies that can occur in the body are found in the oral cavity. In some areas of the world, this percentage is somewhat higher. The majority of that 3% consists of squamous cell carcinomas of the oral mucosa, while the remaining group of tumors is formed by malignant salivary gland tumors, lymphoreticular diseases, bone tumors, malignant melanomas, sarcomas, malignant odontogenic tumors, and metastases from tumors located elsewhere in the body.

## 2. EPIDEMIOLOGY

The incidence of squamous cell carcinomas of the various sites in the oral cavity differs in various parts of the world. The incidence of cancer of the tongue in Bombay, for instance, was 10.2 per 100,000 male population in a certain year, whereas the incidence of cancer of the tongue in Finland in that period was 0.7. Carcinomas of the lower lip were registered in Bombay in 0.3 males per 100,000 population, whereas in Finland that figure was 5.3 [1]. Such differences in incidence for specific sites of the oral cavity are numerous, some of which can be explained on the basis of environmental differences or habits among certain populations. The incidence of oral carcinoma in blacks is somewhat lower than in whites, which is mainly due to the lower incidence of lip cancer in blacks. This can be explained by an apparently better protection of pigmented tissue against actinic rays [2]. However, in a series of patients with head and neck cancer under the age of 45 years, blacks were affected more frequently than whites [3].

In most areas of the world, oral cancer is found mainly after the fourth decade, with a peak in the sixth decade. Carcinomas under the age of 10 years are exceptional [4,5,6]. In a series of 676 patients with a primary squamous cell carcinoma of the oral cavity, 12 (1.8%) were under 35 years of age, the youngest being a 21-year-old female [7].

Some 50 years ago a strong predilection for occurrence of squamous cell carcinomas of the oral cavity in men was recorded. For some locations the male-female ratio was even 20 to 1 or more. In the past 30 to 40 years, however, an impressive change has taken place. In the cancer registry of the Manchester area, for instance, the male-female ratio for tongue cancer was 7.8 to 1 in the 1932–1939 period, while this figure has decreased to 1.7 to 1 in the 1960–1969 period [8]. This change was due mainly to a decrease of oral cancer in men and partly to a slight increase in females. In several parts of the world today, the ratio is 1 to 1 for carcinomas in certain areas in the mouth.

### 3. ETIOLOGY

The excessive use of tobacco in its various forms is generally accepted to result in a much higher risk of developing cancers than is the nonuse of tobacco products [9]. In a study of 214 women with oral carcinomas, 72% had the habit of snuff dipping; for patients with cancer in the gingivobuccal area, the number increased to 90% [10]. In a more recent study of 255 cases of oral and oropharyngeal cancer in women in the southern United States, more or less similar findings were reported [11]. Snuff dipping was also an important etiologic factor in cancer of the anterior vestibular mucosa in a Swedish report [12]. Alcohol probably acts as a local irritant to the oral mucosa, especially in the anterior floor of the mouth. It may also induce oral cancer via a coexistent malnutrition, which in turn may depress the immunological status. There seems to be a synergism between heavy smoking and heavy drinking [13]. Other often-mentioned promoting factors are heredity, poor oral hygiene, chronic mechanic irritation by a poor dentition, and ill-fitting dentures [14]. Worth mentioning is the increased risk of developing oral cancer in textile workers [15]. Patients who have been exposed to ionizing radiation and patients who are immunosuppressed—for instance, in renal and homograft recipients [16]—have a higher incidence of subsequent cancer development. A number of rare conditions predispose to the development of oral cancer, such as xeroderma pigmentosum [17,18,19] and Fanconi's anaemia [20]. Syphilis is another disease that predisposes in its later stages to the development of oral cancer, especially of the tongue. Since this disease is now rather rare and is usually treated effectively in its early stage, its role in the development of oral cancer is at present negligible [21]. The role of sideropenic dysphagia (Plummer-Vinson syndrome) in women, especially in Sweden, seems to be of significance in the development of oral cancer [22]. In recent years the possible role of herpes simplex virus type 1 has been brought forward in the etiology of oral cancer [23].

An important factor of cancer of the lip is probably the excessive exposure to actinic rays as may occur in outdoor workers [24,25]. Trauma, superimposed upon a background of poor oral hygiene, is also thought to be of importance in the etiology of cancer of the lip [26]. Well known, of course, is the possible development of cancer from premalignant lesions such as leukoplakia and erythroplakia (see chapter 1). In this respect oral lichen planus also demands attention [27,28] as well as chronic candidosis [29] and chronic ulcerative diseases [30]. Finally, it should be observed that in many patients with oral cancer, especially in females, none of the forementioned factors or cofactors seem to be present, which makes the development of oral cancer anything but completely understood.

### 4. PREDILECTION SITES: SECOND PRIMARY

Among 14,253 cases of oral carcinomas, including the tonsils, soft palate, and uvula, in the files of the Armed Forces Institute of Pathology, the most common locations were the lower lip (38%), the tongue (22%), and the floor of the mouth (17%), followed by gingiva (6%), palate (5.5%), tonsils (5%), upper lip (4%), buccal mucosa (2%), and uvula (0.5%); it was noticed that in recent years the number of carcinomas of the floor of the mouth has been increasing considerably [31]. By looking at aforementioned data it should be kept in mind that 93% of the cases were from male patients and that the figures of the tongue were for the whole tongue, including the base. The majority of 513 cancers of the oral tongue in another series had originated in the lateral borders, the other cancers being located in the ventral surface and on the tip of the tongue; a surprisingly high number of 37 cases were reported to have originated in the dorsal surface [32]. In a prospective study of 222 early asymptomatic oral carcinomas, an overwhelming proportion of tumors were found in the floor of the mouth (45%); less frequently the tongue was involved (16%), while 31 cases were found in the palate complex. Of those 31 palatal cancers, 30 were located in the soft palate (oropharynx) and only 1 in the hard palate [33]. In what is probably the largest series ever reported on squamous cell carcinoma of the palate, representing 252 patients who had a primary lesion that could be clearly labeled as a hard or soft palate tumor, 62 were located on the hard palate [34].

Cancers of the upper lip are extremely rare. Some authors even wonder whether upper lip cancer is "true" cancer. In Finnish material from the 1953–1974 period, a total number of 28,143 males with cancer of the lower lip were registered and only 69 of the upper lip. Remarkable similarities were found in the epidemiologic parameters between upper lip cancer and skin cancer of the face, a finding that suggests that in terms of etiology upper lip cancer could perhaps be regarded as a separate entity and different from "true" cancer of the lower lip [35].

Slaughter et al. [36] found among 783 patients with oral cancer 88 patients with two or more independent squamous cell carcinomas involving the upper alimentary and respiratory tracts. In about half of those patients, two separate tumors occurred in the same anatomical area of the oral cavity, mostly in the lower lip and the tongue. From that observation the conclusion was drawn that oral carcinoma probably originates by a process of "field cancerization," in which an area of epithelium has been preconditioned by one or more carcinogenic agents [36]. Meyer and Shklar [37] reported their findings in a series of 768 oral carcinomas. Those authors accepted only lesions that appeared in distinct separate sites; when the same region was involved, only cases with carcinomas on opposite sites were accepted. Thus, on the lip and tongue only bilateral lesions were considered. There were 36 cases of multiple separate carcinomas confined to the oral mucosa and 18 cases of malignant tumors of the oral mucosa and other areas of the gastrointestinal tract. In another series 54 patients were found with multiple primary neoplasms among 825 patients with primary carcinomas of the head and neck [38]. The fact was stressed that all 54 patients, 44 males and 10 females, were heavy smokers and drinkers. Gluckmann et al. [39], in 1980, reported their findings of a prospective study, making a distinction between *synchronous* tumors (diagnosed at the same time or within a six-month period) and *metachronous* tumors (diagnosed six months or more after the diagnosis of the primary), with the idea that any neoplasm identified within a six-month period was probably present at the time of the initial cancer. Irrespective of the size or location of the neoplasms, panendoscopy was performed in each patient. In a study of 72 oral cancers, 9 simultaneously presenting second squamous cell carcinomas were identified, all located in the head and neck region. Somewhat similar figures have been reported by others [40].

In conclusion it can be stated that squamous cell carcinomas of the oral cavity show a predilection for occurrence on the lower lip, the borders of the anterior two-thirds of the tongue, and the floor of the mouth. One should be on the alert for a possible second primary in the oral cavity, the lungs, the esophagus, or the gastrointestinal tract, both at the time of the diagnosis of the initial cancer and during the follow-up of that patient. Additionally, heavy smokers and drinkers should vigorously be encouraged to give up their habits in order to minimize their chances of getting a second primary.

## 5. SYMPTOMS

The average duration of symptoms at the time of the first visit to the hospital where definitive treatment is instituted is usually around four to five months, ranging from a few weeks up to one year. Part of the delay in diagnosis and treatment is due to the patient's unawareness of a serious condition or anxiety to be confronted with it. Not infrequently, there is also a considerable doctor's delay, either by the physician, the dentist, or the medical and dental specialist.

Early carcinomas, measuring less than 1 cm, may be completely asymptomatic, being discovered just as an incidental finding during routine dental examination. In larger tumors patients may come in with varying complaints. In a Dutch study on 369 carcinomas of the oral tongue, pain, either local or referred pain to the jaw or the ear, was the first symptom in 44% of all cases, while swelling or ulceration were second (35%), followed by a white or a smooth area (15%) [41]. Reduced mobility of the tongue may be another symptom. It is worth mentioning that 6% of the patients went to seek medical help because of a node in the neck. In 73 patients with a cancer of the floor of the mouth, the majority presented with discomfort or irritation at the site of the tumor [42]. In carcinomas of the alveolar ridge, some discomfort in wearing the denture may be the first complaint, and in advanced cancer of the retromolar area, trismus may actually be the first symptom for the patient. Anesthesia or paresthesia is a rare symptom in oral primaries, even in advanced cases. Those symptoms usually point to an intraosseous lesion, being either a primary or a metastatic growth from a tumor located elsewhere in the body.

## 6. CLINICAL ASPECTS

In a study of the appearance of 158 early asymptomatic squamous cell carcinomas Mashberg et al. [43] emphasized the importance of erythroplastic changes, either smooth or granular in texture. Induration does not have to be a feature of the early and asymptomatic carcinoma. In symptomatic tumors, usually measuring more than 1 to 2 cm, the most frequently encountered aspect is an indurated ulceration (figure 2–1). One is often impressed by the extent of a tumor by carefully palpating, if possible bimanually, the surrounding tissues. In a study of about 1,000 oral cancers, more than 65% were at least 2 cm at the time of admission [31]. A squamous cell carcinoma may also manifest itself as an exophytic, papillary, or verrucous growth without much invasiveness. A special type of carcinoma is the verrucous carcinoma, which will be discussed later. Some of the oral cancers grow submucosally, only to cause ulceration at a late stage of the disease (figure 2–2). It should be remembered that some of the cancers may just look like a leukoplakia with or without intermingled erythroplakia (figure 2–3). It has been mentioned already that second primaries in the oral cavity or head and neck area occur in 5 to 10% of cases [38,39].

Most of the lower lip carcinomas are located on the vermilion border. A carcinoma on the labial mucosa is rare and is usually due to certain chewing habits [44,45]. Crusty lesions on the vermilion border of the lower lip are difficult to diagnose clinically. A harmless looking lesion, clinically diagnosed as actinic keratosis, may actually be a squamous cell carcinoma. A special problem with an elevated, well-circumscribed tumor of the lower lip is the distinction between either a keratoacanthoma or a squamous cell carcinoma. A

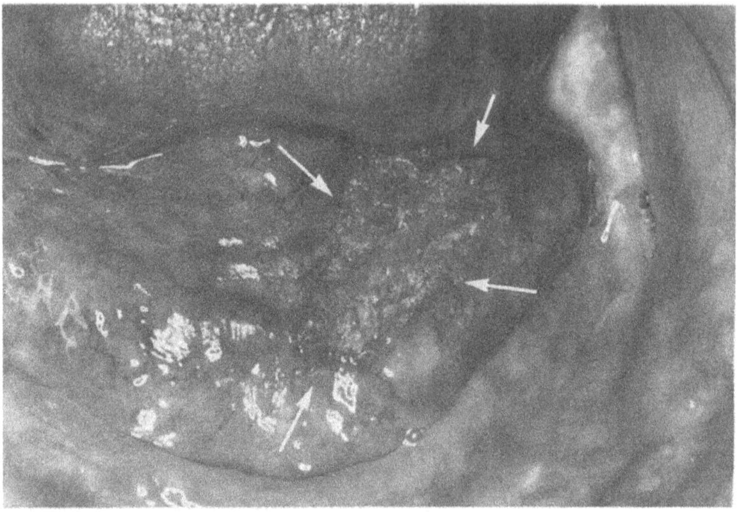

**Figure 2–1.** Asymptomatic, superficial, erosive, and ulcerative changes in the anterior floor of the mouth. Histologically proven squamous cell carcinoma.

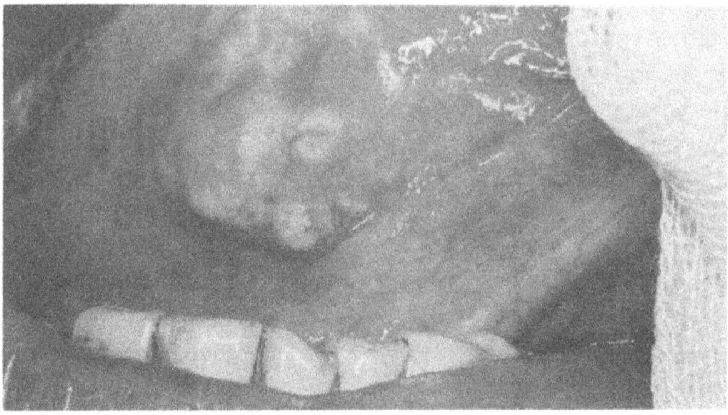

**Figure 2–2.** Submucosal growth of a squamous cell carcinoma in the border of the tongue of a 53-year-old woman.

rapid development of the tumor is in favor of a keratoacanthoma. However, this is not a fully reliable criterion. If possible, an excision should be done in those circumstances to give the best chance for a correct histopathologic diagnosis. Cases remain, however, in which a reliable distinction between keratoacanthoma and well-differentiated squamous cell carcinoma cannot be made histologically. A squamous cell carcinoma in the commissures is rare, but may also be difficult to diagnose clinically as well as histologically because

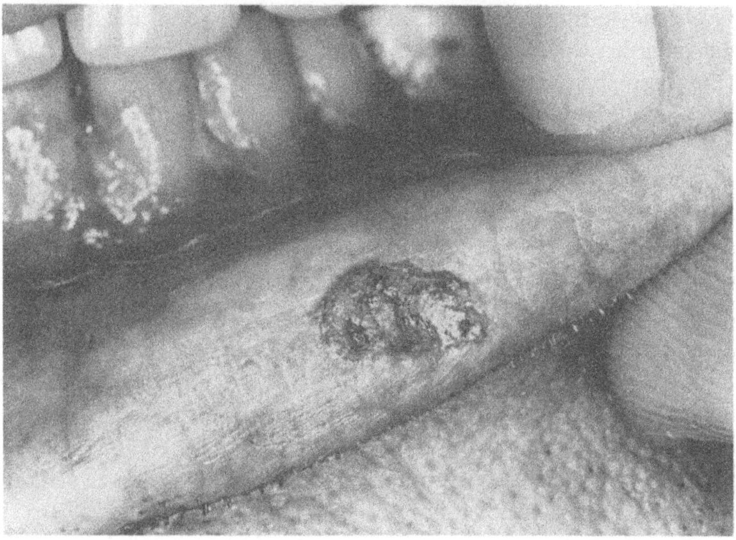

**Figure 2–3.** Ulcerative lesion on the lower lip in a 55-year-old man. Histologically proven squamous cell carcinoma.

of the frequently occurring involvement of that area with Candida albicans. This problem typically arises in elderly male patients who are wearing dentures and who are moderate or heavy smokers. Even when scrapings for Candida are negative, an antifungicide can be applied for some weeks before taking a biopsy. And the patient should be convinced of the need to quit smoking. Some of those lesions will then disappear completely or almost completely. If not, a biopsy should be taken.

Cancers of the floor of the mouth and the borders of the tongue usually do not create problems in the clinical diagnosis. A carcinoma in the anterior part of the floor of the mouth may spread along the epithelial lining of the Wharton's duct. Ulcerations or erosions on the dorsum of the tongue are occasionally misdiagnosed clinically as a cancer, actually being in most instances an expression of candidiasis [46]. Nonindurated ulcers at the borders of the tongue may occur in the course of lichen planus.

Oral cancer rather seldom arises in a dentate part of the alveolar ridge, but more often does so in the mucosa of an edentulous ridge. A radiograph should be taken to examine any possible underlying bone destruction. Changes on the radiographs may be indicative of an invasive or erosive type of bone loss. When teeth are present the picture of "floating teeth" may be seen in advanced bone involvement [47]. When examining a resection specimen, one is often surprised to see invasion by tumor cells in the presence of a "negative" radiograph. Others have stated that invasion of the underlying bone occurs in approximately 50% of the carcinomas in this location [47,48]. The value of bone scanning in the assessment of mandibular invasion in cases of negative findings on either the routine roentgenograms or tomographs is still questionable. The false positive rate can be as high as 53% [49]. When a carcinoma of the mucosa of the alveolar ridge has created destruction of the underlying bone, either by direct invasion of tumor cells or by a secondary inflammatory phenomenon, the T-category of such a tumor should, in our view, not automatically be changed to T-4. In the upper alveolar ridge, palate, and buccal sulcus, it is not uncommon for a carcinoma of the maxillary sinus to break through. Intraosseous or intra-alveolar carcinomas are extremely rare (see chapter 4).

Carcinomas of the buccal mucosa may be of the verrucous type, as will be discussed later. The majority, however, are of the ulceroinfiltrative type, as was shown, for instance, in a series of 85 cases of squamous cell carcinoma of the buccal mucosa [50]. Most of these carcinomas are located at the level of the second and third molars. A simultaneously occurring bilateral carcinoma of the buccal mucosa is an exception [51].

The size, site, and extension of a tumor should be recorded accurately. For the treatment planning it is necessary to have a good impression of the depth of infiltration and the relation of the tumor to other oral structures such as the mandible. In some instances it is worthwhile or even necessary to do the inspection under general anesthesia, which at the same time permits the proper taking of a biopsy and in some cases also the placing of an intra-arterial catheter for chemotherapy.

## 7. EVALUATION OF THE NECK

Although this book is not intended to deal in depth with all kinds of pathology of the neck, attention must be paid to the often occurring lymphatic spread of oral cancers to the cervical lymph nodes. The evaluation of the neck for the possible presence of suspicious nodes requires a proper examining technique by palpation and a vast experience in judgment of whether an enlarged lymph node is suspicious. Moreover, knowledge is required of the chances of metastatic spread and of the lymphatic patterns that oral carcinomas at various sites may take to the neck, as is illustrated in figure 2–4. In midline or near-midline cancers, contralateral and bilateral lymphatic spread is not uncommon. A cytologic puncture, taken by an experienced clinician or cytologist, may considerably increase the reliability of the preoperative staging of the cervical lymph nodes [52]. This technique is, in our experience, of extreme importance in the evaluation and management of the neck. In a preliminary report the possible value of CT in detecting cervical lymph node metastases has been reported [53].

In a series of 898 oral and oropharyngeal carcinomas, Shear et al. [54] were able to predict rather accurately the chance of lymph node metastases by grouping the tumors in three clusters with an increasing tendency for metastatic spread. Cluster 1 consisted of tumors of the lip, floor of mouth, cheek mucosa, hard palate, and gingiva. Cluster 2 consisted of tumors of the anterior two-thirds of the tongue, and cluster 3, with the highest tendency to metastastic spread, was formed by tumors of the posterior third of the tongue and oropharynx. Well-differentiated and moderately differentiated tumors did not show a significantly different tendency to metastasize, whereas poorly differentiated tumors did show a higher incidence of metastases. The same study demonstrated that metastases were present or became manifest in 45% of all carcinomas less than 1 cm in diameter. That figure remained somewhat unchanged for tumors up to 3 cm in diameter and rose to 73% in tumors measuring 4 cm or more. Lindberg [55] found in T-1 carcinomas of the oral tongue and the floor of the mouth suspicious lymph nodes at the time of admission in 14 and 11%, respectively.

Spiro et al. [56] reported on the cervical metastases from 1,069 patients with oral and oropharyngeal cancer, focusing on the assessment of staging of cervical nodes. One of the important findings in that study was a 10% false positive rate (clinically suspicious, but no metastatic involvement demonstrated by histologic examination) and a 15% false negative rate (absence of metastatic nodes clinically, but metastatic involvement demonstrated by histologic examination). In a series of 881 patients with cancer of the head and neck, the false positive rate of the clinical assessment of the neck was somewhat similar to the one of the previously mentioned study. The false negative rate, however, was more than 25% [57]. Jesse et al. [58] reported the findings in 210 patients treated for a node in the neck for which no primary was found. In 37 out of those 210 patients, a tumor became manifest after treatment; just 4 were located in the oral cavity or salivary glands, the remaining primaries being mainly located in the hypopharynx and oropharynx.

Removal of a single suspicious cervical lymph node for diagnostic purposes should be avoided because it may result in a contaminated wound and, moreover, may cause changes in the pattern of lymphatic tumor spread.

## 8. DISTANT METASTASIS

Distant metastasis of oral cancer is rather rare at the time of admission, but does occur with some frequency in a later stage of the disease [59]. In a study of 169 patients with head and neck cancer, bone scans of the skeleton made at the time of admission were positive in only 2% of all cases and all liver scans were negative [60]. In 62 autopsies of patients with primary oral cancer, distant metastases were observed in 13 cases (20%), mostly in the lungs [61]. Other organs involved were the liver, the adrenals, the heart, and the kidneys (figure 2-5). Regional cervical involvement occurred in all those cases as well. In autopsies of 100 patients with cancer of the floor of the mouth, distant metastases were found in 22 patients in the lungs and just occasionally in the long

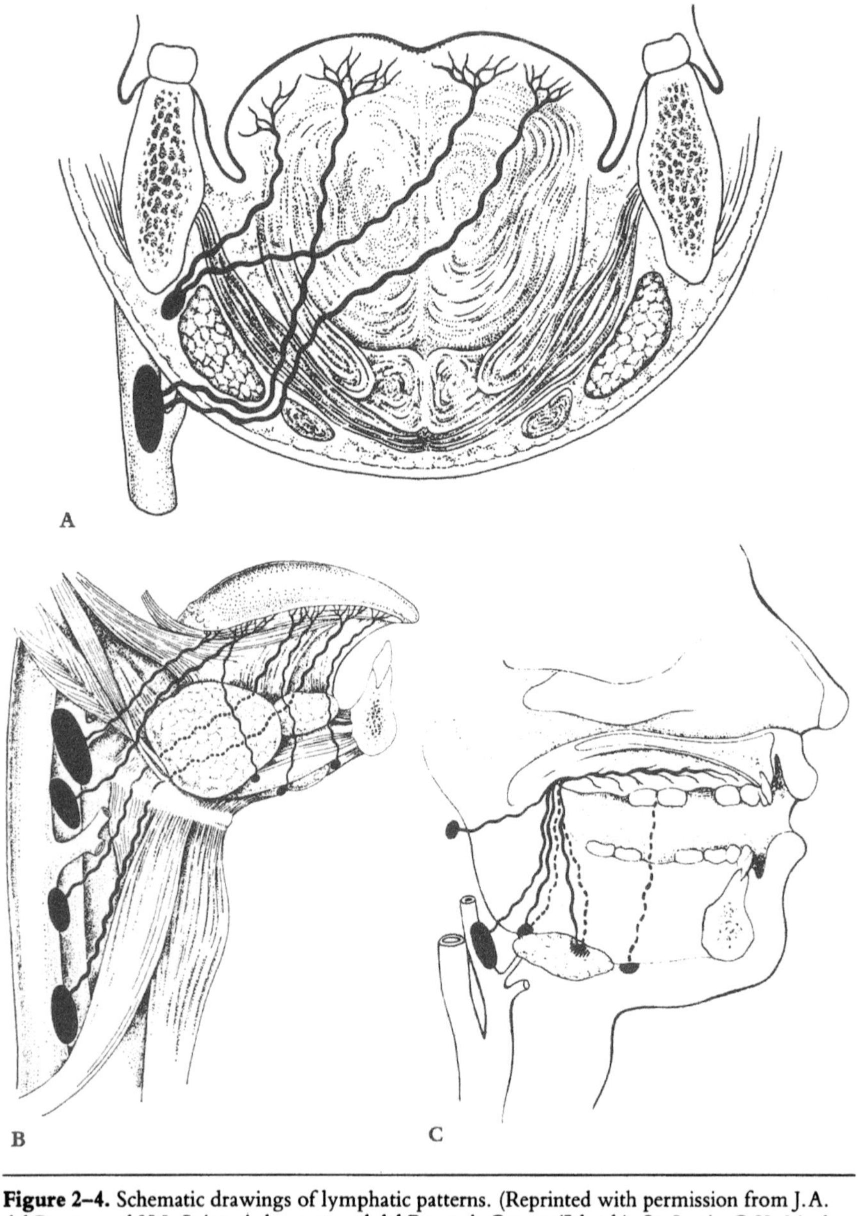



**Figure 2–4.** Schematic drawings of lymphatic patterns. (Reprinted with permission from J.A. del Regato and H.J. Spjut, Ackerman and del Regato's Cancer (5th ed.), St. Louis: C.V. Mosby, 1977).

**A.** Lymphatics of tongue in frontal section illustrating that areas of dorsum are drained by trunks that may cross midline to end in submandibular or cervical lymph nodes in opposite side.

**B.** Lymphatics of tongue illustrating that the more anteriorly they originate in the tongue, the lower may be their draining lymph nodes.

**C.** Lymphatics of upper gingiva which end in submandibular or jugular lymph nodes and rarely in retropharyngeal nodes.

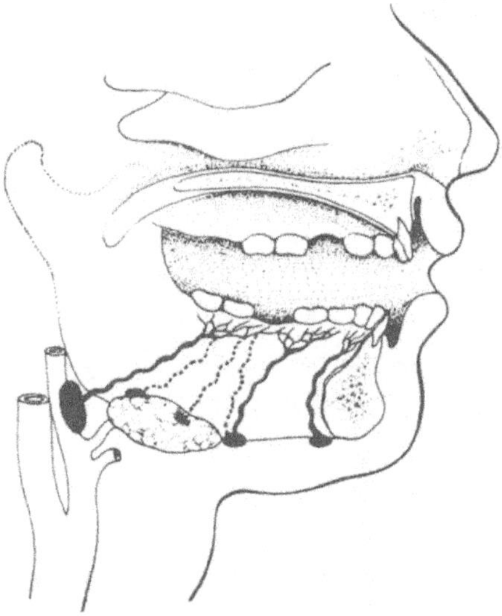

D

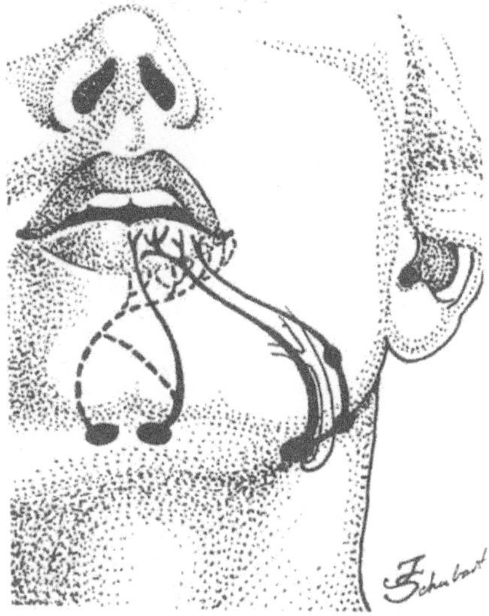

E

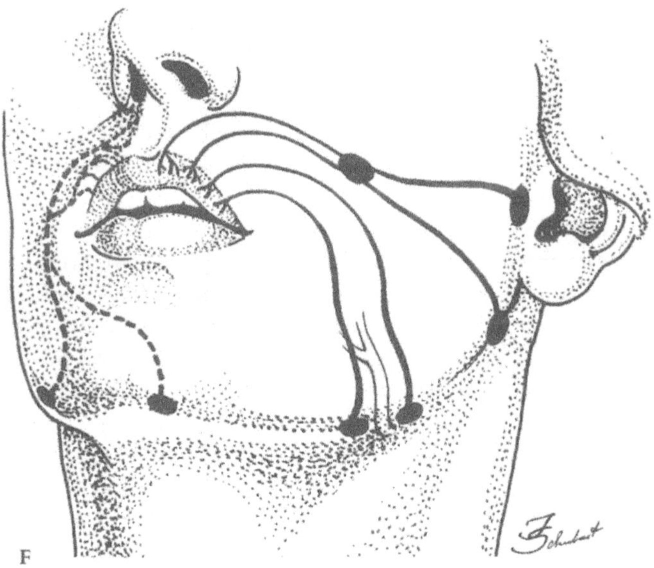

F

**D.** Medial and lateral lymphatics of lower gingiva leading to submental, submandibular, and subdigastric lymph nodes.
**E.** Lymphatics of lower lip which end in submental and prevascular submandibular lymph nodes but sometimes stop in facial nodes. Lymphatics of skin of lower lip (dotted line) may cross midline to end in submental and submandibular nodes of opposite side.
**F.** Lymphatics of upper lip which lead to buccal, parotid, and upper cervical nodes as well as to prevascular and retrovascular submandibular lymph nodes. Lymphatics of skin of upper lip (dotted line) may cross midline to terminate in submental and submaxillary nodes of opposite side.

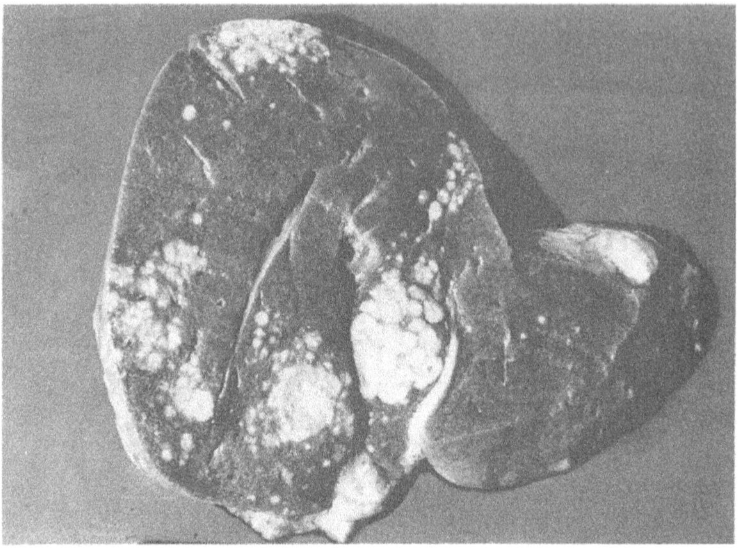

**Figure 2–5.** Multiple metastases in the liver of a 19-year-old man who died from widespread carcinoma of the tongue.

bones, the liver, the adrenal glands, or in the sella turcica [62]. Another study showed that only one of four cases of distant metastases proven at autopsy was diagnosed clinically [63].

In a series of 238 patients with squamous cell carcinomas of the head and neck, hypercalcemia was found in 4.2% of the cases [64]. Another report of hypercalcemia due to bony metastases from tongue cancer observed that a coma may be due to reversible hypercalcemia rather than being the terminal event in the progress of the cancer [65]. Also stressed was that the development of hypercalcemia in a previously normocalcemic patient who has been treated for a cancer is a grave prognostic sign. It has been suggested that the humoral factor responsible for hypercalcemia in patients with head and neck cancer is not parathyroid hormone and that patients with hyperparathyroidism can be distinguished with confidence from those with malignancy-associated hypercalcemia [66].

## 9. DIAGNOSTIC PROCEDURES FOR THE PRIMARY

### 9.1. Toluidine blue application

In the past several authors advocated the use of toluidine blue application in the diagnostic procedure of oral carcinoma. Rather recently the value of such a staining technique has again been emphasized by Mashberg [67], who used a 1% toluidine blue solution containing acetic and alcohol instead of the commonly used 1% aqueous solution. In 83 cases of histologically proven invasive carcinomas, 80 were clinically diagnosed as being suspicious, whereas the staining technique in those 83 patients gave a positive impression in 78 cases. In 118 benign lesions 30 (25.4%) were clinically diagnosed by an experienced clinician as being suspicious, whereas the staining technique in the same group was false positive in only 8 (6.8%) cases. The number of false negative results in a group of 83 histologically proven squamous cell carcinomas was 4.8% just by clinical judgment, 6.7% by using toluidine blue, but less than 2% when both modalities were applied. Moreover, by applying the stain to high-risk areas, second lesions that had been missed during clinical examination were discovered. All authors who have published their experience with this staining technique, including Mashberg, have stressed the fact that in case of positive staining by toluidine blue a biopsy remains mandatory.

### 9.2. Exfoliative cytology

Some authors have demonstrated a high accuracy when using exfoliative cytology in the diagnosis of oral carcinoma [68,69,70]. In those series the number of false negative findings was 10% or less, whereas false positive accounted for less than 4%. Other authors have reported a somewhat less positive experience with this diagnostic aid. Folsom et al [71], for instance, found a false negative rate of 31%, but at the same time admitted to have discovered clinically unsuspected lesions by exfoliative cytology. Payne and Tsaknis [71] reported negative results of the use of a rinse-gargle technique for oral cytologic diagnosis. Although adequate samples were obtained in 18 patients with already biopsy-proven carcinoma, just one smear was interpreted as being suspicious.

All papers dealing with the role of exfoliative cytology in the diagnosis of oral cancer emphasize that exfoliative cytology is not a substitute for an adequate biopsy.

### 9.3. Additional diagnostic aids other than biopsy

In 1972 a screening procedure was described in which cells were collected from ostensibly normal buccal mucosa in about 200 healthy adults, 200 alcoholic persons, 79 patients who had been treated successfully for oral cancer, and 85 patients whose tumor was either untreated as yet, recurrent, or treated within the previous three months [73]. The cells were stained with acriflavine hydrochloride. The widest difference in the dye uptake occurred between the healthy persons and the group of 85 active cancer cases. There was a false positive rate of 25%. In smokers an elevated dye uptake was found, whereas the alcoholic group failed to exhibit an abnormal dye binding.

Carcinomatous oral epithelium loses its isoantigens A, B, or H. That property can be used rather accurately in the specific red cell adherence test, as has been described by George et al. [74], among others, in a group of 124 patients containing 56 healthy persons and 68 with invasive carcinoma or carcinoma in situ. Presently, the test seems mainly of interest for research purposes and is not in use in the daily practice of the pathologist. The use of tumor markers, such as carcinoembryonic agent (CEA), $\alpha_1$-acid glycoprotein ($\alpha_1$-AG), ferritin, soluble immune complexes, and serum immunoglobulins, has proven in several studies to be of some importance, but at this writing does not seem to be of practical value for diagnostic or monitoring purposes in the individual patient.

### 9.4. Biopsy

The clinical suspicion of malignancy should be based on a thorough inspection of the lesion including careful palpation bimanually, if possible. What a suspicious lesion is for an experienced oncologist may not be so for a clinician who is just incidentally involved in the diagnosis of oral cancer. Even in clinically very obvious cases of carcinoma, a biopsy should be taken in order to exclude the slightest chance of misdiagnosis. Besides, the histologic grade of the tumor may be important in the treatment planning.

Myall and Howell [75] strongly suggest, as do the majority of oncologists, that in case of clinically suspected cancer, the patient should be referred for the biopsy directly to the individual or center that will carry out the definitive treatment.

An excisional biopsy is justified only in lesions smaller than 1 cm. As a rule, the margins of the specimen should be at least 1 cm beyond the clinically visible or palpable tumor in all its directions. The specimen should be marked with a suture for proper orientation for the pathologist. A written clinical history and description of the lesion should accompany the specimen to the laboratory; a small drawing of the lesion may be helpful. The specimen can be placed in a regular fixative or, in case of any special interest of the clinician or the pathologist, in another fixative. Some pathologists prefer to have the tissue transported immediately while fresh, whereas others require a special medium during the transportation of the specimen to the laboratory. A small biopsy may be adhered to a piece of cardboard which is then placed upside-down in the fixative, thereby preventing curling of the tissue. In that way the pathologist can make the histologic sections in a proper direction.

In lesions measuring more than 1 cm, an incisional biopsy, taken from the clinically most suspicious area and avoiding necrotic parts, should be done. The measurements of the specimen should be at least $0.5 \times 0.2 \times 0.2$ cm to allow reliable histopathologic examination. It may be helpful to include a small part of clinically normal mucosa in the biopsy. One should realize, however, that by doing so a previously healthy area becomes contaminated with tumor cells, thereby enlarging the tumor field. The same holds true for the taking of multiple biopsies.

Topical anesthesia may be adequate. In some sites a nerve bloc can be applied. Only in unusual circumstances is general anesthesia to be used. Infiltration injection into or close to the tumor area should be avoided at any price.

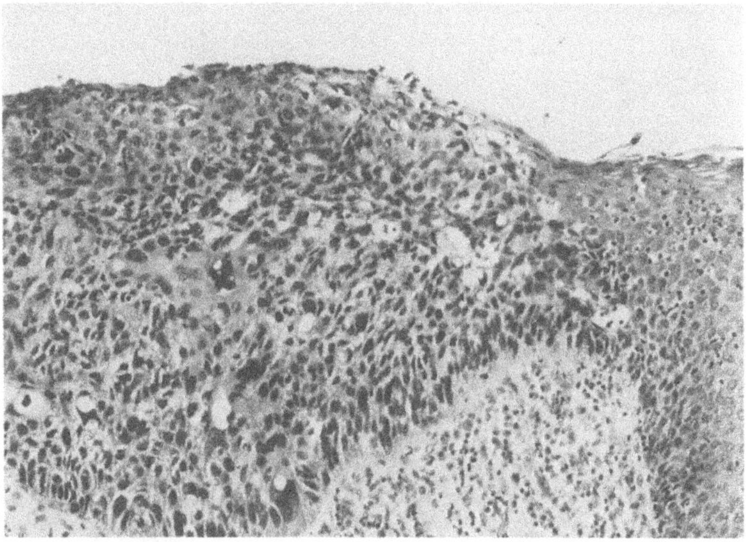

**Figure 2–6.** Biopsy of the mucosa of the floor of the mouth shows cellular and nuclear polymorphism and loss of polarity. The basal membrane is still intact. This picture is compatible with the diagnosis "carcinoma in situ." Notice the rather sharp transition with the adjacent normal epithelium.

## 10. HISTOPATHOLOGY

### 10.1. Carcinoma in situ

Carcinoma in situ can be defined as a lesion in which the epithelium shows the malignant cellular features of a cancer but lacks proven invasive growth (figure 2–6). Shafer [76] has described the findings of 77 carcinomas in situ collected over a period of about 25 years. The fact was stressed that it is actually unknown what percentage of oral carcinomas in situ will finally change into invasive cancer and whether spontaneous regression of oral carcinoma in situ may occur. Carcinomas in situ are especially found in early, asymptomatic lesions. In such a series of 158 oral squamous cell carcinomas, a total number of 46 carcinomas in situ were recorded [43]. In another series of 194 symptomatic oral and oropharyngeal cancers, just 3 such cases were found [77]. Part of that difference in the number of carcinomas in situ is perhaps based upon a different histopathologic appreciation of carcinoma in situ versus severe epithelial dysplasia on one hand and carcinoma in situ versus invasive carcinoma on the other hand.

In spite of aforementioned uncertainty about the behaviour of carcinoma in situ, it is advised to treat a patient with this lesion as having cancer.

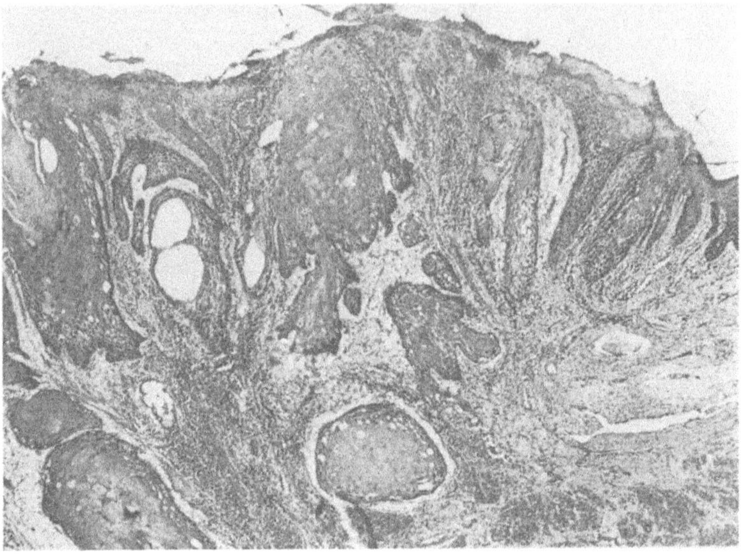

**Figure 2–7.** Low-power view of a well-differentiated squamous cell carcinoma of the floor of the mouth.

### 10.2. Squamous cell carcinoma

Most of the oral squamous cell carcinomas are of the well-differentiated type (figure 2–7). There may be some variation in the pathologist's appreciation of the grade of tumor (see later discussion on histologic grading). The transition between the neoplastic epithelium and the surrounding mucosa may be sharp or rather fluent. Differentiation may be difficult between pseudoepitheliomatous ("pseudocarcinomatous") hyperplasia and invasive well-differentiated carcinoma, especially in small biopsy specimens. Well known is the phenomenon of pseudoepitheliomatous changes in the epithelium overlying a granular cell tumor. Again, when a small biopsy is taken, the underlying benign condition may be missed and a diagnosis of well-differentiated carcinoma may be made erroneously. Hyperplastic candidiasis, either in the commissures, the palate, or the dorsal surface of the tongue, may mimic somewhat the picture of a well-differentiated carcinoma [78]. The presence of candidal hyphae in the PAS-stain is not an unusual finding in a squamous cell carcinoma. Necrotizing sialometaplasia may be diagnosed erroneously as a carcinoma [79]. In these cases, especially, a close contact between pathologist and clinician is of utmost importance for correct diagnosis. Melanotic pigmentation of carcinomas of the skin is not uncommon, in contrast to pigmentation in oral cancer. One such case, on the lateral border of the tongue of a Negro male, was reported in 1974 [80], later followed by a few others [81,82].

Relatively few reports on the ultrastructure of squamous cell carcinoma are available. Chen and Harwick [83] described the electron-microscopic findings in 16 moderately differentiated oral carcinomas, together with some histochemical observations. In a study of 32 cases of oral carcinoma, the possible usefulness of scanning electron microscopy for the early diagnosis of changes in the oral mucosa has been discussed [84].

Lymphatic invasion is quite often seen, especially in carcinomas of the tongue. Invasion of blood vessels, particularly veins, is a rather uncommon phenomenon in primary oral carcinoma, even in the extensive ones (figure 2–8). (In the lungs embolism from gross vascular invasion seems more important in the formation of metastases than is cellular dissemination from microscopic vessels [85]. This is probably also true in oral cancer.) Sometimes perineural spread may be seen, especially in advanced or recurrent disease [86,87]. In that way the cranial cavity may be entered (figure 2–9). Carter et al. [88] studied perineural spread in 35 squamous cell carcinomas of the oral cavity. Perineural spread was found in 9 of the primaries, especially in large, moderately or poorly differentiated tumors, showing signs of lymphatic and/or vascular invasion. Deep infiltration into the substances of the nerves could not be demonstrated. In many of those cases, nerve involvement was detected clinically as well. For a long time lymphatic channels were assumed to be present in association with nerves. An experimental study has demonstrated, however, that no such association exists and that tumor growth along nerves is the result of extension along tissue planes of least resistance [89]. It was also noticed that a nerve may contain tumor cells and still function. The pathologist should be aware of the possible presence of Chievitz's bodies (juxtacortical organ) in the spatium buccotemporale (figure 2–10) since those structures may be misinterpreted as perineural carcinomatous spread [90,91,92]. Somewhat similar pseudocarcinomatous perineural spread of benign epithelium has been reported by Endes and Adler [93] and by Jensen et al. [94].

When a squamous cell carcinoma approaches the underlying bone, there is usually osteoclastic resorption ahead of the invading tumor and replacement of the bone by loose connective tissue and cords or islands of malignant epithelial cells. The tumor may enter the bone through the Haversian system of the cortex and penetrate widely throughout the jaw, or the invasion may be a direct erosion of the cortex of the bone by the advancing tumor. At the margins of the zone of invasion, reactive osteogenesis can usually be seen [95].

Stromal changes in squamous cell carcinomas that have not been radiated or treated by chemotherapy previously are not of much diagnostic importance. In most cases dense infiltrates of lymphocytes and plasma cells are present, both in ulcerative and nonulcerative cancers. A dense lympho-plasmocellular infiltrate is thought by some authors to correlate with a better prognosis [95]. It has been demonstrated that in an area with a dense infiltrate the number of mitoses is decreased [97]. Changes in the blood vessels and in the stromal ground substance may vary from myxomatous changes with an increase of acid mucopolysaccharides, as demonstrated by the use of an Alcian blue stain,

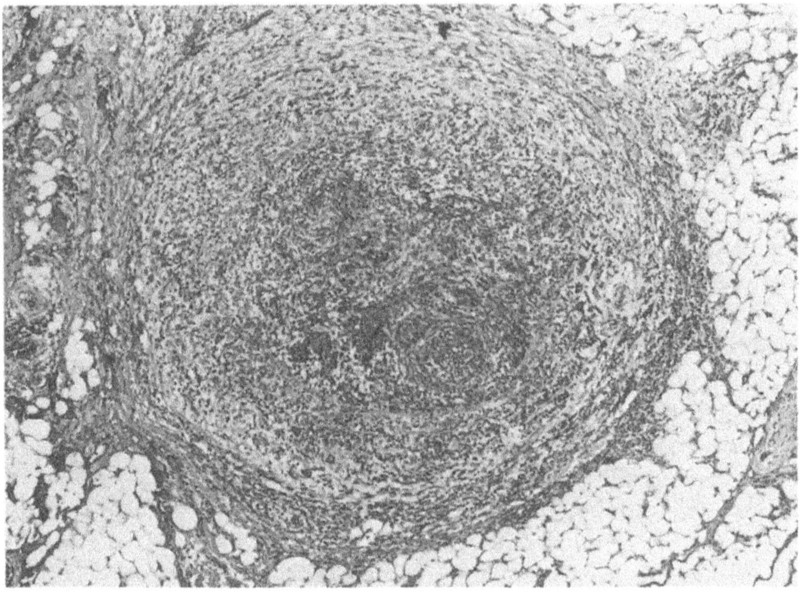

A

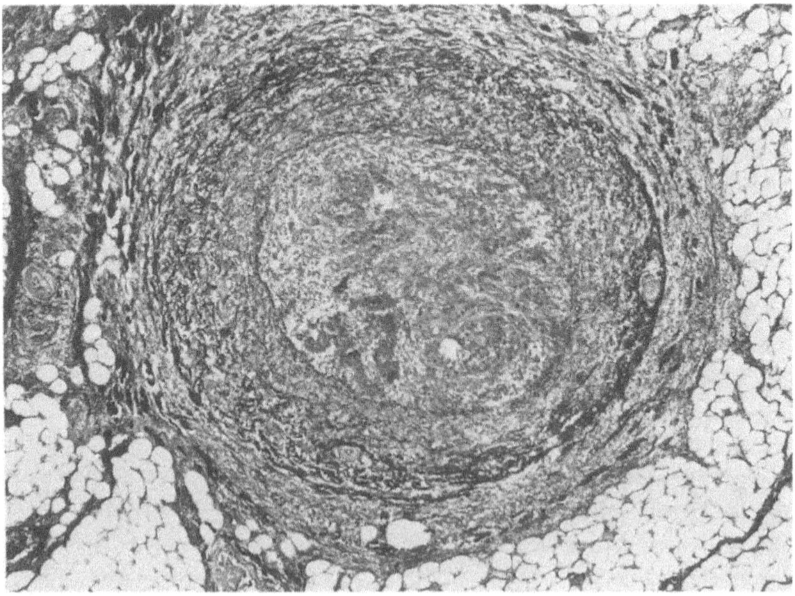

B

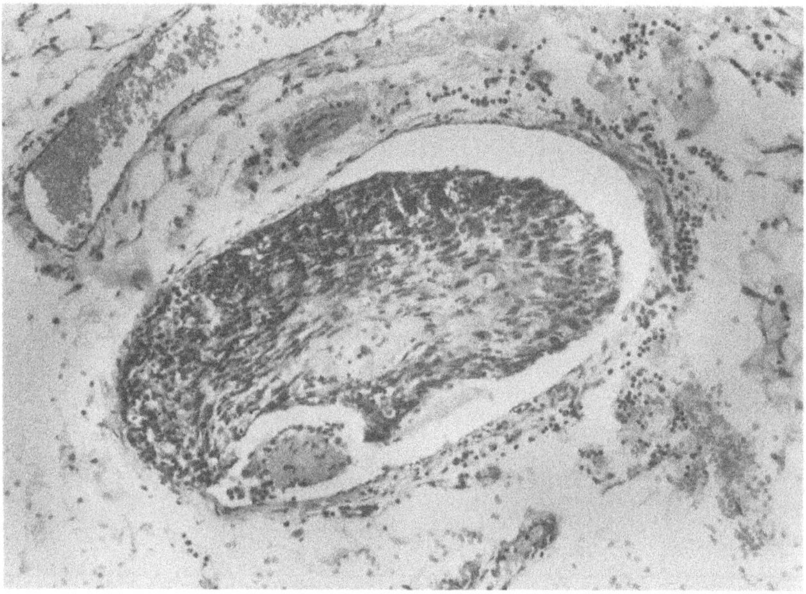

C

**Figure 2–8. A.** Tumor cell located in the center. **B.** In the Van-Gieson-Elastica stain, the structure of a blood vessel is obvious, proving hematogenous spread. **C.** Tumor cells in lymph vessel.

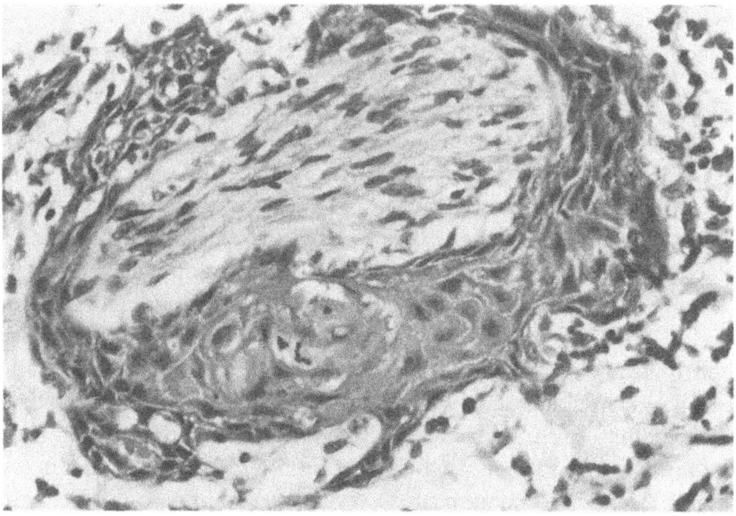

**Figure 2–9.** Perineural spread of a squamous cell carcinoma of the tongue.

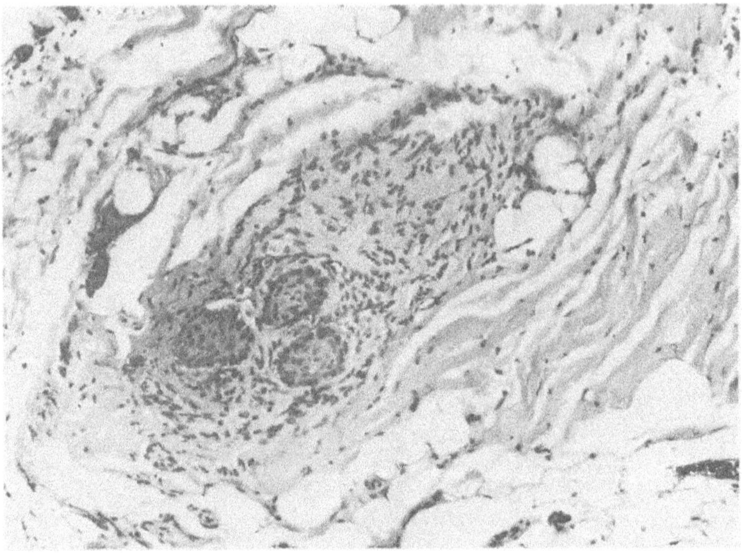

**Figure 2–10.** Epithelial structures in relation to a nerve, the so-called Chievitz bodies. These may be misinterpreted as part of a squamous cell carcinoma.

to hyalinization. It has been shown, both in cancers of the lower lip [98] and of the tongue [99] that a positive Alcian blue reaction correlates with a poor diagnosis.

*10.2.1. Changes due to chemotherapy or radiation*

During treatment with methotrexate or bleomycin, the tumor cells become more or less devitalised by increased keratinization (figure 2–11). Simple necrosis seems to play a minor role. In some cases no vital tumor cells can still be recognized in the specimen. In the stroma a granulomatous reaction occurs in which large numbers of giant cells may be observed [100]. It has been proven that those cells are not giant tumor cells but macrophage polykaryons of monocytic origin. Burkhardt and Gebbers [101] have studied 10 oral squamous cell carcinomas treated by intra-arterial bleomycin therapy and surgery and reported the electron microscopic and ultrahistochemical observations on the genesis and functional activity of the multinucleated giant cells. In a study of 22 patients with extensive squamous cell carcinomas in which polychemotherapy had been used, consisting of methotrexate, bleomycin, and cis-platinum, increased keratinization was observed in well-differentiated carcinomas, while poorly differentiated carcinomas remained more or less unchanged as far as histologic grading was concerned [102]. In another study of 44 tumors of the head and neck, tumor shrinkage after BMV chemotherapy

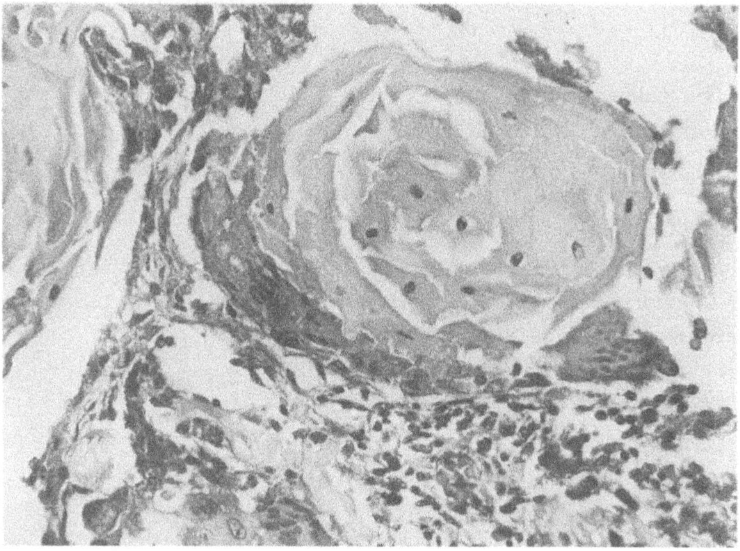

**Figure 2–11.** Squamous cell carcinoma after intra-arterial perfusion with methotrexate. Notice the increased keratinization and the multinucleated giant cells.

was correlated with the histologic grading of the biopsy and showed no relationship [103].

A squamous cell carcinoma that has been preradiated may show bizarre cellular and nuclear aspects. The stroma is usually hyalinized, and the walls of the blood vessels may have become thickened.

*10.2.2. Histologic grading*

Histologic grading has gained considerable popularity since 1920, when Broders introduced a grading system varying from grade I for tumors being 75 to 100% differentiated and cells 0 to 25% de-differentiated. Since then many modifications have been used. Arthur and Fenner [104], for instance, applied a simplified grading system, giving scores for keratinisation, mitotic activity and hyperchromatism, and cell irregularity in 299 carcinomas of the tongue. Eneroth and Moberger [105] applied a more detailed grading system to 110 palatal cancers. Scores were given to characteristics of the tumor cell population, such as structure, differentiation, nuclear polymorphism, and mitosis, and also to characteristics based on tumor-host relationship, such as stage and mode of invasion, presence of vascular invasion, and plasma-lymphocytic response. A similar grading system, applied to 124 squamous cell carcinomas of the gingiva, showed a strong correlation between the degree of histological malignancy and the fatal outcome of the disease [106].

The UICC has devised a histopathological classification of the primary tumor [107]:

G —*Histopathological Grading*
G1 —high degree of differentiation
G2 —medium degree of differentiation
G3 —low degree of differentiation or undifferentiated
GX—grade cannot be assessed

L —*Lymphatic Invasion*
LO—no evidence of lymphatic invasion
L1 —evidence of invasion of superficial lymphatics
L2 —evidence of invasion of deep lymphatics
LX—lymphatic invasion cannot be assessed

V —*Venous Invasion*
VO—veins do not contain tumor
V1 —efferent veins contain tumor
V2 —distal veins contain tumor
VX—venous invasion cannot be assessed

In using histologic grading systems, one should realize that there may be differences from place to place in the same tumor and that both the quality and the amount of tissue determine the reliability of the grading system. To a certain extent there is also some variability in grading between pathologists and in a single pathologist at various times or circumstances. The value of a histological grading system in determining the prognosis or treatment planning in the individual patient remains rather limited since many other apparently much more important factors, such as size and site of the primary tumor and the presence or absence of metastatic spread, are involved.

*10.2.3. Histopathology of lymph node metastases*

On examining a specimen of the neck, the pathologist should take out as many nodes as possible, even the very small ones, recording the level of those nodes in the specimen (see UICC classification 1978, reference 107), the size, the gross encapsulation, and the possible relationship to blood vessels.

Cancerous emboli can get caught within the capsule of a lymph node or in the tissue immediately external to it. This rarely occurs in the absence of deposition within the substance of the node itself [108]. Four patterns of local behaviour in the lymph node can be observed [108]. First, local growth may proceed to a considerable extent before extranodal spread occurs. A second possibility is the extranodal spread in an early stage of the deposit, as evidenced by persistence of much of the nodal architecture. A third possibility consists of local growth in the node and simultaneous tumor growth within capsular or juxtacapsular lymphatics. The fourth pattern is the occurrence of capsular or

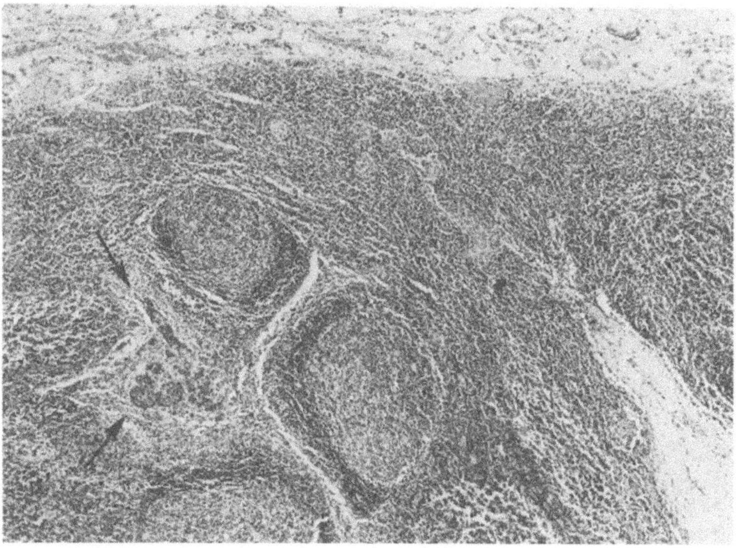

**Figure 2–12.** Metastatic cervical lymph node. The capsule seems to be intact.
**A.** Cervical lymph node with a micrometastatic deposit (arrows).

juxtacapsular emboli in relation to nodes, the substance of which is not involved. The latter possibility seems to be rather exceptional, as has been mentioned. The chance of capsular rupture increases with the size of the metastatic node [109]. That same study showed that the chance of extracapsular spread was not related to the histologic grade of the tumor. In another study of 177 radical neck dissections, 65% of the nodes 2.9 cm or less in diameter were found to demonstrate extracapsular spread [110]. One should realize that the pathologist may have cases that make difficult a black-and-white interpretation of metastatic tumor cells being located either definitely within the node, outside the node, or juxtacapsular (figure 2–12).

In reporting the histologic findings it is important to mention the number and level and/or site of positive nodes, as well as the degree of differentiation, the possible changes induced by previous radiotherapy or chemotherapy, and the presence or absence of rupture of the capsule, since all those factors play a role in the decision for the need of postoperative radiotherapy and/or chemotherapy. In many instances the degree of differentiation of a squamous carcinoma in a node is somewhat higher than in the primary, even to the extent that in some cases a proper classification of the primary cannot be made, being clarified, however, by the histology of the metastasis, with or without ultrastructural study [111]. Shear and Ichilcik [112] have studied the phenomenon of the better differentiation in metastatic lymph nodes, based on 23 oral squamous carcinomas, and suggested that the changes may be due to a kind of an

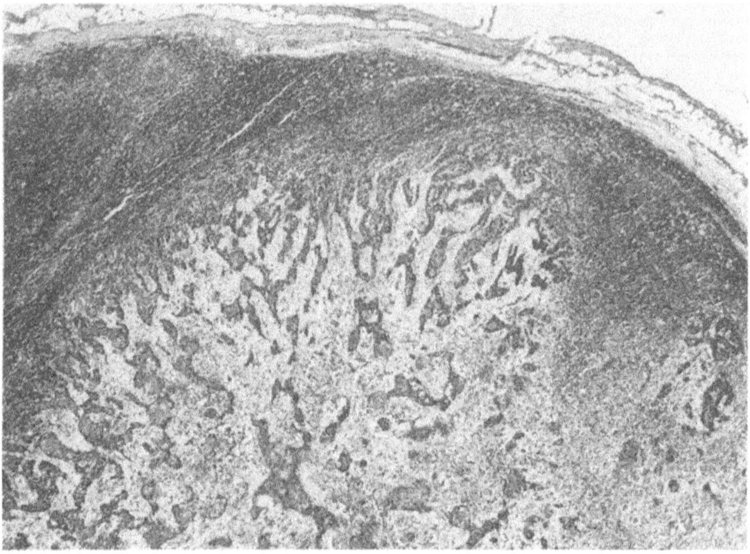

**B.** Cervical lymph node largely replaced by squamous cell carcinoma; the capsule is still intact.

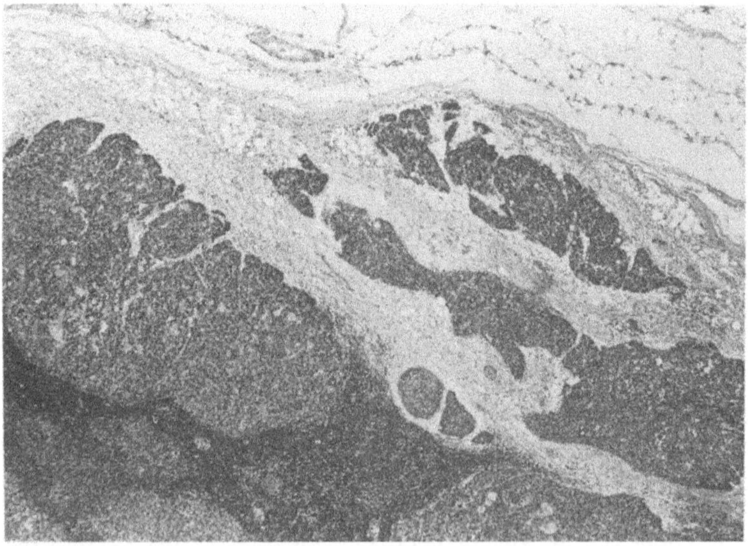

**C.** Cervical lymph node metastasis with extracapsular spread, numerous tumor cells being located in the pericapsular fat.

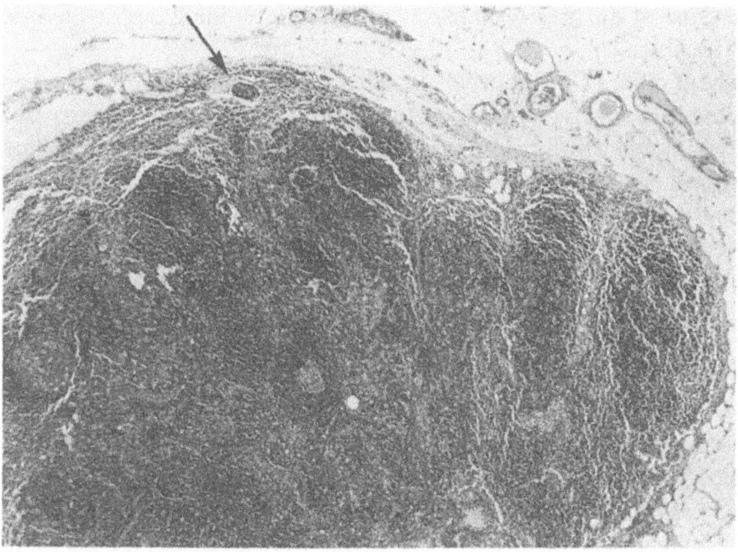

**D.** Cervical lymph node with just one microscopic metastatic deposit located within the capsule.

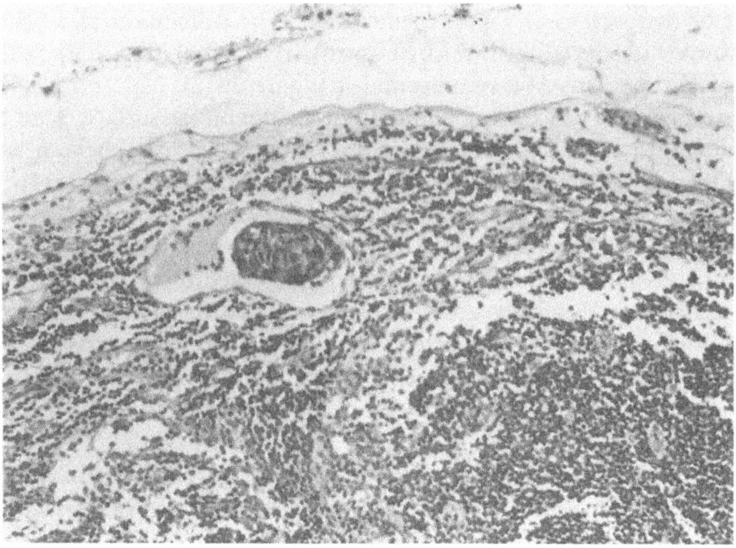

**E.** Detail of figure D.

immune response. The literature contains different opinions about the prognostic value of the host response as manifested by the lymph node morphology [113,114].

Micheau et al. [115] reported six cases of cystic metastases in the neck that presented as a solitary lesion before the primary became manifest. In five of those six cases, a misdiagnosis was made initially, such as branchial cyst, epidermoid cyst, and cyst with carcinomatous change. The question whether a branchial cleft carcinoma exists is still in debate [116,117].

In very rare instances nevus cell aggregates can be found in lymph nodes of the neck. Such aggregates may be diagnosed erroneously as a metastatic spread [118].

### 10.3. Verrucous carcinoma

In 1948 Ackerman [119] introduced the term *verrucous carcinoma* for a variety of squamous carcinoma with characteristic gross and microscopic findings. In his group of 31 patients, there were 26 men and 5 women, all except one above the age of 57 years. Tobacco chewing was thought to be the most important factor in the etiology. The majority of the lesions were located in the buccal mucosa and the alveolar ridge and were of more than one year's duration. Some of the buccal verrucous carcinomas—which can be described grossly as papillary, verrucoid in character, fungating, cauliflowerlike—had grown into the cheek, while others had grown down into the periosteum of the mandible, even to the extent of destruction of a part of the bone. The delineation of a verrucous carcinoma with the adjacent normal mucosa is usually rather sharp, although leukoplakic areas may be seen around it (figure 2–13). Microscopically, the first change in the process is a piling up of keratin on the surface, with beginning downgrowth of club-shaped fingers of hyperplastic epithelium pushing rather than infiltrating their way into the deeper tissues (figure 2–14). Slight dysplasia may be present. Inflammation is always coexistent with the lesion, and, usually, a dense infiltrate of lymphocytes and plasma cells can be observed. Although the tumor may grow in the immediate proximity of lymph nodes, it almost invariably grows around them rather than metastasizing to them. Goethals et al. [120] reported their findings of 55 verrucous carcinomas out of 1,217 oral carcinomas, which is about 5%. McCoy and Waldron [121] reported 49 cases of oral verrucous carcinomas, showing a slight female predominance.

In a series of 77 verrucous carcinomas, locally aggressive behaviour with bone invasion occurred in 15 patients [122]. Lymph node metastases were found in four patients treated by radiation, probably as a result of alteration of the biologic character of the lesion. Prioleau et al. [123] studied one case of verrucous carcinoma of the rectum, one of the plantar surface of the foot, and two cases of the oral cavity by means of light and electron microscopy and autoradiographic and immunofluorescent techniques. Their findings were consistent in all four cases, constituting evidence that verrucous carcinoma is a

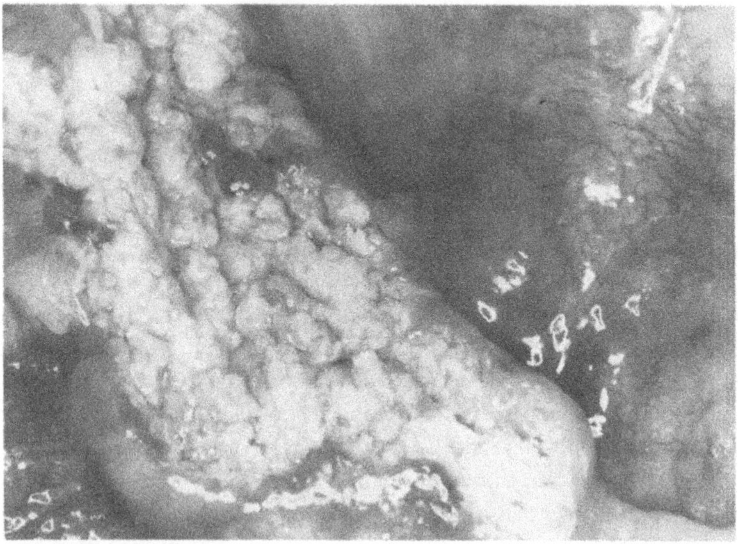

**Figure 2–13.** Verrucous carcinoma of the lower alveolar ridge.

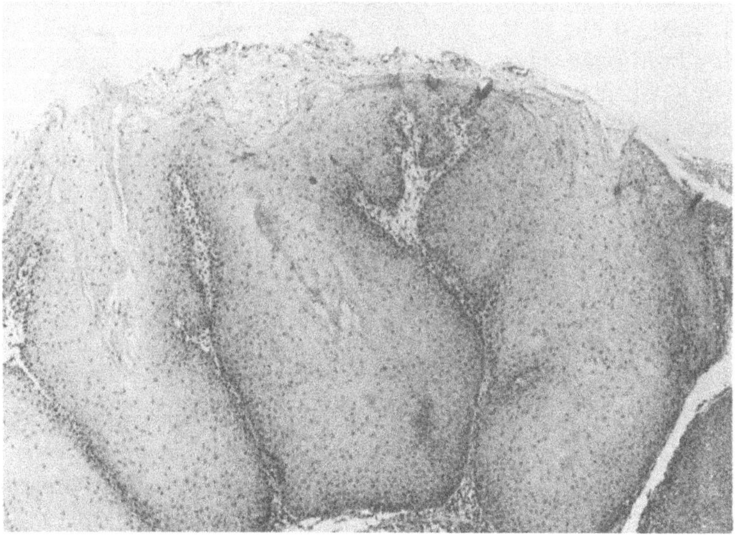

**Figure 2–14.** Histologic picture compatible with the clinicopathologic diagnosis of verrucous carcinoma.

morphologic and cytokinetic entity that may occur in multiple anatomic sites. Shear and Pindborg [124] published on verrucous hyperplasia of the oral mucosa with special reference to verrucous carcinoma. Those authors concluded that verrucous hyperplasia and verrucous carcinoma may be clinically indistinguishable from each other. Microscopically, the verrucous processes and the greater part of the hyperplastic epithelium are superficial to the adjacent normal epithelium in verrucous hyperplasia, whereas in verrucous carcinoma the broad rete processes extend considerably deeper than the adjacent normal epithelium. However, it was noticed that verrucous hyperplasia and verrucous carcinoma may coexist and also may be associated with squamous cell carcinoma. In another series 11 of 37 patients with oral verrucous carcinoma had associated squamous cell carcinoma [125]. In 1982 two very good papers on the subject of verrucous carcinoma were published [126,127].

The diagnosis of verrucous carcinoma requires both examination of the lesion in the patient and careful histologic study. An adequate biopsy, including an appropriate amount of connective tissue, must show a well-differentiated hyperkeratotic warty surface and an equally well-differentiated bulbous rete-ridge pattern at the base of the lesion. The biopsy may be underestimated as being hyperplasia.

### 10.4. Basal cell carcinoma

Intraoral basal cell carcinomas are rare [128,129]. Most of the cases described were located on one of the alveolar ridges, and some of those tumors have probably been reported as a peripheral ameloblastoma, which, according to Simpson [130], may actually be considered an identical lesion. In sites other than the alveolar mucosa, it may be difficult to differentiate between a basal cell carcinoma and a salivary gland tumor. Fresko and Lazarus [131] described a case of oral carcinoma in situ progressing to squamous, basosquamous, and basal cell carcinoma and suggested that the terms *basal cell carcinoma, basosquamous carcinoma,* and *squamous carcinoma* are descriptive rather than of histogenetic significance. Indeed, most pathologists seem to reject the existence of basal cell carcinoma of the oral cavity as a separate entity (figure 2–15).

### 10.5. Spindle cell carcinoma (Sarcomatoid squamous cell carcinoma)

The spindle cell tumor is a rather exceptional malignancy in the oral cavity. Ellis and Corio [132] reported the findings of 59 cases collected at the AFIP. Their histologic criteria to accept a tumor in the reported group were the demonstration of epithelial changes ranging from prominent dysplasia to frank squamous cell carcinoma in conjunction with a dysplastic spindle cell element or evidence of direct transition of epithelial cells to dysplastic spindle cells. These tumors were believed to represent a variant of squamous cell carcinoma, also a proposal of Wahi et al. [133]. In a few cases osteoid-appearing material within the spindle cell component was found (figure 2–16). Multinucleated giant cells were often present. The supporting stroma was scant. No cross

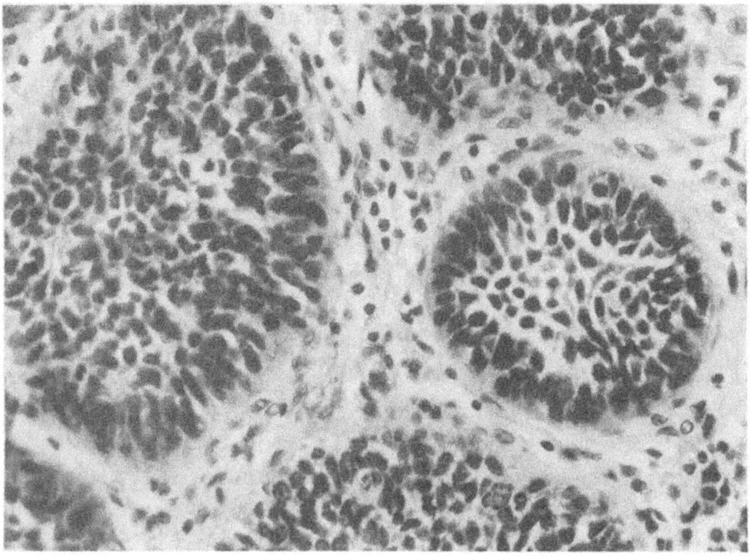

**Figure 2–15.** Basaloid appearance of an otherwise "normal" well-differentiated squamous cell carcinoma of the floor of the mouth.

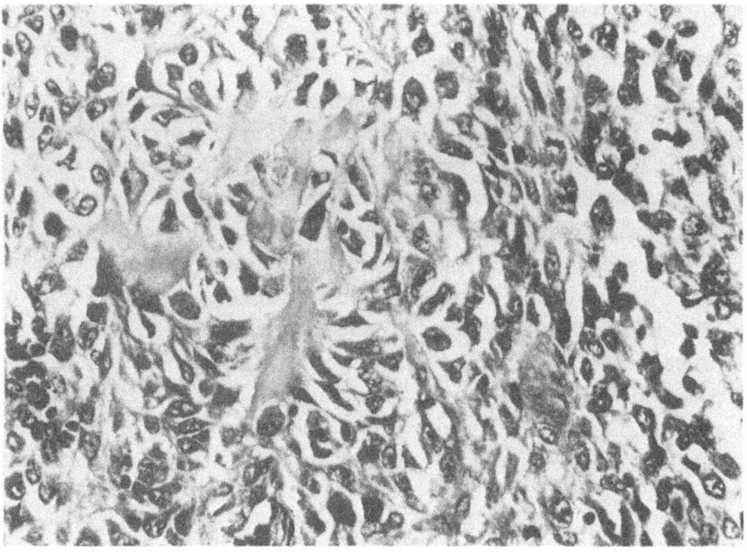

**Figure 2–16.** Detail from a spindle cell variant of a squamous cell carcinoma of the palate with formation of osteoid like structures.

striations or melanin pigment could be demonstrated. Tissue from metastatic foci was available in just six cases, four of them showing only the spindle cell elements and two both squamous cell carcinoma and spindle cells. The lower lip, the tongue, and the alveolar ridges were the favorite sites. Half of the lesions were polypoid, the other half consisting of sessile, nodular, and endophytic lesions. Surgery seems to be the treatment of choice since radiotherapy proved to be rather ineffective [134].

The term *sarcomatoid squamous cell carcinoma,* or *carcinoma sarcomatodes,* is perhaps a better one since in most cases the sarcomatous component is the most obvious one, whereas spindling is not always very distinct [135].

### 10.6. Adenoid squamous cell carcinoma

A few cases have been reported by adenoid squamous cell carcinomas in the oral cavity, especially on the lower lip [136,137] and the tongue [138]. In two autopsy cases of adenoid squamous cell carcinoma of the gingiva and of the lateral border of the tongue, pseudoglandular changes were clearly demonstrated to have taken place in an otherwise regular squamous cell carcinoma. It was observed that the adenoid pattern was reproduced in the lymph node metastases in both cases [139]. The adenoid structure results from loss of cohesion of the epidermoid tumor cells (figure 2–17). There is no sialomucin production. The biologic behaviour of this type of carcinoma, when located on the lip, seems rather mild. For other oral locations, insufficient data are available to comment on the prognosis.

### 10.7. Adenosquamous carcinoma

In 1968 three cases of so-called adenosquamous carcinoma of the tongue have been reported [140]. The patients were males, varying in age from 53 to 60 years. At the time of biopsy, none of the tumors was larger than 1.0 cm in diameter. Histologically, four basic components were classified: ductal carcinoma in situ, adenocarcinoma, squamous cell carcinoma, and a mixed carcinoma. Tumors biopsied early in their development showed only ductal epithelium. Although the histopathologic picture showed some resemblance to the adenoidsquamous cell carcinoma, it was suggested that the adenosquamous carcinoma represented a separate entity [140]. For instance, varying numbers of cells containing intracellular epithelial mucins were found in each case of adenosquamous carcinoma, a feature lacking in adenoidsquamous cell carcinoma. Separation of adenosquamous carcinoma from mucoepidermoid carcinoma may be difficult.

The adenosquamous carcinoma was found to be highly malignant, with a high percentage of metastatic spread.

### 10.8. Transitional-cell carcinoma and lymphoepithelioma

The terms *transitional-cell carcinoma* and *lymphoepithelioma* are used synonymously to describe a variant of a squamous cell carcinoma in which a lym-

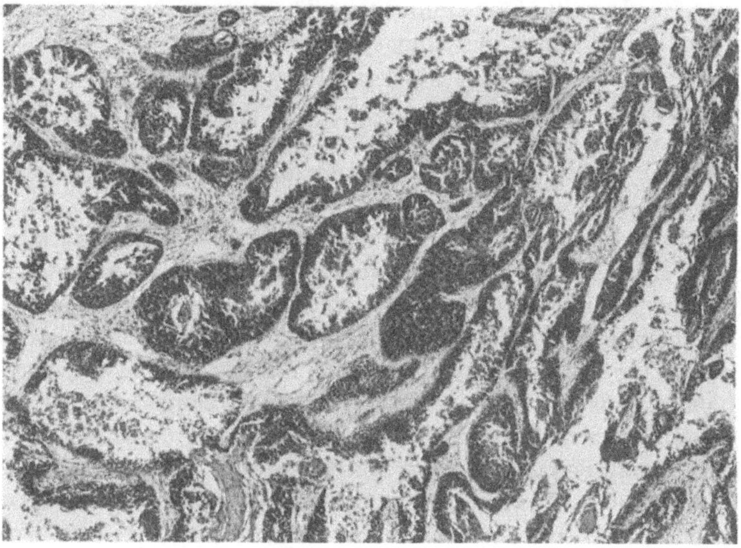

**Figure 2–17.** Adenoid squamous cell carcinoma, resulting from loss of cohesion of the tumor cells.

phoid stroma is often found. Since this tumor very seldom arises in the oral cavity itself, it will not be discussed here [141].

### 10.9. Undifferentiated carcinoma

At times it may be difficult to diagnose a tumor histologically, even after repeated biopsies. A poorly differentiated carcinoma of the oral mucosa may be indistinguishable in routine sections from a salivary gland carcinoma, a malignant lymphoma, a malignant melanoma, or a metastatic growth of a tumor located elsewhere in the body. In spite of the additional help of enzyme histochemistry and even electron-microscopic examination, all pathologists come across tumors that they cannot diagnose with certainty. In those instances the responsibility for the patient remains with the clinician, who has the complete history of that patient and who knows the clinical and possible radiographic aspects of the tumor and the results of all other diagnostic examinations.

## 11. HANDLING OF THE SURGICAL SPECIMEN

The surgical specimen should be sent to the laboratory immediately upon removal, properly marked, and accompanied by a brief clinical description of the lesion, previous treatment, and so forth. Additionally, the surgeon should mention the clinical staging of the primary tumor and the regional nodes. Before placing the specimen in a fixative, the pathologist should write a descriptive report and delineate all resection margins to prevent any misunderstanding of final results of the examination. The clinician should realize the fact that proper decalcification of a bony specimen may take several weeks.

### 12. FRESH-FROZEN SECTION

The use of fresh-frozen sections has its limitations. The histologic picture may be too difficult to diagnose in a few minutes. One should also be aware of the fact that the quality of a fresh-frozen section is usually not as good as a paraffin-embedded section. A patient may be biopsied in one hospital and be referred to another center for the definitive surgery. In such cases the biopsy should be revised by the pathologist in the center where the definitive treatment will be instituted beforehand and the histologic slides should be kept at hand during the surgery and until the time that the surgical specimen is received and examined microscopically. This allows comparison between the biopsy and the resected tumor, facilitates the possible use of a fresh-frozen section, and may reveal a different appraisal of the histologic picture before and not after the performance of major surgery. In fresh-frozen sections of lymph nodes, both false positive and false negative diagnoses may occur.

### 13. REGISTRATION AND CLASSIFICATION

When dealing with a cancer patient, the exact site of the tumor should be recorded as accurately as possible. In large tumors, extending into several anatomical regions, knowledge of the precise site of origin of the particular tumor is not always possible. The several anatomic regions in the mouth, as proposed by Roed-Petersen and Renstrup [142] and used in Pindborg's book on oral cancer and precancer [143] and also in the WHO "Guide to Epidemiology and Diagnosis of Oral Mucosal Diseases and Conditions" [144], are somewhat different than those used by the UICC [107] and the American Joint Committee for Cancer Staging and End Results [145]. For a detailed description see the appendix to this chapter.

#### 13.1. TNM classification UICC, 1978 [107]

It is somewhat confusing that the Union Internationale Centre le Cancer (103) has separated the lips from the oral cavity and that the vermilion border and the mucosal surface of the lips are grouped in different anatomical sites and subsites. The UICC division is shown in table 2–1. The value of the UICC division of the different anatomical sites may be enhanced by a more accurate definition of the floor of the mouth and the boundary between the termination of the oral cavity and the commencement of the oropharynx [147].

The UICC has developed a TNM classification for 28 "sites" in the body, including the oral cavity, in which it is only applied to squamous cell carcinoma (table 2–2). The three symbols of the classification refer to the extent of the primary (T), the presence or absence of suspicious regional lymph node (N), and distant metastases (M). Minimum requirements are given for assess-

**Table 2–1.** UICC categorization of lip and oral cavity sites[1]

| |
|---|
| *Lip* |
| upper lip: vermilion surface (140.0) |
| lower lip: vermilion surface (140.1) |
| commissures: (140.6) |
| *Oral cavity* |
| buccal mucosa |
| mucosal surfaces of upper and lower lip (140.3.4) |
| mucosal surfaces of cheeks (145.0) |
| retromolar areas (145.6) |
| buccoalveolar sulci, upper and lower (145.1) |
| upper alveolus and gingiva (143.0) |
| lower alveolus and gingiva (143.1) |
| hard palate (145.2) |
| tongue |
| dorsal surface and lateral borders anterior to vallate papillae (anterior two-thirds) (141.1.2) |
| floor of mouth (144) |

[1]The numbers in parentheses refer to the codes of the International Classification of Diseases to Dentistry and Stomatology, ICD-DA, issued by the WHO in 1978 [146].

**Table 2–2.** UICC TNM classification of malignant tumors

T —*Primary Tumor*
Tis —preinvasive carcinoma (carcinoma in situ)
TO —no evidence of primary tumor
T1 —tumor 2 cm or less in its greatest dimension
T2 —tumor more than 2 cm but not more than 4 cm in its greatest dimension
T3 —tumor more than 4 cm in its greatest dimension
T4 —tumor with extension to bone, muscle, skin, antrum, neck, etc.
TX —the minimum requirements to assess the primary tumor cannot be met

N —*Regional Lymph Nodes*
NO—no evidence of regional lymph node involvement
N1 —evidence of involvement of movable homolateral regional lymph nodes
N2 —evidence of involvement of movable contralateral or bilateral regional lymph nodes
N3 —evidence of involvement of fixed regional lymph nodes
NX—the minimum requirements to assess the regional lymph nodes cannot be met

*Level 1.* lymph nodes palpable in the submandibular and/or submental regions.
*Level 2.* lymph nodes palpable distal to level 1 and confined to the region above the skin crease at or just below the level of the thyroid notch.
*Level 3.* lymph nodes palpable distal to level 2 and confined to the anterior cervical triangle including those deep to the sternomastoid muscle.
*Level 4.* lymph nodes palpable distal to level 3 and confined to the posterior cervical triangle below the skin crease at or just below the level of the thyroid notch.

M —*Distant Metastases*
MO—no evidence of distant metastases
M1 —evidence of distant metastases
MX—the minimum requirements to assess the presence of distant metastases cannot be met

ment of the several parts of the classification. For the T category clinical examination and radiography (not for the lips) are required, for the N category only clinical examination, and for the M category clinical examination and radiography.

If there is doubt concerning the correct T, N, or M category to which a case should be allotted, the lower category should be chosen.

There are two classifications: a pretreatment clinical classification (TNM) and a postsurgical histopathological classification (p.TNM). When the definitive surgery is preceded by other treatment, the prefix "y" is added. In recurrent tumors the letter "r" should be placed before the TNM or p.TNM classification.

Of the clinical and postsurgical histopathological classifications, the clinical is the most important one for purposes of reporting and evaluation. Usually four stages are grouped:

*Stage I:* T1; NO; MO
*Stage II:* T2; NO; MO
*Stage III:* T3; NO; MO
  T1; T2, T3; N1; MO
*Stage IV:* T4; NO, N1; MO
  any T; N2, N3; MO
  any T; any N; M1

### 13.2. TNM classification AJC, 1978 [145]

The T and M categories of the AJC classification are the same as in the UICC classification, but the N categories are different (table 2–3). The use of subgroups a, b, and c in cervical node classification is not required, but just recommended. Stage grouping is done exactly the same way as in the UICC classification:

**Table 2–3.** AJC classification for TNM categories

| Designation | Description |
|---|---|
| NO | No clinically positive nodes. |
| N1 | Single clinically positive homolateral node less than 3 cm in diameter. |
| N2 | Single clinically positive homolateral node 3 to 6 cm in diameter or multiple clinically positive homolateral nodes; none over 6 cm in diameter. |
| N2a | Single clinically positive homolateral node 3 to 6 cm in diameter. |
| N2b | Multiple clinically positive homolateral nodes; none over 6 cm in diameter. |
| N3 | Massive homolateral node(s), bilateral nodes, or contralateral node(s). |
| N3a | Clinically positive homolateral node(s); none over 6 cm in diameter. |
| N3b | Bilateral clinically positive nodes (in this situation, each side of the neck should be staged separately; that is, N3b: right, N2a; left, N1). |
| N3c | Contralateral clinically positive node(s) only. |
| NX | Nodes cannot be assessed. |

### 13.3. STNMP classification

In 1977 Rapidis et al. [148] used an alternative TNM system in 136 patients by taking the site (S) and the pathology (P) into account since those factors are generally accepted to be important for the prognosis. That system, for instance, rated the labial mucosa with 4 points and the tongue with 8 points. A carcinoma in situ counted for 5 points, as did a verrucous carcinoma, but a moderately differentiated squamous cell carcinoma counted for 15 points. Using these additional credits and also changing somewhat the T, N, and M categories, applying points to them as well, four stages, I to IV, were made, ranging from I (0 to 30 points) to IV (71 to 155 points). Those authors claimed that their system was considerably more accurate than the UICC and AJC classifications. Another variable, velocity of tumor growth, has recently been shown to be of prognostic significance [149].

In conclusion, it can be said that the registration and classification of oral cancers on an international level is not uniform and is in some areas somewhat confusing. This is well demonstrated by a publication in which both the UICC classification of 1973 and 1978 and the AJC classification of 1978 have been applied to 1,022 cases. The authors of that study felt that the three T categories of the UICC classification of 1973 were much more useful than the more recent four T categories from both the UICC and the AJC classifications [150]. Others have stated that improvements in the T and N categories are possible and that multidimensional analyses of prognostic relevant factors are necessary [151,152].

## 14. PROGNOSIS

Apart from the several treatment modalities, the prognosis for a patient with an oral carcinoma depends largely on the size and the site of the primary tumor as well as on the presence or absence of metastatic spread and to some degree also on the grade of differentiation of the tumor. In the last decades much interest has been placed on the possible influence of immunologic mechanisms on the development of cancer of the head and neck and on the possibilities of immunotherapy [153].

The prognosis for squamous cell carcinomas of the lower lip is rather good. A five-year cure of about 80 to 90% can be expected either with radiation therapy or surgery [154], at least in the absence of metastatic spread at the time of admission. For lesions under 1 cm in diameter, that percentage is even higher [155]. In the presence of regional nodes, the overall curability drops down to about 50% [156]. The five-year survival rate for patients with upper lip carcinomas is considerably worse compared with that of the lower lip. In a series of 154 of such cases, this percentage was somewhat less than 60% [157]. The prognosis for commissure lesions is not as good as for carcinomas located elsewhere in the lip. Actually, those tumors behave similarly to tumors involving the buccal mucous membrane [26].

The prognosis for cancer of the tongue depends largely on the size of the primary and the presence or absence of metastatic nodes. Five-year cure rates vary from almost 70% in stage I to about 35% in stage III lesions [158]. In a study of 99 squamous cell carcinomas of the oral tongue in which a histologic grading was used applying separate scores for the growth pattern, no significant correlation could be demonstrated between the grade of differentiation and the size, the frequency of local recurrences, the frequency of lymph node metastases, and the cure of the patient [159]. The only correlation found was a higher frequency of metastatic spread in carcinomas growing in nests and cords as compared with growth in compact tumor fields. Such a growth pattern in nests and cords was not correlated with the size, the frequency of local recurrences, and the cure of the patient.

For the prognosis of cancers of the floor of the mouth, somewhat similar figures are applicable as for cancers of the tongue [160].

Cancers of the alveolar ridges have a rather favorable prognosis [161]. In localized cases, the five-year survival rate is about 80%. In stages II, III, and IV, the percentages show a considerable decrease to about 60, 35, and 15%, respectively. Somewhat similar percentages are applicable to cancers of the buccal mucosa [162, 163].

Carcinomas of the hard palate are rather rare, as mentioned before. The stage of disease at the time of initial treatment has a distinct influence on prognosis, with the five-year survival rates ranging from 70% in stage I to 45, 32, and 6% in stages II, III, and IV, respectively [34].

Patients who continue heavy smoking and drinking habits after having been treated for oral cancer risk a fair chance of getting a second primary either in the head and neck region or elsewhere in the body [164].

The assumption has been made that changes in serum zinc and copper levels are useful indicators of prognosis and response to treatment of epidermoid cancers of the head and neck [165]. Others, however, have not been able to substantiate that assumption [166]. In a series of 37 patients with oral cancer, serum immunoglobulins were elevated (IgA) or depressed (IgG and IgM) in a considerable percentage. Those values were almost always normal one month after successful operative or cytostatic therapy [167], making this phenomenon perhaps a useful parameter for monitoring the course of the disease.

## APPENDIX

### A.1. Anatomic regions (WHO, 1980) [144]

The several anatomic sites are defined as follows (figure 2A–1):

vermilion border: the "lipstick" area between the labial mucosa and the skin of the lip; upper *1*, lower *2*.

labial commissures: a square of approximately 1.5 cm of mucous membrane extending about 1.5 cm distally from the corner of the mouth (angula oris); right *3*, left *4*.

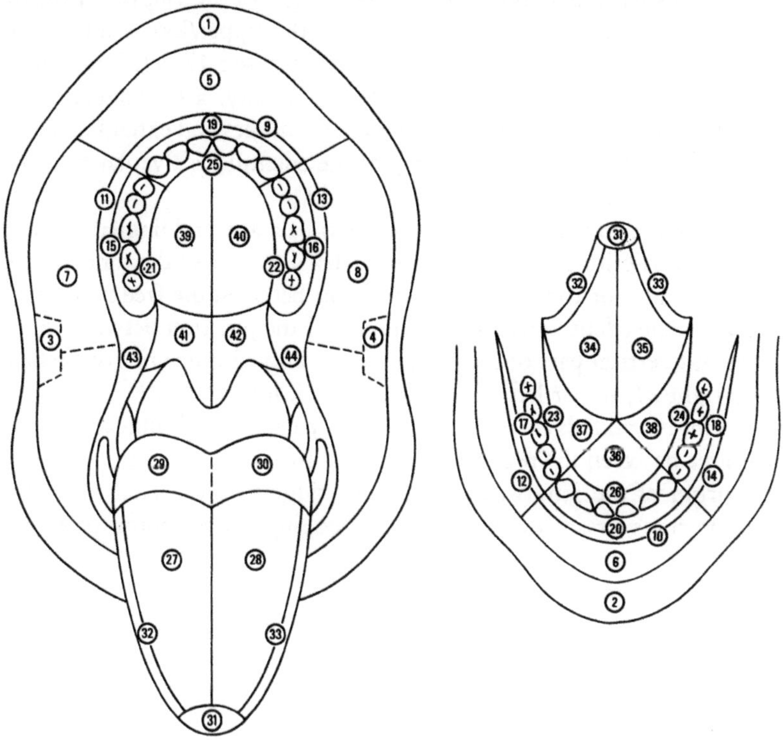


**Figure 2A–1.** Schematic drawing of the oral mucous membranes. The figures refer to the different anatomic regions as explained in the text.

labial mucosa: a rectangular area extending from the vermilion border to 1 cm from the deepest part of the labial sulcus, and laterally to a line drawn vertically from the angles of the mouth; upper *5*, lower *6*.

labial sulci: a rectangular area mesial to the distal surfaces of the upper/lower canines and extending from the mucogingival reflexion to the deepest part of the sulcus and then approximately 1 cm toward the mucosa of the lip; upper *9*, lower *10*.

cheek (buccal mucosa): lies between the upper and lower buccal sulci, and extends forward to a line drawn vertically from the angles of the mouth. The areas defined as labial commissures are excluded; right *7*, left *8*.

buccal sulcus: a rectangular area posterior to the regions of the distal surfaces of the canines, back to the anterior tonsillar pillar and extending from the mucogingival reflexion to the deepest part of the sulcus and then approximately 1 cm toward the mucosa of the cheek; right upper *11*, right lower *12*, left upper *13*, left lower *14*.

posterior gingiva and alveolar ridge (process) bucally: a rectangular area posterior to the regions of the distal surfaces of the canines extending to the anterior tonsillar pillar and from the free margin of the gingiva or the top of the edentulous alveolar ridge (process) to the upper/lower mucogingival reflexion; right upper *15,* left upper *16,* right lower *17,* left lower *18.*

anterior gingiva and alveolar ridge (process) labially: a rectangular area between the regions of the distal surfaces of the canines and extending from the free margin of the gingiva or the top of the edentulous alveolar ridge to the mucogingival reflexion; upper *19,* lower *20.*

posterior gingiva and alveolar ridge (process) palatally and lingually: a rectangular area posterior to the regions of the distal surface of the canines extending to the anterior tonsillar pillar and lying between the free margin of the gingiva or the edentulous alveolar ridge and the junction between the horizontal and vertical part of the palate, or the lingual mucogingival reflexion; upper right *21,* upper left *22,* lower right *23,* lower left *24.*

anterior gingiva and alveolar ridge (process) palatally and lingually: a rectangular area between the regions of the distal surfaces of the canines and from the margin of the gingiva or edentulous ridge to the palatal rugae (plicae palatinae transversae) or the lingual mucogingival reflexion; palatally *25,* lingually *26.*

dorsum of the tongue: a triangular area posterior to the tip back to the terminal sulcus and between the margin and the midline; right *27,* left *28.*

base of the tongue (region belongs to oropharynx, not to oral cavity): a rectangular area posterior to the terminal sulcus and between the two anterior tonsillar pillars; right *29,* left *30.*

tip of the tongue: a circular area with a radius of 1 cm with the centre at the tip of the tongue, *31.*

margin of the tongue: a rectangular area starting 1 cm posterior to the tip of the tongue, extending back to the anterior tonsillar pillar and covering 1 cm of the dorsal and ventral edge of the tongue; right *32,* left *33.*

ventral (inferior) surface of the tongue: a triangular area from the reflexion of the tongue following the midline to 1 cm posterior to the tip of the tongue and following an imaginary line lying 1 cm from the edge of the tongue; right *34,* left *35.*

floor of the mouth, *frontal:* a triangular area between lines drawn from the regions of the distal surfaces of the lower canines to the lingual frenulum and the anterior lower alveolar ridge (process) lingually, *36.*

floor of the mouth, *lateral:* triangular areas posterior to area between the lingual mucogingival reflexion and the reflexion of the tongue; right *37,* left *38.*

hard palate: a triangular area between the upper alveolar ridge (process) palatally, the midline, and the junction of the hard and soft palates; right *39,* left *40.*

soft palate (region belongs to oropharynx, not to oral cavity): a rectangular area posterior to the junction of the hard and soft palate and between the anterior tonsillar pillar and the midline, and including half the uvula; right *41,* left *42.*

anterior tonsillar pillar (region belongs to oropharynx, not to oral cavity): the fold of tissue that forms the margin of the tonsillar fossa; right *43*, left *44*.

**A.2. Anatomic regions (AJC, 1978) [145]**

The American Joint Committee for Cancer Staging and End Results Reporting (1978) has issued a manual in which the several anatomic regions are defined somewhat differently than by the WHO. Furthermore, the division in sites and subsites in the oral cavity differs from that used by the UICC:

lip: the lip begins at the junction of the vermilion border with the skin and includes only the vermilion surface or that portion of the lip that comes into contact with the opposing lip. It is well defined into an upper and lower lip joined at the commissures of the mouth.

buccal mucosa: this includes all the membrane lining of the inner surface of the cheeks and lips, from the line of contact of the opposing lips to the line of attachment of mucosa of the alveolar ridge (upper and lower) and pterygomandibular raphe.

lower alveolar ridge: this ridge includes the alveolar process of the mandible and its covering mucosa, which extends from the line of attachment of mucosa in the buccal gutter to the line of free mucosa of the floor of the mouth. Posteriorly, it extends to the ascending ramus of the mandible.

upper alveolar ridge: the upper ridge is the alveolar process of the maxilla and its covering mucosa, which extends from the line of attachment of mucosa in the upper gingival buccal gutter to the junction of the hard palate. Its posterior margin is the upper end of the pterygopalatine arch.

retromolar gingiva (retromolar trigone): this is the attached mucosa overlying the ascending ramus of the mandible from the level of the posterior surface of the last molar tooth to the apex superiorly, adjacent to the tuberosity of the maxilla.

floor of the mouth: this is a semilunar space over the mylohyoid and hypoglossus muscles, extending from the inner surface of the lower alveolar ridge to the undersurface of the tongue. Its posterior boundary is the base of the anterior pillar of the tonsil. It is divided into two sides by the frenulum of the tongue and contains the ostia of the submaxillary and sublingual salivary glands.

hard palate: this is the semilunar area between the upper alveolar ridge and the mucous membrane covering the palatine process of the maxillary palatine bones. It extends from the inner surface of the superior alveolar ridge to the posterior edge of the palatine bone.

anterior two-thirds of the tongue (oral tongue): this is a freely mobile portion of the tongue that extends anteriorly from the line of circumvallate papillae to the undersurface of the tongue at the junction of the floor of the mouth. It is composed of four areas: the tip, the lateral borders, the dorsum, and the undersurface (nonvillous surface of the tongue).

## REFERENCES


1. Waterhouse J, Shanmugaratnam K, Muir C, Powell, J (eds). Cancer Incidence in Five Continents, vol. IV. Intern. Lyon: Agency for Research on Cancer, 1982.
2. Lefall LD, White JE. Cancer of the oral cavity in Negroes. Surg Gynaecol Obstet (120): 70–72, 1965.
3. Slotman GJ, Swaminathan AP, Rush BF. Head and neck cancer in a young age group: High incidence in black patients. Head & Neck Surgery (5): 293–298, 1983.
4. Boenninghaus H-G. Oberkieferkarzinom bei einem Kleinkind. Ztsch Laryngol (40): 860–863, 1961.
5. Frank LW, Enfield CD, Miller AJ. Carcinoma of the tongue in a newborn child: Report of case. Am J Cancer (26): 775–777, 1936.
6. Lancaster L, Fournet LF. Carcinoma of the tongue in a child: Report of case. J Oral Surg (27): 269–270, 1969.
7. Amsterdam JT, Strawitz JG. Squamous cell carcinoma of the oral cavity in young adults. J of Surg Oncol (19): 65–68, 1982.
8. Easson EC, Palmer MK. Prognostic factors in oral cancer. Clin Oncol (2): 191–202, 1976.
9. Wynder EL, Stellman SD. Comparative epidemiology of tobacco-related cancers. Cancer Res (37): 4608–4622, 1977.
10. Rosenfeld L, Callaway J. Snuff dipper's cancer. Am J Surg (106): 840–844, 1963.
11. Wimm DM, Blot WJ, Shy CM, Pickel LW, Toledo A, Fraumeni JF. Snuff dipping and oral cancer among women in the southern United States. N Engl J Med (304): 745–749, 1981.
12. Sundström B, Mörnstad H, Axéll T. Oral carcinomas associated with snuff dipping; some clinical and histological characteristics of 23 tumours in Swedish males. J Oral Pathol (11): 245–251, 1982.
13. Schmidt W, Popham RE. The role of drinking and smoking in mortality from cancer and other causes in male alcoholics. Cancer (47): 1031–1041, 1981.
14. Binnie WH, Rankin KV, Mackenzie IC. Etiology of oral squamous cell carcinoma. J Oral Path (12): 11–29, 1983.
15. Moss E, Lee WR. Occurrence of oral and pharyngeal cancers in textile workers. Br J Ind Med (31): 224–232, 1974.
16. Mullen DL, Silverberg SG, Penn I, Hammond WS. Squamous cell carcinoma of the skin and lip in renal homograft recipients. Cancer (37): 729–734, 1976.
17. Plotnick H. Xeroderma pigmentosum and mucocutaneous malignancies in three black siblings. Cutis (25): 311–313, 1980.
18. Harper JI, Copeman PWM. Carcinoma of the tongue in a boy with xeroderma pigmentosum. Clin Exp Dermatol (6): 601–604, 1981.
19. Yagi K, Ali AEGE, Abbas KED, Prabha SR. Carcinoma of the tongue in a patient with xeroderma pigmentosum. Int J Oral Surg (10): 73–76, 1981.
20. Schofield IDF, Worth AT. Malignant mucosal change in Fanconi's anemia. J Oral Surg (38): 619–622, 1980.
21. Meyer I, Abbey LM. The relationship of syphilis to primary carcinoma of the tongue. Oral Surg (30): 678–681, 1970.
22. Wynder EL, Hultberg S, Jacobsson F, Bross IJ. Environmental factors in cancer of the upper alimentary tract: A Swedish study with special reference to Plummer-Vinson (Patterson-Kelly) syndrome. Cancer (10): 470–487, 1957.
23. Shillitoe EJ, Greenspan D, Greenspan JS, Hansen LS, Silverman S. Neutralizing antibody to herpes simplex virus type I in patients with oral cancer. Cancer (49): 2315–2320, 1982.
24. Ju DMC. On the etiology of cancer of the lower lip. Plast Reconstr Surg (52): 151–154, 1973.
25. Bailey BJ. Management of carcinoma of the lip. Laryngoscope (87): 250–260, 1977.
26. Cross JE, Guralnick E, Daland EM. Carcinoma of the lip; a review of 563 case records of carcinoma of the lip at the Pondville Hospital.
27. Fulling H-J. Cancer development in oral lichen planus. A follow-up study of 327 patients. Arch Dermatol (108): 667–669, 1973.
28. Pogrell MA, Weldon LL. Carcinoma arising in erosive lichen planus in the midline of the dorsum of the tongue. Oral Surg (55): 62–66, 1968.
29. Eyre J, Nally FF. Oral candidiasis and carcinoma. Br J Derm (85): 73–75, 1971.
30. Faraci RP, Schour L, Graykowski EA. Squamous cell carcinoma of the oral cavity; chronic oral ulcerative disease as a possible etiologic factor. J Surg Oncol (7): 21–26, 1975.

31. Krolls SO, Hoffman S. Squamous cell carcinoma of the oral soft tissues: A statistical analysis of 14,253 cases by age, sex and race of patients. JADA (92): 571–574, 1976.
32. Flamant R, Hayem M, Lazar Ph, Denoix P. Cancer of the tongue; a study of 904 cases. Cancer (17): 377–385, 1964.
33. Mashberg A, Meyers H. Anatomical site and size of 222 early asymptomatic oral squamous cell carcinomas; a continuing prospective study of oral cancer, II. Cancer (37): 2149–2157, 1976.
34. Evans JF, Shah JP. Epidermoid carcinoma of the palate. Am J Surg (142): 451–455, 1981.
35. Lindqvist C, Teppo L. Is upper lip cancer "true" lip cancer? J Cancer Res Clin Oncol (97): 187–191, 1980.
36. Slaughter DP, Southwick HW, Smejkal W. "Field cancerization" in oral stratified squamous epithelium; clinical implications of multicentric origin. Cancer (6): 963–968, 1953.
37. Meyer I, Shklar G. Multiple malignant tumors involving the oral mucosa and the gastrointestinal tract. Oral Surg (13): 295–307, 1960.
38. Weichert KA, Schumrick D. Multiple malignancies in patients with primary carcinomas of the head and neck. Laryngoscope (89): 988–991, 1979.
39. Gluckmann JL, Crissman JD, Donegan JD. Multicentric squamous cell carcinoma of the upper aerodigestive tract. Head & Neck Surgery (3): 90–96, 1980.
40. McGuirt WF, Matthews B, Koufman JA. Multiple simultaneous tumors in patients with head and neck cancer. A prospective, sequential panendoscopic study. Cancer (50): 1195–1199, 1982.
41. Steensma DJ. Het plaveiselcelcarcinoom van de tong. Thesis. University Groningen, the Netherlands, 1971.
42. Crismann JD, Gluckman J, Whiteley J, Quenelle D. Squamous cell carcinoma of the floor of the mouth. Head & Neck Surgery (3): 2–7, 1980.
43. Mashberg A, Morissey JB, Garfinkel L. A study of the appearance of early asymptomatic oral squamous cell carcinoma. Cancer (32): 1436–1445, 1973.
44. Pape H-D. Grösse der malignen Mundschleimhauttumoren zum Zeitpunkt der Primärdiagnostik. Dtsch zahnärztl Z (36): 689–692, 1981.
45. Tournier-Lasserve C, Sun SH, Tol Y, et al. Le cancer des lèvres chez les "chiqueuses de betel" au Cambodge. Med Trop (36): 255–261, 1976.
46. Ogus HD, Bennett MH. Carcinoma of the dorsum of the tongue: A rarity or misdiagnosis. Br J Oral Surg (16): 115–124, 1978.
47. Whitehouse GH. Radiological bone changes produced by intraoral squamous carcinomata involving the lower alveolus. Clinical Otolaryngol (1): 45–52, 1976.
48. Byars LT. Extent of mandibular resection required for treatment of oral cancer. Arch Surg (70): 914–922, 1955.
49. Weisman RA, Kimmelman CP. Bone scanning in the assessment of mandibular invasion by oral cavity carcinomas. Laryngoscope (92): 1–4, 1982.
50. Vegers JWM, Snow GM, van der Waal I. Squamous cell carcinoma of the buccal mucosa; a review of 85 cases. Arch Otolaryng (105): 192–195, 1979.
51. Tan KN, Medak H, Cohen L, Burlakow P. Extensive simultaneous bilateral carcinomas of the buccal mucosa; report of a case. J Oral Med (27): 54–57, 1972.
52. Zajicek J. Monographs in Clinical Cytology, vol. 4. Aspiration Biopsy Cytology, part 1. Cytology of Supradiaphragmatic Organs, 90–124. Basel: S. Karger, 1974.
53. Mancuso AA, Maceri D, Rice D, Hanafee W. CT of cervical lymph node cancer. AJR (136): 381–385, 1980.
54. Shear M, Hawkins DM, Farr HW. The prediction of lymph node metastases from oral squamous carcinoma. Cancer (37): 1901–1907, 1976.
55. Lindberg R. Distribution of cervical lymph node metastases from squamous cell carcinoma of the upper respiratory and digestive tracts. Cancer (29): 1446–1449, 1972.
56. Spiro RH, Alfonso AE, Farr HW, Strong EW. Cervical node metastasis from epidermoid carcinoma of the oral cavity and oropharynx; a critical assessment of current stating. Am J Surg (128): 562–567, 1974.
57. DeSanto LW, Holt JJ, Beahrs OH, O'Fallon WM. Neck dissection: Is it worthwhile? Laryngoscope (92): 502–509, 1982.
58. Jesse RH, Perez CA, Fletcher GH. Cervical lymph node metastasis: Unknown primary cancer. Cancer (31): 854–859, 1973.

59. Viadana E. The metastatic spread of "head and neck" tumors in men (autopsy study of 371 cases). Z Krebsforsch (83): 293–304, 1975.
60. Belson ThP, Lehman RH, Chobanian SL, Malin ThC. Bone and liver scans in patients with head and neck carcinoma. Laryngoscope (90): 1291–1296, 1980.
61. Topazian DS. Distant metastasis of oral carcinoma. Oral Surg (14): 705–711, 1961.
62. Ballard BR, Suess GR, Pickren JW, Greene GW, Shedd DP. Squamous cell carcinoma of the floor of the mouth. Oral Surg (45): 568–579, 1978.
63. Ju DMC. A study of the behaviour of cancer of the head and neck during its late and terminal phases. Am J Surg (108): 552–557, 1964.
64. Goodwin JR, Chandler JR. Hypercalcemia in epidermoid carcinoma of the head and neck. Am J Surg (132): 444–448, 1976.
65. Liston SL. Hypercalcemia and head and neck cancer; bony metastases from tongue cancer. Arch Otolaryng (104): 597–600, 1978.
66. Angel MF, Stewart A, Pensak ML, Pillsbury HRC, Sasaki CT. Mechanisms of hypercalcemia in patients with head and neck cancer. Head & Neck Surg (5): 125–129, 1982.
67. Mashberg A: Reevaluation of toluidine blue application as a diagnostic adjunct in the detection of asymptomatic oral squamous carcinoma; a continuing prospective study of oral cancer, III. Cancer (46): 758–763, 1980.
68. Sandler HC, Stahl SS, Cahn LR, Freund HR. Exfoliative cytology for detection of early mouth cancer. Oral Surg (13): 994–1009, 1960.
69. Umiker WO, Lampe I, Rapp R, Hinikerr JJ. Oral smears in the diagnosis of carcinoma and premalignant lesions. Oral Surg (13): 897–907, 1960.
70. Schwarz K, Böcking A, Lehmann W, Hahn W. Möglichkeiter und Grenzen der Exfoliativzytologie zur Beurteilung der Dignität von Mundschleimhaut-veränderungen. Dtsch zahnärztl Z (36): 701–703, 1981.
71. Folsom TC, White CP, Bromer L, Canby HF, Garrington GE. Oral exfoliative study. Review of the literature and report of a three-year study. Oral Surg (33): 61–74, 1972.
72. Payne ThF, Tsaknis PJ. An evaluation of the rinse technique for oral cytologic diagnosis. Oral Surg (40): 382–384, 1975.
73. Roth D, Hayes RL, Ross NM, Gitman L, Kissin B. Effectiveness of acridine-binding method in screening for oral, pharyngeal and laryngeal cancer. Cancer (29): 1579–1583, 1972.
74. George DI, Burzynski NJ, Miller RL. Reactive properties of oral lesions to the specific red cell adherence test. Oral Surg (47): 51–57, 1979.
75. Myall RWT, Howell RM. A rational approach to biopsy. J Oral Med (26): 71–74, 1974.
76. Shafer WG. Oral carcinoma in situ. Oral Surg (39): 227–238, 1975.
77. Langdon JD, Harvey PW, Rapidis AD, Patel MF, Johnson NW. Oral cancer; the behaviour and response to treatment of 194 cases. J Max Fac Surg (5): 221–237, 1977.
78. Van der Waal I, Beemster G, van der Kwast WAM. Median rhomboid glossitis caused by Candida? Oral Surg (47): 31–35, 1979.
79. Gad A, Willén R, Thorstensson S, Ekman L. Necrotizing sialometaplasia of the lip simulating squamous cell carcinoma. Histopathology (4): 111–121, 1980.
80. Patakas B, Hecker R, Kramer HS. Report on an oral, pigmented, squamous cell carcinoma. Int J Oral Surg (3): 445–448, 1974.
81. Ide F, Kusukara S, Ohnuma H, Miyake T, Nakajima T, Kimura T. Pigmented squamous cell carcinoma of the oral mucosa—With special reference to the role of nonkeratinocytes in tumors and tumorous conditions. J Nih Univ Dent (23): 1–9, 1980.
82. Dunlap CL, Tomich CE. Melanocyte colonization of oral squamous cell carcinoma. Oral Surg (52): 524–530, 1981.
83. Chen S-Y, Harwick RD. Ultrastructure of oral squamous cell carcinoma. Oral Surg (44): 744–753, 1977.
84. Reichart PA, Althoff J. The surface cell structure of oral carcinoma: A scanning electron microscope study of 32 cases. Int J Oral Surg (10): suppl. 1: 11–15, 1981.
85. Pryce DM, Walter JB. The frequency of gross vascular invasion in lung cancer with special reference to arterial invasion. J Path Bact (79): 141–146, 1960.
86. Ballantyne AJ, McCarten AB, Ibanez ML. The extension of cancer of the head and neck through peripheral nerves. Am J Surg (106): 651–667, 1963.

87. Dodd GD, Dolan PA, Ballantyne AJ, Ibanez ML, Chau P. The dissemination of tumors of the head and neck via the cranial nerves. Radiol Clin North Am (8): 445–461, 1970.
88. Carter RL, Tanner NSB, Clifford P, Shaw HJ. Perineural spread in squamous cell carcinomas of the head and neck: A clinicopathological study. Clin Otolaryngol (4): 271–281, 1979.
89. Larson DL, Roberts DK, O'Steen WK, Rapperport AS, Lewis SR. Perineural lymphatics: Myth or fact. Am J Surg (112): 488–492, 1966.
90. Danforth RA, Baughman RA. Chievitz's organ: A potential pitfall in oral cancer diagnosis. Oral Surg (48): 231–236, 1979.
91. Mikó T, Molnár P. The juxtaoral organ; a pitfall for pathologists. J Pathol (133): 17–23, 1981.
92. Zenker W. Juxtaoral Organ (Chievitz' Organ). Morphology and Clinical Aspects. Baltimore-Munich: Urban & Schwarzenberg, 1982.
93. Endes P, Adler P. Nonmalignant perineural spread of epithelial tissue in the orofacial region. Virchows Arch A Path Anat and Histol (374): 81–86, 1977.
94. Jensen JL, Wuerker RB, Correll RW, Erickson JO. Epithelial islands associated with mandibular nerves. Oral Surg (48): 226–230, 1979.
95. Schwartz S, Shklar G. Reaction of alveolar bone to invasion of oral carcinoma. Oral Surg (24): 33–37, 1967.
96. Seifert G, Burkhardt A. Neuere morphologische Gesichtspunkte bei malignen Tumoren der Mundschleimhaut. Dtsch med Wsch (102): 1596–1601, 1977.
97. Ioachim HL. The stromal reactions of tumors: An expression of immune surveillance. J Natl Cancer Inst (57): 465–475, 1976.
98. Jones JH, Coyle JI. Squamous carcinoma of the lip: A study of the interface between neoplastic epithelium and the underlying mesenchym. J Dent Res (48): 702–708, 1969.
99. Paavolainen M, Tarkkanen J, Saksela E. Stromal reactions as prognostic factors in epidermoid carcinoma of the tongue. Acta Otolaryngol (75): 316–317, 1973.
100. Burkhardt A, Höltje W-J. The effects of intra-arterial bleomycin therapy on squamous cell carcinomas of the oral cavity. J Max Fac Surg. (3): 217–230, 1975.
101. Burkhardt A, Gebbers J-O. Giant cell stromal reaction in squamous cell carcinomata. Virchows Arch A Path Anat and Histol (375): 263–280, 1977.
102. Böheim K, Mikuz G, Böheim C. Pathohistologische veränderungen nach zytostatischer induktionstherapie mit methotrexat (M), bleomycin (B) und cis-platinum (P)-(MBP). Laryng Rhinol Otol (61): 246–250, 1982.
103. Jørgensen K, Schlichting J. Relationship between histologic grading of head and neck tumours and regression after chemotherapy. Acta Radiologica Oncology (19): 357–359, 1980.
104. Arthur JF, Fenner ML. The influence of histological grading on prognosis in carcinoma (a computer analysis of 299 cases). Clin Radiol (17): 384–396, 1966.
105. Eneroth C-M, Moberger G. Histological malignancy grading of squamous cell carcinoma of the palate. Acta Otolaryngol (75): 293–295, 1973.
106. Willén R, Nathanson A, Moberger G, Anneroth G. Squamous cell carcinoma of the gingiva; histological classification and grading of malignancy. Acta Otolaryngol (79): 146–154, 1975.
107. Harmer MH (ed). TNM-Classification of Malignant Tumors, 3rd ed. Geneva: Union Internationale Contre le Cancer, 1978.
108. Toker C. Some observations on the deposits of metastatic carcinoma within cervical lymph nodes. Cancer (16): 364–374, 1963.
109. Cachin Y, Sancho-Garnier H, Micheau C, Marandas P. Nodal metastasis from carcinomas of the oropharynx. Otolaryng Clin N Amer (12): 145–154, 1979.
110. Johnson JT, Barnes L, Myers EN, Schramm VL, Borochowitz D, Sigler BA. The extracapsular spread of tumors in cervical node metastasis. Arch Otolaryngol (107): 725–729, 1981.
111. Wheelis RF, Hammar SP, Yarington CT. The ultrastructural diagnosis of tumors of the head and neck. Laryngoscope (89): 234–243, 1979.
112. Shear M, Ichilcik E. Morphologic changes in lymph code deposits of oral squamous carcinoma. Int J Oral Surg (2): 1–12, 1973.
113. Gilmore BB, Repola DA, Batsakis JG. Carcinoma of the larynx: Lymph node reaction patterns. Laryngocope (88): 1333–1338, 1978.

114. Berlinger NT, Tsakraklides V, Pollak K, Adams GL, Yang M, Good RA. Prognostic significance of lymph node histology in patients with squamous cell carcinoma of the larynx, pharynx, or oral cavity. Laryngoscope (86): 792–803, 1976.
115. Micheau C, Cachin Y, Caillou B. Cystic metastases in the neck revealing occult carcinoma of the tonsil; a report of six cases. Cancer (33): 228–233, 1974.
116. Katubig C, Damjanov I. Branchial cleft carcinoma. Arch Otolaryng (89): 92–93, 1969.
117. Martin H, Morfit HM, Ehrlich H. The case for branchiogenic cancer (malignant branchioma). Ann Surg (132): 867–887, 1950.
118. Jensen JL, Correll RW. Nevus cell aggregates in submandibular lymph nodes. Oral Surg (50): 552–556, 1980.
119. Ackerman LV. Verrucous carcinoma of the oral cavity. Surgery (23): 670–678, 1948.
120. Goethals PL, Harrison EG, Devine KD. Verrucous squamous carcinoma of the oral cavity. Am J Surg (106): 845–851, 1963.
121. McCoy JM, Waldron CA. Verrucous carcinoma of the oral cavity; a review of forty-nine cases. Oral Surg (52): 623–629, 1981.
122. Kraus FT, Perez-Mesa C. Verrucous carcinoma; clinical and pathologic study of 105 cases involving oral cavity, larynx and genitalia. Cancer (19): 26–38, 1966.
123. Prioleau PhG, Santa Cruz DJ, Meyer JS, Bauer WC. Verrucous carcinoma; a light and electron microscopic, autoradiographic, and immunofluorescence study. Cancer (45): 2849–2857, 1980.
124. Shear M, Pindborg JJ. Verrucous hyperplasia of the oral mucosa. Cancer (46): 1855–1862, 1980.
125. Burns HP, van Nostrand AWP, Palmer JA. Verrucous carcinoma of the oral cavity; management by radiotherapy and surgery. Canad J Surg (23): 19–22, 1980.
126. Batsakis JG, Hybels R, Crissman JD, Price DH. The pathology of head and neck tumors: Verrucous carcinoma, part 15. Head & Neck Surg (5): 29–38, 1982.
127. McDonald JS, Crissman JD, Gluckman JL. Verrucous carcinoma of the oral cavity. Head & Neck Surg (5): 22–28, 1982.
128. Edmonson HD, Browne RM, Potts AJC. Intra-oral basal cell carcinoma. Br J Oral Surg (20): 239–247, 1982.
129. Hume WJ, Turner EP. Basal cell carcinoma of lip mucosa. Br J Oral Surg (20): 248–255, 1982.
130. Simpson HE. Basal-cell carcinoma and peripheral ameloblastoma. Oral Surg (38): 233–240, 1974.
131. Fresko D, Lazarus SS. Oral carcinoma in situ; its progression to squamous, baso-squamous and basal-cell carcinoma. Arch Pathol Lab Med (105): 15–19, 1981.
132. Ellis GL, Corio RL. Spindle cell carcinoma of the oral cavity; a clinicopathological assessment of fifty-nine cases. Oral Surg (50): 523–534, 1980.
133. Wahi PN, Cohen B, Luthra UK, Torloni H. Histological typing of oral and oropharyngeal tumours. International Histological Classification of Tumours, no. 4, WHO, Geneva, 1971.
134. Batsakis JG, Rice DH, Howard DR. The pathology of head and neck tumors: Spindle cell lesions (sarcomatoid carcinomas, nodular fasciitis, and fibrosarcoma) of the aerodigestive tracts, part 14. Head & Neck Surg (4): 499–513, 1982.
135. Leventon GS, Evans HL. Sarcomatoid squamous cell carcinoma of the mucous membranes of the head and neck: A clinicopathologic study of 20 cases. Cancer (48): 994–1003, 1981.
136. Weitzer S. Adenoid squamous-cell carcinoma of vermilion mucosa of lower lip. Oral Surg (37): 589–593, 1974.
137. Jacoway JR, Welson JF, Boyers RC. Adenoid squamous-cell carcinoma (adenoacanthoma) of the oral labial mucosa. A clinicopathologic study of fifteen cases. Oral Surg (32): 444–449, 1971.
138. Goldman RL, Klein HZ, Sung M. Adenoid squamous cell carcinoma of the oral cavity; report of the first case arising in the tongue. Arch Otolaryng (103): 496–498, 1977.
139. Takagi M, Sakota Y, Takayama S, Ishikawa G. Adenoid squamous cell carcinomas of the oral mucosa; report of two autopsy cases. Cancer (40): 2250–2255, 1974.
140. Gerughty RM, Henniger GR, Brown FM. Adenosquamous carcinoma of the nasal, oral and laryngeal cavities; a clinicopathologic survey of ten cases. Cancer (22): 1140–1155, 1968.
141. Smith JF. Transitional-cell carcinoma and lympho-epithelioma; review of eighteen cases. Oral Surg (15): 965–969, 1962.

142. Roed-Petersen B, Renstrup G. A topographical classification of the oral mucosa suitable for electronic data processing: Its application to 560 leukoplakias. Acta Odontol Scand (27): 681–695, 1969.
143. Pindborg JJ. Oral Cancer and Precancer. Bristol: Wright & Sons, 1980.
144. World Health Organization. Guide to epidemiology and diagnosis of oral mucosal diseases and conditions. Community Dent and Oral Epidem (8): 1–26, 1980.
145. American Joint Committee. Manual for Staging of Cancer. Chicago, Illinois, 1978.
146. World Health Organization. Application of the International Classification of Diseases to Dentistry and Stomatology (ICD-DA), 2nd ed. Geneva, 1978.
147. Lederman M. Cancer of the oral cavity: Observations on classification and natural history. Int J Radiation Oncology Biol Phys (6): 1559–1565, 1980.
148. Rapidis A, Langdon JD, Patel MF, Harvey PW. STNMP, a new system for the clinicopathological classification and identification of intra-oral carcinomata. Cancer (39): 204–209, 1977.
149. Evans SJW, Langdon JD, Rapidis D, Johnson NW. Prognostic significance of STNMP and velocity of tumor growth in oral cancer. Cancer (49): 773–776, 1982.
150. Platz H, Fries R, Hudec M, Tjoa AM, Wagner RR. Kritische Beurteilung der T-Klassifizierung von Karzinomen der Mundhöhle nach den Regeln der UICC von 1978. Dtsch Z Mund-Kiefer-Gesichts-Chir (4): 4S–10S, 1980.
151. Platz H, Fries R, Hudec M, Tjoa AM, Wagner RR. Retrospektive DOSAK-Studie ueber Karzinome der Mundhöhle. Analyse verschiedener prätherapeutischen Klassifizierungen. Dtsch Z Mund-Kiefer-Gesichts-Chir (6): 5–20, 1982.
152. Platz H, Fries R, Hudec M, Tjoa M, Wagner RR. Carcinomas of the oral cavity: Analysis of various pretherapeutic classifications. Head & Neck Surgery (5): 93–107, 1982.
153. Scully C. The immunology of cancer of the head and neck with particular reference to oral cancer. Oral Surg (53): 157–169, 1982.
154. Ashley FL, McConnel DV, Machida R, Sterling HE, Galloway D, Grazer F. Carcinoma of the lip: A comparison of five-year results after irradiation and surgical therapy. Am J Surg (110): 549–551, 1965.
155. Ward GE, Hendrick JW. Results of treatment of carcinoma of the lip. Surg (27): 321–342, 1950.
156. Jørgensen K, Elbrønd O, Andersen AP. Carcinoma of the lip: A series of 869 cases. Acta Radiologica (12): 177–190, 1973.
157. Molnar L, Ronay P, Tapolcsanyi L. Carcinoma of the lip: Analysis of the material of 25 years. Oncology (29): 101–121, 1974.
158. Spiro RH, Strong EW. Surgical treatment of cancer of the tongue. Surg Clin N Amer (54): 759–765, 1974.
159. van der Waal I. Het tongcarcinoom. Thesis, Amsterdam, 1973.
160. Ildstad ST, Bigelow ME, Remensnyder JP. Intra-oral cancer at the Massachusetts General Hospital; squamous cell carcinoma of the floor of the mouth. Ann Surg (197): 34–41, 1983.
161. Byers RM, Newman R, Russell N, Yue A. Results of treatment for squamous carcinoma of the lower gum. Cancer (47): 2236–2238, 1981.
162. MacComb WS, Fletcher GH. Cancer of the Head and Neck. Baltimore: Williams & Wilkins, 1967.
163. Cummings BJ, Clark RM. Squamous cell carcinoma of the oral cavity. J of Otolaryngology (1): 359–364, 1982.
164. Silverman S, Greenspan D, Gorsky M. Tobacco-usage in patients with head and neck carcinomas: A follow-up study on habit changes and second primary oral/oropharyngeal cancers. JADA (106): 33–35, 1983.
165. Abdulla M, Björklund A, Mathur A, Wallenius K. Zinc and copper levels in whole blood and plasma from patients with squamous cell carcinoma of head and neck. J Surg Oncol (12): 107–113, 1979.
166. Garofalo JA, Erlandson E, Strong EW, Lesser M, Gerold F, Spiro R, Schwartz M, Good RA. Serum zinc, serum copper and the Cu/Zn ratio in patients with epidermoid cancers of the head and neck. J Surg Oncol (15): 381–386, 1980.
167. Jung H, Mondorf W, Frenkel G. Veränderungen der serumimmunglobulin-konzentrationen bei patienten mit plattenepithelkarzinomen im mundhöhlenbereich nach operation und zytostasetherapie. Dtsch Z Mund-Kiefer-Gesichts-Chir (7): 138–142, 1983.

# 3. TUMOURS OF THE MINOR SALIVARY GLANDS: CLINICAL AND HISTOLOGICAL ASPECTS

R.B. LUCAS
A.C. THACKRAY

## 1. CLASSIFICATION AND NOMENCLATURE

Tumours of the salivary glands are nearly all of epithelial origin, only a very small proportion deriving from nonepithelial tissues. The nomenclature used here for the epithelial tumours follows the World Health Organization's scheme [1] and is shown in table 3–1. Nonepithelial tumours of the major glands appear as distinct clinical lesions that are localised to one or other of the glands. The minor glands, however, unlike the major glands, are not organised into anatomically discrete entities, so that tumours of adjacent connective or other nonepithelial tissue present simply as fibromas, neuromas, or the like of palate, lip, or other area, and are not especially identifiable with the glands. They are not considered further in this chapter.

## 2. EPIDEMIOLOGY

Incidence figures for salivary gland tumours in general are scanty; such reports as are available indicate that they occur in 3 or less per 100,000 of the population [2–4]. Major gland tumours have been estimated to account for 5% of all benign and malignant tumours, apart from skin tumours, and for up to 2% of all neoplasms [5]. Minor gland tumours are much less common, accounting for only about one-fifth of all salivary gland tumours [6]. However, some

*I. van der Waal and G.B. Snow (eds), ORAL ONCOLOGY.* 

**Table 3–1.** Percentage distribution of 481 tumours in the minor salivary glands

| | Palate | Lip | Cheek | Gingiva | Retromolar | Tongue | Floor of mouth | Total |
|---|---|---|---|---|---|---|---|---|
| Pleomorphic adenoma | 33.8 | 9.0 | 6.4 | 0.4 | 1.0 | 0.2 | 0.3 | 51.1 |
| Monomorphic adenoma | | | | | | | | |
| Adenolymphoma | — | — | — | — | — | — | — | — |
| Oxyphilic adenoma | — | — | — | — | — | — | — | — |
| Other types | 2.7 | 5.1 | 1.9 | — | — | — | — | 9.7 |
| Mucoepidermoid tumour | 5.6 | 0.2 | 1.3 | — | 1.3 | 0.9 | — | 9.3 |
| Acinic cell tumour | 0.2 | 0.4 | — | — | — | — | — | 0.6 |
| Adenoid cystic carcinoma | 9.2 | 0.6 | 1.7 | 0.4 | — | 1.9 | 1.4 | 15.2 |
| Adenocarcinoma | 6.8 | 0.6 | 0.8 | 0.2 | 0.4 | 1.4 | 0.2 | 10.4 |
| Epidermoid carcinoma | — | — | — | — | — | — | — | — |
| Undifferentiated carcinoma | 0.4 | 0.4 | 0.2 | — | — | 0.4 | — | 1.4 |
| Carcinoma in pleomorphic adenoma | 1.3 | 0.2 | 0.4 | — | — | — | 0.4 | 2.3 |
| Total | 60.0 | 16.5 | 12.7 | 1.0 | 2.7 | 4.8 | 2.3 | 100.0 |

reports have indicated a rather greater relative frequency in parts of Africa and India [7–9].

Tumours of the minor salivary glands occur over a wide age range. Although the predominant decades of incidence for all varieties of tumour are the fourth to the sixth, there are some differences for the various tumour types. Thus, the mean age for patients presenting with pleomorphic adenoma is between 45 and 50 years, whereas for the carcinomas the mean age is about 10 years greater. At the upper end of the range, therefore, there is a somewhat greater likelihood for a tumour to be malignant rather than benign. At the lower end of the range, in children and adolescents, pleomorphic adenoma is again the commonest tumour, but adenoid cystic carcinoma is distinctly rare and adenocarcinoma a little less so. Mucoepidermoid tumours, however, do occur from time to time in these younger age groups.

Although the cited sex ratios for minor salivary gland tumours are variable, there is usually a preponderance of females, taking all varieties of tumour into consideration. Pleomorphic adenoma accounts for much of this preponderance in most series; in only a few do males outnumber females for this tumour. The figures for adenoid cystic carcinoma are variable; in some series females preponderate, in other males are in excess. Adenocarcinomas and the remaining carcinomas have an equal sex incidence or a preponderance of males.

The frequency of the various tumour types in the different minor glands is shown in table 3–1, which is based on a series of personally observed cases. The figures are generally comparable with those reported in some other series of minor gland tumours. However, a close correspondence cannot be expected from any of the published series for a number of reasons. Some of the earlier series employ rather different terminologies than are commonly in use today, which makes comparison difficult, and tumours that have only relatively recently been recognized as separate entities do not of course appear as such. Many tumours belonging to the group of monomorphic adenomas are examples. Other factors affecting the comparability of reported series include variability of criteria for histological diagnosis and the fact that series of salivary gland tumours, like many other groups of pathological conditions, are very often subject to a high degree of selection. Thus, they frequently emanate from special hospitals or departments to which have been referred the more difficult cases, or perhaps malignant rather than benign lesions with a view to radiotherapy or other specialized treatment. Consequently, a report from a particular institution may give a picture of the situation that should not be taken as accurately reflecting that in the population in general. Nor should such a report be expected to be strictly comparable to reports from other sources. Nevertheless, despite all these reservations, certain generalisations concerning the frequency and distribution of tumours of the minor salivary glands emerge from the published series.

Although there are reports in which pleomorphic adenoma accounts for less than 30% and even as little as 9% of all tumours of the minor glands [10–

13], the majority of reports indicate that in the major glands pleomorphic adenoma is the commonest tumour. But whereas in the major glands this tumour accounts for 70 to 75% of all neoplasms, it constitutes only around 50 to 60% of minor gland tumours. Correspondingly, the figures for the remaining tumour types vary in the two gland groups; this effectively means that all types of carcinoma are commoner in the minor glands than in the major glands, with adenoid cystic carcinoma and adenocarcinoma being the most important tumours in this category. Thus, in those series in which the proportion of pleomorphic adenoma is low, the figures for the carcinomas and sometimes mucoepidermoid tumour are correspondingly high. The lowest figures given in the literature for adenoid cystic carcinoma are in the region of 3 to 5% [14,15], while the highest is about 50% [10]. The low figures are the exceptions rather than the rule; in most series the figure is well over 10%. The mean from a number of recent reports was 25%. Adenoid cystic carcinoma thus occurs much more frequently in the minor than in the major glands, where it accounts for some 5% of all tumours.

Adenocarcinoma likewise shows considerable variation in the reported figures, from 7 to 8% to over 30% [9,10,12]. An average figure would appear to be about 15%. The figure for the major glands is about 5%.

The four neoplasms just dealt with—pleomorphic adenoma, adenoid cystic carcinoma, adenocarcinoma and mucoepidermoid tumour—account for over 90% of all tumours of the minor glands in the great majority of series. Thus, all remaining types of tumours account for 10% or less of minor gland tumours, with the exception of the monomorphic adenomas. Since the relatively recent recognition and delineation of many members of this group, these tumours have been increasingly reported and have appeared in some of the more recent series, where they have accounted for up to 15% of all minor gland tumours [14,16]. Presumably, in some earlier reports, tumours of this type have for the most part been counted as pleomorphic adenomas or possibly in some cases as adenoid cystic carcinoma. The group of monomorphic adenomas, using the WHO terminology, is comprised of adenolymphoma, oxyphilic adenoma, and adenomas of "other types." The first two, although very rare in the minor glands, have long been recognised as major gland tumours. There are very few reported cases of adenolymphoma in the minor glands and only occasional instances of oxyphilic adenoma [17,18]. It is the adenomas of "other types" that have been more recently recognised and that have now begun to appear as such in the published series.

The residue of tumours that remain to be accounted for includes acinic cell tumour and carcinomas of other types. Acinic cell tumour is not very common in the major glands and rare in the minor glands. In the major glands it accounts for 5% or less of all tumours; in the minor glands fewer than 60 cases have been reported [19–21]. The other carcinomas include epidermoid carcinoma and undifferentiated carcinoma, equally rare in both major and minor glands. Carcinoma in pleomorphic adenoma is also uncommon but is being increasingly recognised.

## 3. ETIOLOGY

Very little is known about possible causal factors concerned in salivary gland neoplasia. Major gland carcinomas have been found to have some association with mammary carcinoma, although the extent of this relationship is disputed. Radiation has also been implicated; evidence has been adduced from instances of salivary tumors following radiotherapy of the head and neck [22,23] and from the increased frequency of salivary gland tumours in atomic bomb survivors [24,25]. Here again, there is some doubt as to the exact significance of the findings, but in any event they can relate only to a very small area of tumour genesis. Otherwise, almost nothing is known about the etiology of salivary neoplasia, either in the major or the minor glands.

## 4. DISTRIBUTION OF TUMOURS IN THE ORAL GLANDS

Like the figures for the frequencies of the different histological types of minor gland tumours, those for the frequencies of tumour occurrence in the various oral glands show considerable differences in the published series. However, all reports agree that the palatal glands are much more often the site of tumour formation than any of the other glands. In 12 recent series published in the 1970–80 period, palatal tumours ranged between 45 and 69% of the total, with an average of 57%. The range here is much less wide than the range in histological types in the same reports with pleomorphic adenoma, for example, varying between 12 and 52% of all tumours. In all probability, while observer variation could, at least in part, account for the frequency differences in histological types, this factor could hardly play more than a minor role in deciding the anatomical site of tumours. Other factors, including those mentioned previously, are more likely to be concerned.

After the palate the upper lip and the cheek or buccal mucosa are the most frequent sites for tumours, with an average occurrence rate of 10 to 15% for each. But the figures are variable; in one series lip tumours accounted for 23% of all tumours and buccal mucosa tumours for 7% [16], while in another lip tumours were 5% and buccal mucosa tumours 23% [26]. The lower lip is an infrequent site for tumours.

The remaining oral glands are involved in some 10 to 15% of tumours, again variable figures, depending possibly on the treatment policy of the department or hospital from which a particular report emanates. Thus, some reports exclude tonsillar or tongue tumours, whereas others take in tumours of the nasal cavity and sinuses as well as those of the oral glands. In part, also, the variation may depend on differing designations for the situation of tumours, with possibly an overlap between gingival, alveolar ridge and retromolar designations.

A small number of tumours occur as intraosseous growths within the mandible or, even less commonly, within the maxilla.

The frequency of the various histological types of tumour in the minor glands is roughly comparable in most reported series, with most types of tumours occurring in each gland situation. As would be expected, in the palatal glands most tumours—between 60 and 80%—are pleomorphic adenomas, and this preponderance affects most other gland groups, although to a much lesser extent. Again, as expected, adenoid cystic carcinoma, adenocarcinoma and mucoepidermoid tumour are the next most frequent neoplasms in the palatal glands, the proportions varying somewhat in different reports. Carcinoma in pleomorphic adenoma has also been reported most often in the palatal glands.

In the lip, pleomorphic adenoma is again the most frequent tumour, but the next most frequent is monomorphic adenoma, which occurs more often in the lip than in any other gland. These adenomas account for the great majority of lip tumours [27]. Carcinomas of various types occur but are uncommon. Adenoid cystic carcinoma has been reported in the lip more often than adenocarcinoma, which is uncommon in this situation [28,29], but it is not likely that there has been some variance of histological criteria in connection with these tumours and also, perhaps especially, with the papillary cystadenoma type of monomorphic adenoma. It is probable that the last named has been misdiagnosed as adenoid cystic carcinoma on occasion. Acinic cell tumours, when they do occur in the minor glands, are seen most frequently in the upper lip, followed by the lower lip and the other minor glands [19].

The glands of the buccal mucosa and cheek also have pleomorphic adenoma as the commonest tumour. Monomorphic adenomas and carcinomas occur in much smaller numbers.

The retromolar glands and the glands of the floor of the mouth and tongue give rise to a relatively small number of tumours compared with those of the palate, lip, and buccal mucosa, and of this small number pleomorphic adenoma is only an occasional member. Mucoepidermoid tumour, adenoid cystic carcinoma, and adenocarcinoma are more likely to be seen in these situations [30,31].

Intraosseous tumours are mostly mucoepidermoid. Some 50 cases have now been reported, but many of them are of questionable identity either because they have not been shown conclusively to be of intraosseous origin or because the histology is not convincing [32,33]. These remarks apply even more cogently to the small number of tumours, other than mucoepidermoid tumour, that have been reported as intraosseous growths. They include pleomorphic adenoma, adenoid cystic carcinoma and acinic cell tumour.

## 5. CLINICAL ASPECTS

### 5.1. Duration of symptoms

Owing to their naturally slow rate of growth and, very often, absence of pain or other symptoms, tumours of the salivary glands have been prominent among those conditions that patients have tolerated for long periods, frequently many years, before seeking advice. In one extensive survey of the

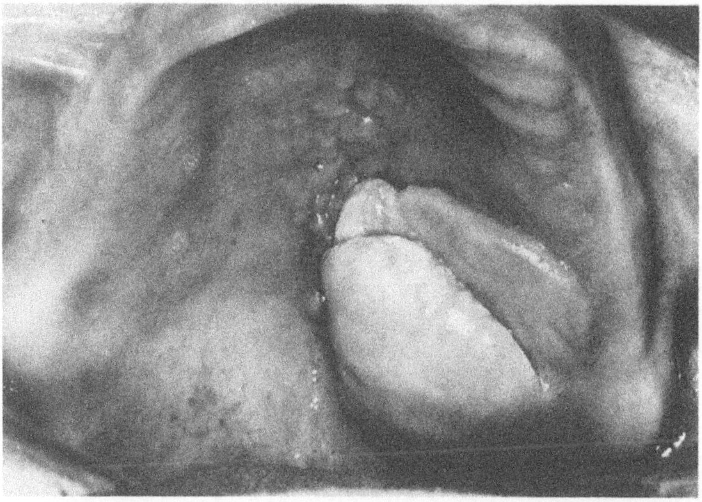

**Figure 3–1.** Pleomorphic adenoma of palate. The tumour forms a smooth dome-shaped mass situated to one side of the palate.

literature, for example, the duration of the lesion prior to diagnosis varied from one week to 39 years in the case of pleomorphic adenoma. Despite these extremes, however, nearly half the patients had had their tumours for one year or less [34]. Most other surveys that give figures for duration of symptoms prior to diagnosis show similar findings, but clearly the patients with long-standing lesions first had their symptoms at a time when public health provisions and social and health awareness were much less developed than they are now. Today, long delays in seeking treatment are relatively uncommon; most patients report the presence of untoward oral manifestations within weeks or months if painless and within a very much shorter period if pain is present.

Similar considerations apply to the other tumour types, but with the average duration of symptoms before diagnosis being rather shorter than for pleomorphic adenoma.

Much the commonest complaint, in the majority of patients and irrespective of the type of tumour, is the presence of a painless swelling (figure 3–1). Frequently, its presence is the only complaint, but even this may be absent since occasionally the existence of a tumour is discovered in the course of routine oral examination by the dentist or physician, having been hitherto unrecognized by the patient. Less often, there are also concomitant symptoms due to the physical presence of the swelling. Thus, dentures may cease to fit when the tumour involves a denture-bearing area, or there may be dysphagia or dysphonia where tumours involve the soft palate or the tongue. It is remarkable, however, how frequently tumours have attained considerable di-

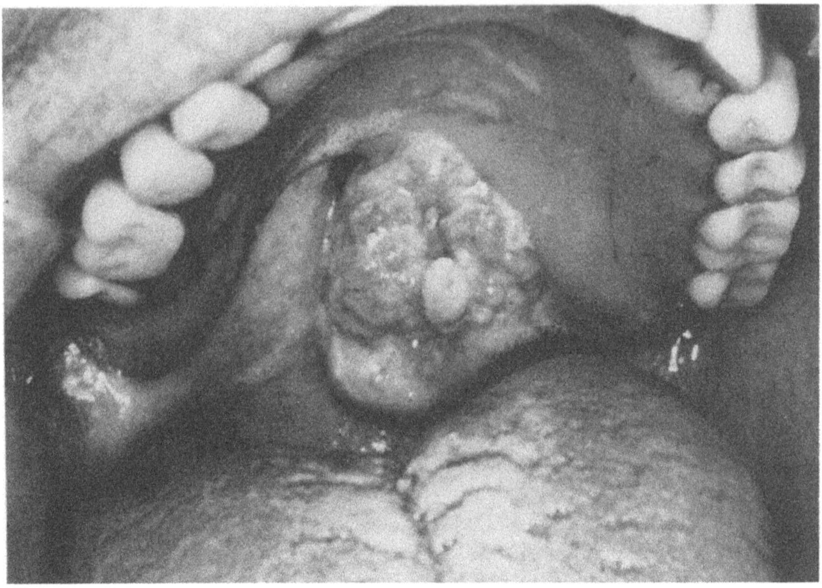

**Figure 3–2.** Adenocarcinoma of palate. The tumour has a rather irregular outline and is ulcerated.

mensions without apparently causing very much, or even any, discomfort to the patient.

The absence of pain or discomfort in many patients is due to the slow rate of growth that is so characteristic of many salivary gland tumours and that allows patients to accommodate themselves gradually to the almost imperceptibly changing conditions. However, some tumours do grow more rapidly, and although it is the malignant ones that tend to behave in this way, this is by no means a constant feature. Benign tumours can also grow more rapidly than usual in the absence of any suggestion of malignant change. Moreover, a tumour that has been present for some time with little perceptible change may take on a period of accelerated growth, again without any threat of malignancy, although the possibility does exist and should always be considered when this type of growth pattern occurs. It is very characteristic of carcinoma arising in pleomorphic adenoma to find that a tumour has been present for a long time, perhaps 10 years or more, during which little change has occurred. It then begins to grow more rapidly, and this is the signal of malignant change.

Similar considerations apply to pain and ulceration (figure 3–2). When present, the question of malignancy arises, but benign tumours can show both features. The presence of pain with malignant tumours, when it does occur, is rather less common in minor gland tumours than in those of the corresponding type in the major glands. Numbness is an occasional symptom in malignant tumours that have involved regional nerves.

**5.2. Clinical presentation**

On examination a swelling is apparent in one or another of the sites previously discussed. In the commonest situation, the palate, the tumour is often dome-shaped and found to either side of the midline in the posterior part of the palate. Tumours at or near the palatal midline do occur but are very uncommon since glands are practically absent from this area, although plentiful on either side [35,36]. Most tumours measure less than 2.5 to 3 cm in their longest axis, but larger masses are occasionally seen [37]. The overlying mucosa frequently appears normal although ulceration may be evident, and not only in malignant tumours, as already mentioned. However, in benign tumours the ulceration is primarily due to local trauma, perhaps from dentures, and this or some other cause may be evident.

On palpation most palatal tumours feel smooth and firm, and the overlying mucous membrane is not fixed. The tumour itself is not mobile, due to its being kept firmly against the bone by the thin yet rather tough and fibrous soft tissues. This lack of mobility applies equally to benign and malignant tumours. In the latter there is the element of invasion and infiltration, which also leads to fixity of the growth, and it may be possible to appreciate the indefinite borders and lack of circumscription on palpation. However, it may be said in general terms that neither this nor any of the other clinical features is sufficiently distinctive to allow more than a provisional diagnosis of malignancy or otherwise. With regard to consistency most tumours are firm, as just mentioned, but some are softer and some are hard, again without consistent relationship to the tumour type. A rather softer than average and possibly fluctuant tumour, however, may be a mucoepidermoid tumour of the low-grade type in which mucus-containing cysts are prominent. Rarely, a sinus may form discharging mucus into the oral cavity.

Like tumours of the palate, tumours of the alveolar ridge tend to be firmly held to the adjacent bone and to be immobile. Tumours of the lips, buccal mucosa, and floor of mouth, on the other hand, are generally mobile (figure 3–3).

Intraosseous tumors are characterised by swelling of the jaw, which may be accompanied by pain, but this symptom is not invariable. When pain is complained of, it has been described as dull and persistent or intermittent. The swelling itself is not a constant finding; cases have been reported in which there were no symptoms, the lesion being discovered only on radiotherapy. In most cases the lesion is situated in the mandibular molar region. Maxillary lesions are rare and are also situated in the molar region. If criteria of acceptable histology, radiographic evidence of osteolysis and intact cortical plates are adopted, the number of cases acceptable as salivary gland tumours of intraosseous origin is very small, probably in single figures only.

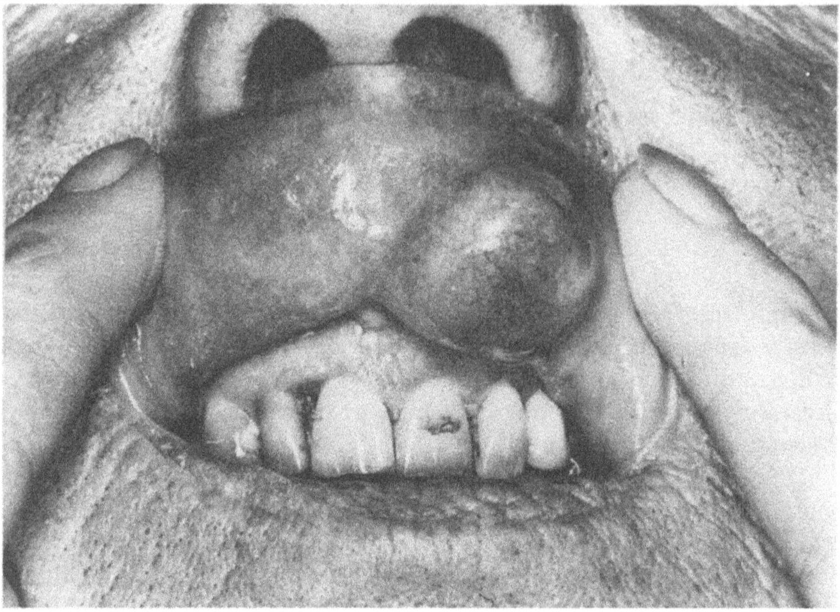

**Figure 3–3.** Monomorphic adenoma of lip. The tumour forms a well-defined and circumscribed swelling in the upper lip.

Tumours in any of the situations just discussed may be associated with enlargement of the regional lymph nodes, which will be evident on physical examination. Evidence may also be found of more distant dissemination, the lungs being a relatively common site for metastatic deposits from malignant salivary gland tumours.

### 6. RADIOGRAPHIC ASPECTS

Although no specific radiographic features are associated with tumours of the minor salivary glands that point to a positive diagnosis, radiographic examination is nevertheless helpful in assembling the total clinical picture, not only by showing some features but also by excluding others.

Benign lesions situated in proximity to bone—for example, pleomorphic or monomorphic adenoma of the palate—may give rise to pressure resorption. This usually appears as a well-defined shallow or saucer-shaped depression. Some authors describe the appearance as cystlike [34]. It has also been pointed out that tomography will show that the edges of the bony defect are bevelled upward, a radiographic sign denoting pressure resorption by an expanding intraoral mass. It also demonstrates that the tumour is confined within the actual bony defect and that there is no periosteal reaction adjacent to the radiolucent defect [38].

These radiographic signs are not of course found in association with every benign tumour in proximity to bone. Many such tumours, in fact, produce no effect on the bone that is radiographically detectable. And equally important, the same may apply to malignant tumours, which do not always show evidence of invasion radiographically. However, when this is present, it shows as an irregular radiolucent defect with ill-defined edges. A particular feature has been noted in the case of adenoid cystic carcinoma. This tumour tends to spread through the marrow spaces as well as invading bone by direct destruction of the calcified tissue. Since there is less resistance to the former type of spread than to the latter, the extent of invasion by the tumour in bone is often appreciably greater than is apparent from the radiograph.

Intraosseous tumours are characterised by a radiolucency of variable nature. In some of the reported cases the defect has been multilocular, in others unilocular, with irregular and diffuse borders or with well-demarcated outline. Association with unerupted teeth has also been noted.

## 7. BIOPSY

Although a provisional diagnosis of minor salivary gland tumour may be made on clinical grounds, the definitive diagnosis always depends on histological examination. Tumours in readily accessible areas such as the lip or cheek, and in which the majority of tumours are benign may, if they appear to be circumscribed and present no unusual features, be removed with a margin of surrounding tissue without preliminary biopsy. Many surgeons would deal similarly with palatal tumours, again provided that the lesion appeared to be well circumscribed. Since the excision would include as wide a zone of surrounding tissue as feasible, it might well be effective treatment also for small low-grade carcinomas that may have deceptively appeared circumscribed. Others always carry out incision biopsy for palatal tumours, and certainly this should be the rule for suspected tumours in the remaining sites.

Ill-defined lumps and ulcerated tumours suspected of malignancy are always biopsied both for diagnosis and as a guide to the extent of the subsequent definitive surgery or radiotherapy. Since there are so many tumour types and the histological features can be so diverse, even in some cases with both benign and malignant areas in different parts of the same tumour, it is important that the biopsy should be of adequate size. Also, it should be so placed that the whole of the biopsy wound will be removed at the ensuing operation.

Since minor gland tumours are within easy reach of the surface, needle biopsy is not indicated, although cytological examination of a needle aspirate may suffice for a diagnosis of malignancy. Negative results, however, cannot be relied upon. Frozen section diagnosis is not always reliable, although once the diagnosis has been made with paraffin sections of a preliminary biopsy, frozen sections at the time of definitive operation may be of value in checking to ensure that the limits of excision are tumour free.

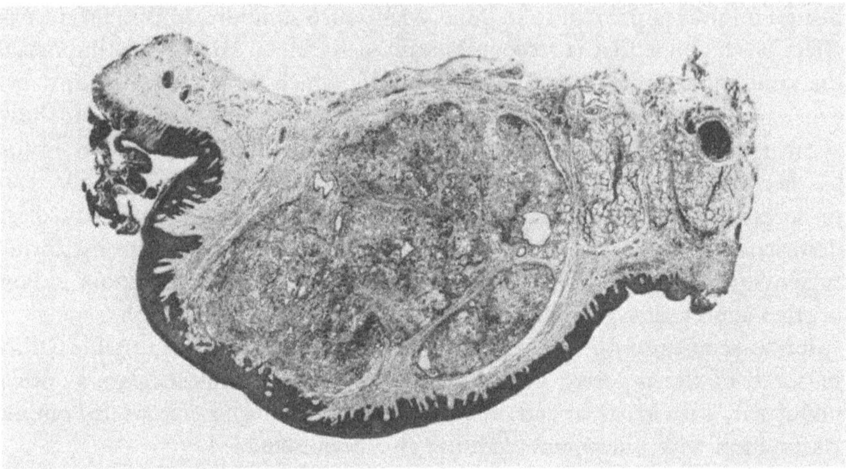

**Figure 3–4.** Pleomorphic adenoma of palate. This complete cross section of an operation specimen shows the lobulated but well-defined and encapsulated tumour forming a swelling that protrudes into the mouth. There is a margin of normal tissue deep to the tumour and some normal mucous glands are seen to one side. (× 10).

## 8. HISTOPATHOLOGY

The epithelial tumours of the salivary glands, with the possible exception of the acinic cell tumour, are derived from the salivary ducts. These ducts are lined by a double layer of cells, those of the inner layer being columnar or cubical while those of the outer layer are flattened. These flattened outer layer cells, the myoepithelial cells, are of epidermal origin but have developed myofibrils and become contractile. In the normal gland the myoepithelial cells are inconspicuous, but they play a prominent part in several of the tumours and take a variety of forms [4,39].

### 8.1. Pleomorphic adenoma

The commonest benign tumour of both the major and minor glands characteristically displays a slow growth rate. This permits the progressive compression of the surrounding tissues to form a capsule, which is generally complete (figure 3–4). In addition growth is also uneven, with the formation of localised extensions, so that tumours often acquire a lobulated outline. However, this is a less prominent feature of minor than of major gland tumours. In an appropriately situated tumour, a tonguelike outgrowth may extend through a natural anatomical aperture and, continuing to enlarge on the other side, result in a dumbbell- or hourglass-shaped growth. A tumour of the deep portion of the parotid may in this way extend medially between the styloid process and the mandible into the lateral pharyngeal space, where it then enlarges and pushes

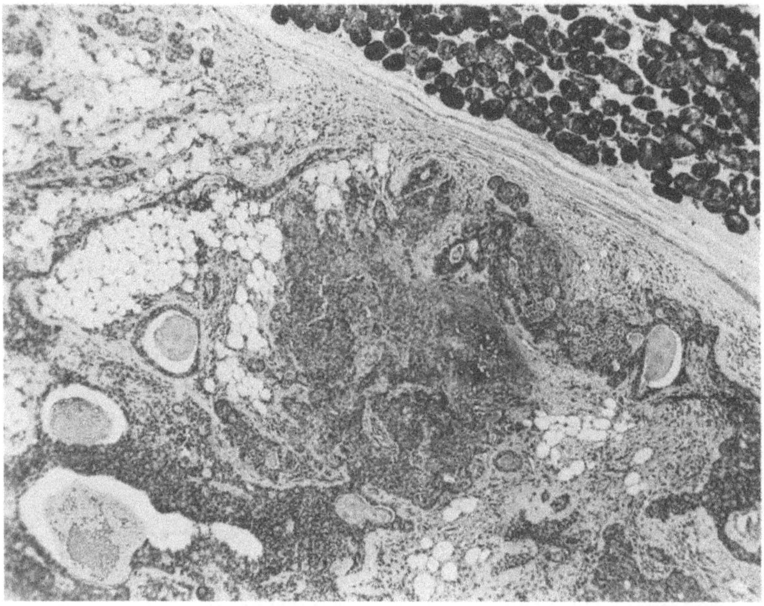

**Figure 3–5.** Edge of a typical palatal pleomorphic adenoma. There is clear demarcation between tumour and the adjacent deeply staining normal mucous glands. The tumour consists of ducts, cysts, and sheets of darkly stained cells. There are some fat cells in the fibrous stroma. (× 45).

the tonsil inward as the first sign of its presence, the parotid swelling not always being noticed. There are minor salivary glands normally situated deep to the tonsil from which pleomorphic adenomas may occasionally arise, and it is important to distinguish the two conditions.

Microscopically, the tumour shows such a wide variety of histological appearances in different areas that it is aptly termed pleomorphic. In some parts there are to be found ducts lined by a single layer of cubical or columnar cells. Around these, often making up the greater part of the tumour, are numerous spindle-shaped myoepithelial cells (figure 3–5). These are usually small and darkly staining, but in some areas they may be larger and with eosinophilic cytoplasm. In other areas of the tumour, the myoepithelial cells may give rise to a mucoid intercellular substance so that a myxoid appearance results. The cells lying in this basophilic background may take on an appearance very similar to cartilage cells (hence the term *mixed tumour* formerly applied to these growths). These myxoid and chondroid areas are often extensive in tumours of the major salivary glands, but are usually less prominent in minor gland tumours.

Squamous metaplasia is a not uncommon feature, and quite large keratin-filled cysts may develop. Less often, there may be groups of goblet cells in the

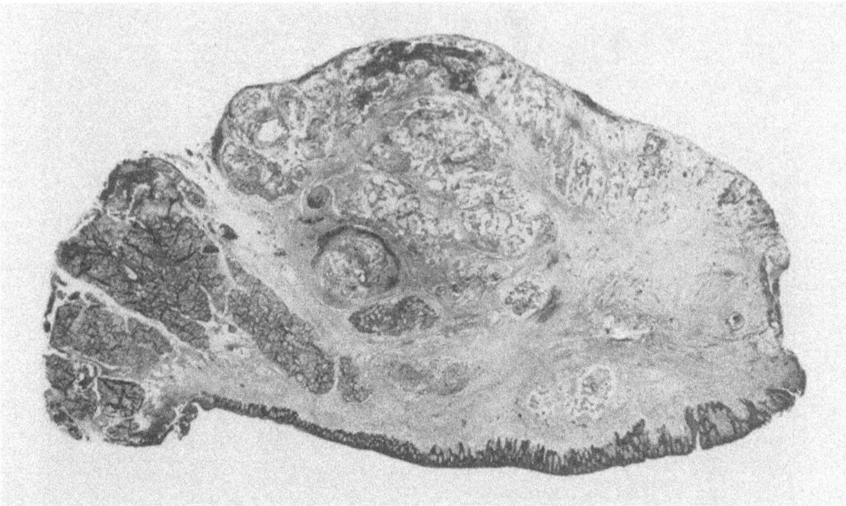

**Figure 3–6.** Recurrent pleomorphic adenoma of palate. The excised portion of palate contains numerous separate nodules of recurrent tumour which extend to the deep surface and also to within a short distance of the epithelium. Normal mucous glands are seen to one side. × 5.

duct linings, with associated mucus production. Long-standing tumours may undergo hyaline degeneration centrally, with elastic fibres developing in the walls of the ducts as the epithelium atrophies. Calcification may eventually take place.

Particularly myxoid and soft tumours may occasionally rupture in the course of removal, spilling tumour tissue into the wound, while any attempt at localised removal or shelling out of the tumour may leave surface projections behind. Either of these events is likely to be followed by recurrence. Although a local recurrence of pleomorphic adenoma may take the form of a single tumour not unlike the original, in most instances it is multifocal, each separate nodule resulting from a group of tumour cells left behind or implanted in the wound at operation (figure 3–6). It is important to remember that these nodules vary in size, depending to some extent on the size of the remnant from which they grew. Only the largest nodule may be apparent clinically, but small tumour deposits are liable to be situated anywhere in the field of operation. If at a subsequent attempt at excision only the obvious recurrent tumour is removed, there may well be further recurrences as small remnants from the original attempt at removal grow and become manifest. Not surprisingly, therefore, recurrence after a second operation is more likely than after the first. Because the recurrent tumour may take years to develop, these patients must be followed for a long time.

## 8.2. Monomorphic adenoma

### *8.2.1. Adenolymphoma*

Adenolymphoma is a not uncommon tumour in the parotid gland, but it is rare in the submandibular and quite exceptional in the minor glands. There are two elements in the tumour: epithelial and lymphoid. The epithelium, which consists of tall columnar cells with a strikingly eosinophilic cytoplasm that contains numerous mitochondria, lines cystic spaces and fills them with papillary ingrowths. The stroma between the spaces is densely infiltrated by lymphocytes, and germinal centres are often present. Although the literature contains a number of case reports of minor gland adenolymphomas, very few indeed record lesions that really resemble the characteristic histopathological structure of the parotid tumour [17,18].

### *8.2.2. Oxyphilic adenoma*

Oxyphilic adenoma is a very rare tumour in the minor salivary glands. It is composed of oncocytes in compact masses, with only occasional tubular formations. Oncocytes are transformed epithelial cells that are much larger than normal and that have a characteristic granular eosinophilic cytoplasm which, like that of the cells of adenolymphoma, is packed with mitochondria. They are not uncommonly seen in the minor salivary glands and in many other tissues in the elderly, where their presence may be considered a normal aging phenomenon. In the minor glands they are usually noted incidentally on microscopy of tissue removed for other reasons, but occasionally some dilatation of oncocyte-lined ducts may occur that produces an expansion large enough to be detected clinically and that may be provisionally diagnosed as a neoplasm. This condition is termed *oncocytosis*. It is harmless.

### *8.2.3. Other types*

Other types of monomorphic adenoma all form circumscribed, usually encapsulated, tumours less likely to be lobulated than pleomorphic adenoma (figure 3–7). Some of them, particularly in the lip, may be quite extensively cystic, with only a few nodules of solid tumour in the cyst wall or sometimes with papillary ingrowths. Microscopically, these tumours show a variety of histological appearances, but the picture is more or less uniform in any given tumour, and there are no myxochondroid areas such as characterise pleomorphic adenoma [40]. The tumours are composed of duct-lining and myoepithelial cells, some of them almost exclusively of one or the other type of cell, but more often of varying proportions of both. If duct-lining cells predominate, the tumour may be termed a tubular or canalicular adenoma (figure 3–8). This is a common lip tumour [41]. Where myoepithelial cells predominate, the tumour has been designated as *myoepithelioma* by some writers [42], although others, unconvinced of the identity of the constituent small

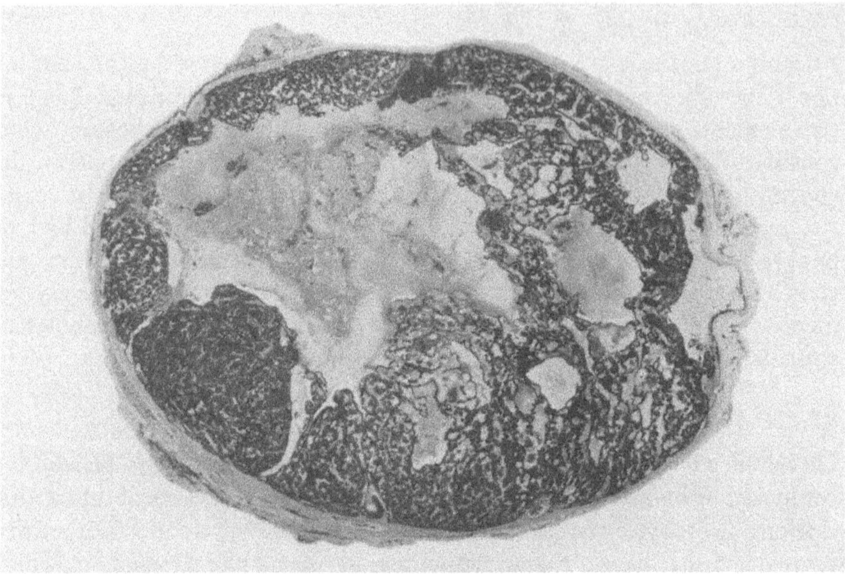

**Figure 3–7.** Monomorphic adenoma of lip. This tumour of the upper lip shows extensive cyst formation. It has a thin rim of surrounding normal tissue. (× 13).

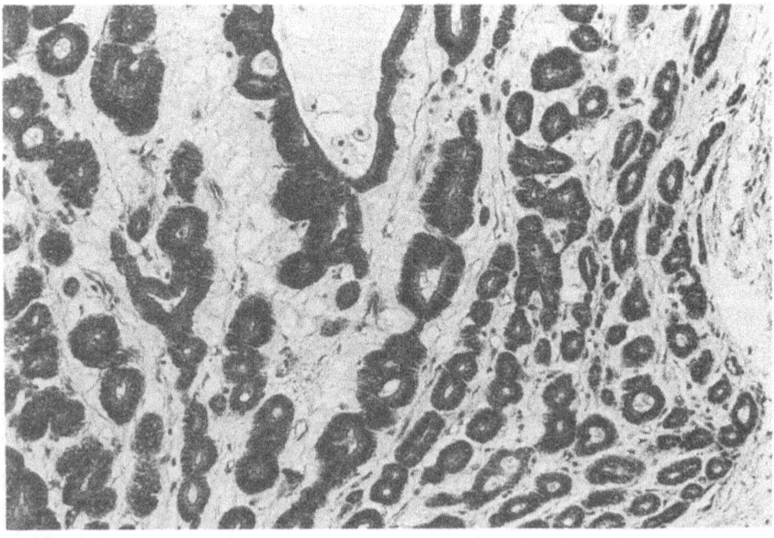

**Figure 3–8.** High-power field from the tumour in figure 3–7. The tumour consists of tubules lined by a single layer of tall columnar cells. (× 120).

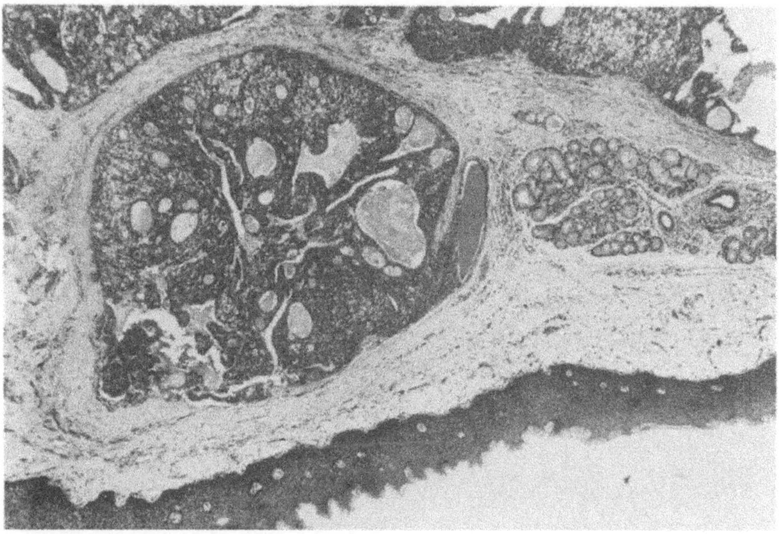

**Figure 3–9.** Mucoepidermoid tumour of palate. One large islet of tumour and part of others are lying in the subepithelial connective tissue. Note the mucus-filled spaces in the tumour epithelium. A group of normal mucous glands lies to the side of the larger tumour islet. (× 30).

darkly staining cells, term such tumours *basal cell adenomas*. The tumour cells may sometimes be arranged in branching and interlacing columns (trabecular adenoma), while in one less common type the myoepithelial cells become clear from the accumulation of glycogen within them (clear cell adenoma). Tumours with much cystic change are sometimes termed *cystadenomas,* or papillary cystadenomas if papillary ingrowths are also a feature. These different cellular patterns are of interest to the histopathologist but are of no special behavioural significance.

**8.3. Mucoepidermoid tumour**

The mucoepidermoid tumour is frequently a fairly well localised growth in its earlier stages, but it is only partially if at all encapsulated, and as it grows it infiltrates locally (figure 3–9). Microscopically, the tumour is composed of three cell types—squamous, mucus-producing, and smaller intermediate cells—the relative numbers of which vary from tumour to tumour. Some tumours may be almost wholly epidermoid with only a few scattered goblet cells, or mucus production may predominate with cystic spaces full of mucus, only occasional epidermoid areas being present. Between these extremes all combinations can occur (figure 3–10). In mainly epidermoid tumours prickle cells are not always easy to find, although the tumour tissue has a typical squamous arrangement. Where mucous cysts are formed, extravasation of mucus into the stroma may occur, with a consequent inflammatory reaction.

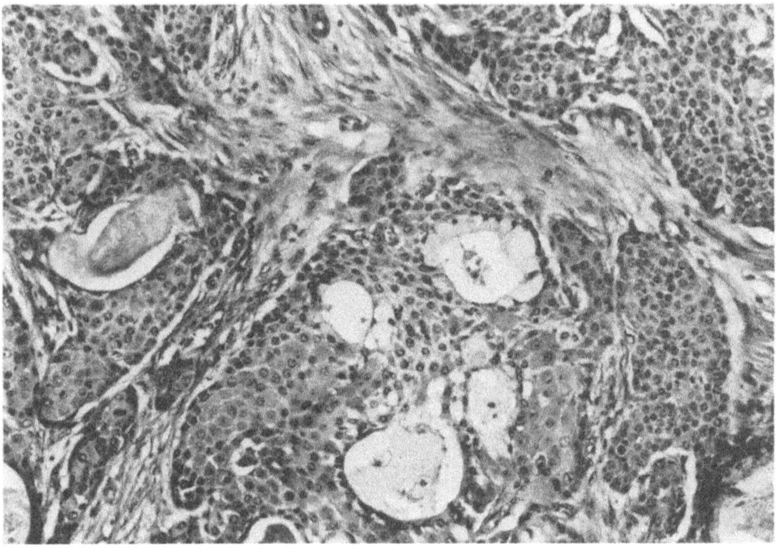

**Figure 3–10.** High-power field from a mucoepidermoid tumour. Most of the cells in this field are epidermoid or intermediate cells. Some spaces lined by goblet cells and filled with mucus are present.

Most mucoepidermoid tumours are well differentiated, and local infiltrative growth does not usually extend beyond the limits of the macroscopic swelling. They are unlikely to recur after local surgical removal. The less common poorly differentiated tumours are usually mainly squamous, with some pleomorphism and mitotic activity, and these are less well defined and more widely infiltrative. Lymph node metastasis is unlikely but a possibility with the well-differentiated tumours. It is much more likely with the poorly differentiated neoplasms [12].

### 8.4. Acinic cell tumour

Since the minor salivary glands are almost entirely mucus-secreting, with only very occasional serous cells, not surprisingly tumours composed of cells resembling those of serous acini are rare. Serous acinar cells are characterised by the presence of basophilic secretory granules that are strongly PAS-positive and cells of this type, forming solid masses or acinar groupings, are typical of acinic cell tumour. Small cystic spaces may be present, but ducts or ductlike structures are practically never seen. Many acinic cell tumours are well differentiated with very little if any cellular atypia. They are well circumscribed and do not recur if removed intact and entire. The risk of metastasis is small. Nearly all the reported minor gland tumours are of this well-differentiated type [19], but the possibility of the occurrence of a more aggressive tumour, such as is seen in the major glands, should be kept in mind. Tumours of this type show varying degrees of differentiation, and the typically granulated cells may be identified only with difficulty.

**8.5. Adenoid cystic carcinoma**

This distinctive type of carcinoma consists essentially of cells that are similar to the two types of cells that line normal salivary ducts. In the majority of tumours the myoepithelial-type cells predominate, those of the inner lining type usually being less numerous. Mucoid material is often present, but instead of accumulating among the myoepithelial cells and separating them widely from one another, as in the myxoid areas of pleomorphic adenoma, it fills multiple microscopic cysts between which the myoepithelial cells, together with occasional tubular structures, remain compact. These multiple cysts give to the tumour a netlike or cribriform appearance (figure 3–11). Sometimes the mucoid material, which is apparently a product of the myoepithelial cells, is replaced by a structureless hyaline substance that forms sheaths around the cell masses. These hyaline sheaths around the columns of tumour tissue are the cylinders that gave rise to the original name, *cylindroma*.

Although adenoid cystic carcinoma is a malignant tumour there are few cytological features indicative of this, there being practically no mitotic activity or pleomorphism or other evidence of cellular atypia. But infiltrative activity is a characteristic feature, and columns of tumour tissue extend into the surroundings, often with little fibrous or other reaction. Cross sections of such columns of tumour tissue with their typical cribriform pattern may be seen on microscopy well beyond the macroscopic limits of the tumour. In addition, adenoid cystic carcinoma has a special predilection for growth in perineural spaces, and nerve fibres surrounded by tumour can often be seen.

After a number of years of slow local infiltration, an occasional tumour may begin to grow rapidly and extend widely. Tumours of this type have the features of an anaplastic spindle cell growth.

The microscopic diagnosis of adenoid cystic carcinoma is frequently a matter of no great difficulty since the histological appearances are so often characteristic, particularly when the typical cylindromatous and cribriform patterns are present. However, the pathologist must remember that superficially similar patterns may appear in other tumours. Some monomorphic adenomas, for instance, have cystic areas that can simulate quite closely the cribriform pattern of adenoid cystic carcinoma, particularly when they are extensive, as occurs not infrequently in lip tumours. Adenocarcinoma may also at times show a cribriform type of pattern, as may the occasional acinic cell tumour.

**8.6. Adenocarcinoma**

Adenocarcinoma is an ill-defined and infiltrative tumour, often showing necrosis and ulceration, with the possibility of early metastasis to the regional lymph nodes (figure 3–12). It is composed of a single type of cell analogous to

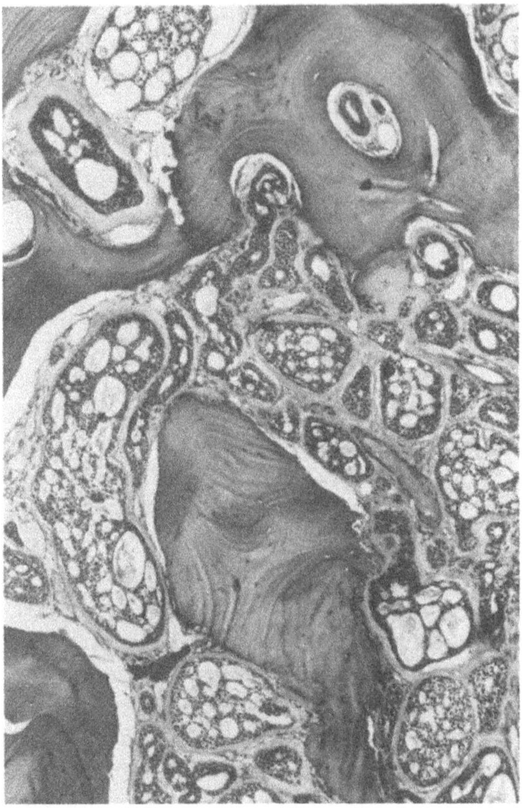

**Figure 3–11.** Section of palatal bone permeated by adenoid cystic carcinoma. The tumour shows its characteristic cribriform or netlike pattern. (× 50).

the inner duct lining type, being thus unlike adenoid cystic carcinoma in which myoepithelial-type cells are also present (figure 3–13). However, a cribriform pattern may also be seen in some adenocarcinomas, as noted above. In other growths there may be a papillary arrangement with or without cyst formation [43], while in some tumours or other areas of the same tumour there may be mucus production. These structural variations suggest that they might represent the malignant counterparts of the various "other types" of monomorphic adenoma. However, these variations do not seem to affect prognosis, which depends rather on the degree of differentiation of the tumour. Well-differentiated tumours, which may be very similar to adenomas and only with difficulty distinguished from them microscopically, may be curable by wide surgical excision. Tumours at the other end of the scale may be so anaplastic that areas of tubular formation justifying the designation of adenocarcinoma are few and far between. They grow quickly and metastasise early.

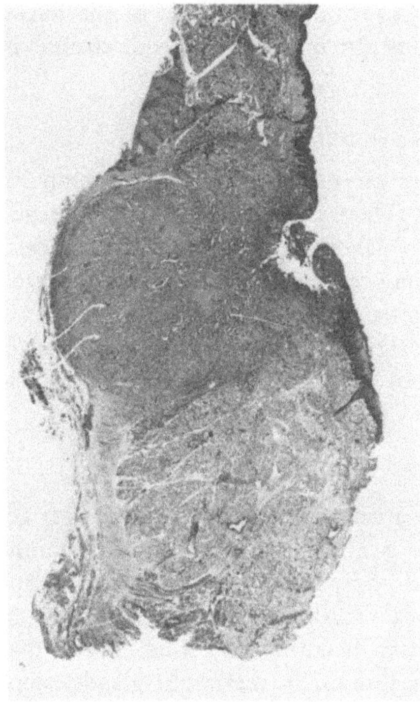

**Figure 3–12**

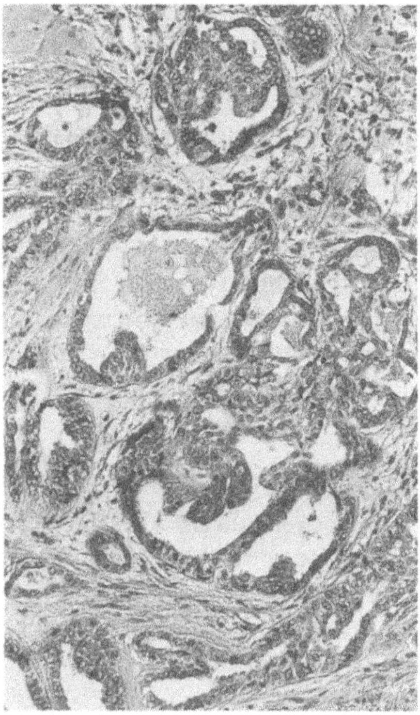

**Figure 3–13**

**Figure 3–12.** Adenocarcinoma of palate. The ulcerated palatal epithelium is on the right of the section. The tumour tissue, which stains more deeply than the adjoining normal mucous glands, extends from the epithelial surface where it forms the floor of the ulcer to the deep limit of the specimen. (× 4).

**Figure 3–13.** Higher power field from the tumour in figure 3–12. The tumour consists of irregular tubules lined by pleomorphic columnar and cubical epithelial cells. (× 120).

## 8.7. Squamous cell carcinoma

Squamous cell carcinoma is a rare but well-recognised malignant tumour of the major salivary glands, probably arising in areas of squamous metaplasia of the ducts consequent on chronic inflammation or the presence of a calculus. In the minor glands this tumour is seldom if ever identified. In these glands the necks of the larger ducts are lined by squamous epithelium, which may proliferate and extend inward in chronic inflammation. However, if carcinoma did develop in this hyperplastic epithelium, it could hardly be distinguished from a tumour of the surface epithelium by the time it had been noticed and removed.

The lesions of *necrotizing sialometaplasia* have occasionally been misdiagnosed on microscopy as squamous cell carcinoma or as mucoepidermoid tumour [44]. This condition, which usually affects the palate, presents as a unilateral or bilateral swelling or ulceration, which may resemble carcinoma clinically. Although the lesion heals spontaneously in a few weeks, biopsy during the active phase shows marked squamous metaplasia of the ductal epithelium of the minor salivary glands and also infarctlike necrotic changes in the acinar epithelium [45,46].

### 8.8. Undifferentiated carcinoma

Tumours of this type consist of masses of cells that show no attempt to reproduce glandular or other structures. There are usually areas of necrosis, and the cells vary in size and staining, often showing many mitoses. Tumours that have probably derived from duct-lining cells or their forerunners are made up of solid masses of spheroidal or polygonal cells. Other tumours, composed of spindle cells, suggest a myoepithelial origin. The possibility of a spindle cell undifferentiated tumour developing from an adenoid cystic carcinoma has already been mentioned.

### 8.9. Carcinoma in pleomorphic adenoma

In the major salivary glands, carcinoma arising in pleomorphic adenoma accounts for some 4% of tumours [4]. It is even less common in the minor glands. The malignant change, characterised by rapid infiltrative growth, appears in a pleomorphic adenoma or its local recurrence usually after it has been slowly growing for at least 10 to 15 years. It is this long time interval that accounts for the lesser frequency of the tumour in the minor glands, since patients with oral tumours are less likely than those with parotid tumours to tolerate them untreated long enough for malignant change to become a risk.

The carcinoma that supervenes on a pleomorphic adenoma may be an adenocarcinoma, a squamous or undifferentiated carcinoma, or more than one of these patterns may be present in the same tumour. To substantiate the diagnosis of carcinoma in pleomorphic adenoma, areas of frank malignancy and of benign pleomorphic adenoma must both be identified (figures 3–14 and 3–15).

## 9. COURSE AND PROGNOSIS

The outlook for patients with salivary gland tumours depends essentially on two factors: the histological type of the tumour and the possibility of complete surgical removal. Of these two factors, the second has the greater influence on the outcome. The reason is that although at least half of all tumours of the minor salivary glands may be described histologically as malignant, the great majority do not metastasise until relatively late. If they can be completely removed, therefore, at a reasonably early stage, the prognosis should be good. Complete removal of growths that are locally infiltrative, however, is frequently a very difficult task in the confined area of the oral region, where restricted space, the presence of important anatomical structures and the necessity of inflicting the least possible degree of mutilation combine to present formidable problems for the surgeon.

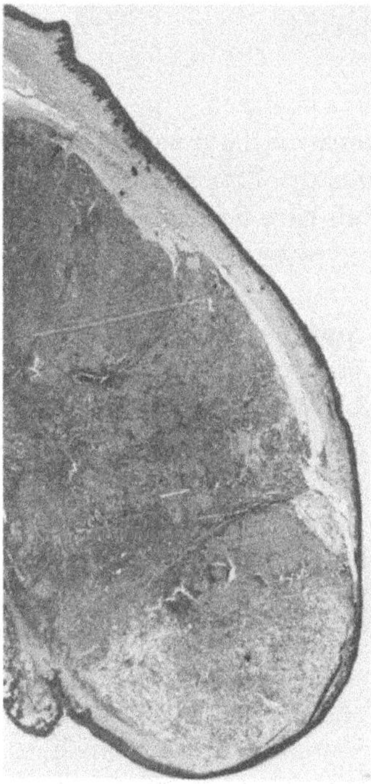

**Figure 3–14**

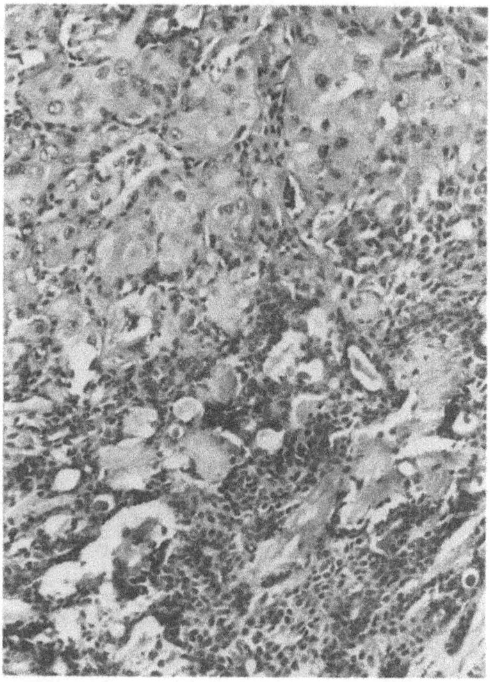

**Figure 3–15**

**Figure 3–14.** Carcinoma in a palatal pleomorphic adenoma. The palatal surface is to the right. The pleomorphic adenoma is the smaller and more palely staining mass; the carcinoma that has developed from it is seen as the more deeply staining tissue that is now extending widely into the palate and is replacing most of the original adenoma. (× 7).

**Figure 3–15.** High-power field from tumour in figure 3–14 shows the contrast between the small dark myoepithelial cells and tubules of the original adenoma, seen in the lower part of the illustration, and the much larger and pleomorphic cells of the carcinoma in the upper part. (× 120).

### 9.1. Pleomorphic adenoma

Untreated, pleomorphic adenoma may have a very long natural history, as already mentioned. The danger in such cases is that after many years carcinoma may develop, but the frequency of such an event is not definitely known. It should become very rare, in the future, in view of the current emphasis on early diagnosis and adequate treatment.

Recurrent pleomorphic adenoma, resulting either from enucleation or from inadequate excision, has a poorer prognosis than a primary tumour that has been treated adequately, since it is very likely to consist of multiple nodules of growth that will be more difficult to excise than the unicentric mass of a primary tumour. For this reason second and subsequent recurrences are not unusual, once the pattern has been established. Apart from the ever-increasing difficulty in dealing with these recurrences surgically, there exists also the danger of carcinomatous change in one of the nodules.

### 9.2. Monomorphic adenoma

The rare adenolymphomas and oxyphilic adenomas of the minor glands are benign tumours, and the extremely rare carcinomas that have been reported in association with these tumours in the major glands have not been reported in the minor glands, although a locally aggressive oxyphilic tumour of the palate has been recorded [47].

The monomorphic adenomas of other types appear to behave in the same way as pleomorphic adenoma, although the literature contains few long-term reports. Undoubtedly, incomplete removal can be followed by multinodular recurrence, and some carcinomas of the minor glands have appearances suggesting an origin in a preceding monomorphic adenoma.

### 9.3. Mucoepidermoid tumour

Low-grade tumours that have been completely excised have a good prognosis, and high-grade tumours also may be treated with good results if they are dealt with before metastasis or extensive local invasion has occurred. However, only a small minority of tumours in the minor glands are of high-grade malignancy. Although most series of mucoepidermoid tumours are quite small, the cumulative indications are that most low-grade tumours can be cured. In high-grade tumours cervical node metastases are likely to appear sooner or later. In one of the largest series of minor gland tumours there was one treatment failure in 13 cases of low-grade tumour and 20 failures in 39 higher grade tumours [12]. These were due to persistence of disease at the primary site, nodal metastases, or a combination of these features.

### 9.4. Acinic cell tumour

The largest series of minor gland tumours comprises 19 cases [19]. Follow-up of 11 of these cases showed local recurrence in three patients, in one of them nine years after initial treatment and in the other two after two years. Regional or distant metastases were not found. This would seem to reflect in general the follow-up findings, where these have been available, of the other cases in the literature, which amount to less than 40. In the minor glands, therefore, acinic cell tumour appears to be mainly a slow-growing and locally invasive tumour, although regional metastases can occur [21].

### 9.5. Adenoid cystic carcinoma

Although like most of the other salivary tumours adenoid cystic carcinoma grows slowly, it is a notably infiltrative neoplasm that invades adjacent tissues to a greater extent than the clinical appearance would seem to indicate and can invade bone despite the absence of radiographic changes. A palatal tumour, for example, may infiltrate the bone of the hard palate in the absence of radiographic evidence, and similarly a tumour of antral mucous glands may infiltrate through the palate and produce a palatal swelling as its first sign.

Recurrence after excision is frequent, and of all the commoner salivary neoplasms it is the most persistent and difficult to eradicate. Untreated, or recurrent after incomplete excision, it can spread widely, tending to follow the course of cranial nerves, and may ultimately invade the skull. As a result of the rather slow rate of growth in the majority of cases, and the relatively late occurrence of metastases, the five-year survival rate may be as high as 80% for palatal tumours, but by 15 years the rate has dropped to 38% [48]. For oral tumours in general, a 10-year determinate cure rate of 23% has been reported in a large series [49], indicating that tumours in the palate have a better prognosis than those in other intraoral sites. Metastases occur in about 30% of patients, the lungs being the commonest site [50]. Despite the fact that perineural infiltration is such a characteristic feature of the tumour, lymph node metastases are much less common than visceral metastases and are due to direct extension rather than true embolic dissemination, which has been shown to be rare [51,52].

### 9.6. Adenocarcinoma

Well-differentiated tumours that can be completely excised may very well have a good prognosis. Those that are less well differentiated and have extensive local infiltration may metastasise to the regional nodes relatively early. The prognosis for an adenocarcinoma of this type is therefore poor. However, many adenocarcinomas of the minor glands are of low-grade malignancy, and the higher-grade tumors that grow rapidly are in a definite minority. Variations in criteria for the histological diagnosis of adenocarcinoma, with possibly in some cases inadequate distinction of this tumour from adenoid cystic carcinoma or from carcinoma in pleomorphic adenoma, have resulted in a lack of any clear consensus in the literature.

### 9.7. Carcinoma in pleomorphic adenoma

Since carcinoma arising in pleomorphic adenoma is a relatively recently defined entity, little guidance is available from previously published series of minor gland tumours. For primary cases, that is to say, those cases in which carcinoma has developed in a previously untreated pleomorphic adenoma, the prognosis is likely to be similar to that for adenocarcinoma. Where the carcinoma has developed in a recurrent pleomorphic adenoma, the outlook is even less favourable.

## REFERENCES

1. Thackray AC, Sobin L. Histological Typing of Salivary Gland Tumours. Geneva: World Health Organization, 1972.
2. Eneroth C-M. Histological and clinical aspects of parotid tumours. Acta Otolaryngol, Suppl 1–191 (99): 1964.

3. Doll R, Nuir C, Waterhouse J. Cancer in Five Continents, Vol 2. New York: UICC and Springer, 1970.
4. Thackray AC, Lucas RB. Tumors of the Major Salivary Glands. Atlas of Tumor Pathology, 2nd series. Fascicle 10. Washington, D.C.: Armed Forces Institute of Pathology, 1974.
5. Frazell EL. Clinical aspects of tumors of the major salivary glands. Cancer (7): 637–659, 1954.
6. Eneroth C-M. Salivary gland tumors in the parotid gland, submandibular gland, and the palate region. Cancer (27): 1415–1418, 1971.
7. Davies JNP, Dodge OG, Burkitt DP. Salivary gland tumors in Uganda. Cancer (17): 1310–1322, 1964.
8. Thomas KM, Hutt MSR, Borgstein J. Salivary gland tumors in Malawi. Cancer (46): 2328–2334, 1980.
9. Potdar GG, Paymaster JC: Tumors of minor salivary glands. Oral Surg (28): 310–319, 1969.
10. Luna MA, Stimson PG, Bardwil JM. Minor salivary gland tumors of the oral cavity. A review of sixty-eight cases. Oral Surg (25): 71–86, 1968.
11. Stuteville OH, Corley RD. Surgical management of tumors of intraoral minor salivary glands. Report of eighty cases. Cancer (20): 1578–1586, 1967.
12. Spiro RH, Koss LG, Hajdu SI, Strong EW. Tumors of minor salivary origin. A clinicopathologic study of 492 cases. Cancer (31): 117–129, 1973.
13. Epker BN, Henny FA. Clinical, histopathologic, and surgical aspects of intraoral minor salivary gland tumors: Review of 90 cases. J Oral Surg (27): 792–804, 1969.
14. Pogrel MA. Tumours of the salivary glands: A histological and clinical review. Brit J Oral Surg (17): 47–56, 1979.
15. Crocker DJ, Calalaris CJ, Finch R. Intraoral minor salivary gland tumors. Report of 38 cases. Oral Surg (29): 60–68, 1970.
16. Stene T, Koppang HS. Carcinomas of intraoral salivary glands. Histopath (2): 19–29, 1978.
17. Baden E, Pierce M, Selman AJ, Roberts TW, Doyle JL. Intraoral papillary cystadenoma lymphomatosum. J Oral Surg (34): 533–541, 1976.
18. Fantasia JE, Miller AS. Papillary cystadenoma lymphomatosum arising in minor salivary glands. Oral Surg (52): 411–416, 1981.
19. Chen S-Y, Brannon RB, Miller AS, White DK, Hooker SP. Acinic cell adenocarcinoma of minor salivary glands. Cancer (42): 678–685, 1978.
20. Abrams AM, Melrose RJ. Acinic cell tumors of minor salivary gland origin. Oral Surg (46): 220–233, 1978.
21. Ferlito A. Acinic cell carcinoma of minor salivary glands. Histopath (4): 331–343, 1980.
22. Rice DH, Batsakis JG, McClatchey KD. Postirradiation malignant salivary gland tumor. Arch Otolaryngol (102): 699–701, 1976.
23. Schneider AB, Favus MJ, Stachura ME, Arnold MJ, Frohman LA. Salivary gland neoplasms as late consequence of head and neck irradiation. Ann J Int Med (87): 160–164, 1977.
24. Belsky JL, Takeichi N, Yamamoto T, Cihak RW, Hirose F, Ezaki H, Inove S, Blot WJ. Salivary gland neoplasms following atomic radiation: Additional cases and reanalysis of combined data in a fixed population, 1957–1970. Cancer (35): 555–559, 1975.
25. Takeichi N, Hirose F, Yamamoto T. Salivary gland tumors in atomic bomb survivors, Hiroshima, Japan. 1. Epidemiologic observations. Cancer (38): 2462–2468, 1976.
26. Main JHP, Orr JA, McGurk FM, McComb RJ, Mock D. Salivary gland tumors: Review of 643 cases. J Oral Path (5): 88–102, 1976.
27. Fantasia JE, Neville BW. Basal cell adenomas of the minor salivary glands. Oral Surg (50): 433–440, 1980.
28. Heidelberger KP, McClatchey K, Batsakis JG, Van Wieren CR. Primary adenocarcinoma of the lip. J Oral Surg (35): 68–69, 1977.
29. Byers RM, Boddie A, Luna MA. Malignant salivary gland neoplasms of the lip. Amer J Surg (134): 528–530. 1977.
30. Burbank PM, Dockerty MB, Devine KP. A clinicopathologic study of 43 cases of glandular tumors of the tongue. Surg Gynec Obstet (109): 573–582, 1959.
31. Goepfert H, Giraldo AA, Byers RM, Luna MA. Salivary gland tumors of the base of the tongue. Arch Otolaryngol (102): 391–395, 1976.
32. Silverglade LB, Alvares OF, Olech E. Central mucoepidermoid tumors of the jaws. Review of the literature and case report. Cancer (22): 650–653, 1968.

33. Alexander RW, Dupuis RH, Holton H. Central mucoepidermoid tumor (carcinoma) of the mandible. J Oral Surg (32): 541–547, 1974.
34. Chaudhry AP, Vickers RA, Gorlin RJ. Intraoral minor salivary gland tumors. An analysis of 1,414 cases. Oral Surg (14): 1194–1226, 1961.
35. Hjertman L, Eneroth C-M. Tumours of the palate. Acta Otolaryngol Suppl. (263): 179–182, 1970.
36. Coates HLC, Devine KD, Desanto LW, Weiland LH. Glandular tumors of the palate. Surg Gynec Obstet (140): 589–593, 1975.
37. Frable WJ, Elzay RP. Tumors of minor salivary glands. A report of 73 cases. Cancer (25): 932–941, 1970.
38. Pinto RS, Kelly DE, George AE. Radiologic features of benign pleomorphic adenoma of the hard palate. Oral Surg (39): 976–981, 1975.
39. Lucas RB. Pathology of Tumours of the Oral Tissues. Edinburgh, London, and New York: Churchill Livingstone, 4th ed, 1984.
40. Crumpler C, Scharfenberg JC, Reed RJ: Monomorphic adenomas of salivary glands. Trabecular-tubular, canalicular, and basaloid variants. Cancer (38): 193–200, 1976.
41. Anderson JH, Provencher RF, McKean TW. Basal cell adenoma: Review of the literature and report of case, J Oral Surg (38): 844–846, 1980.
42. Sciubba JJ, Brannon RB. Myoepithelioma of salivary glands: Report of 23 cases. Cancer (49): 562–572, 1982.
43. Allen MS, FitzHugh GS, Marsh WL. Low-grade papillary adenocarcincoma of the palate. Cancer (33): 153–158, 1974.
44. Grillon GL, Lally ET. Necrotizing sialometaplasia: Literature review and presentation of five cases. J Oral Surg (39): 747–753, 1981.
45. Lynch DP, Crago CA, Martinez MG. Necrotizing sialometaplasia. A review of the literature and report of two additional cases. Oral Surg (47): 63–69, 1979.
46. Birkholz H, Minton GA, Yuen YL. Necrotizing sialometaplasia: Review of the literature and report of non-ulcerative case. J Oral Surg (37): 588–599, 1979.
47. Briggs J, Evans JNG. Malignant oxyphilic granular-cell tumor (oncocytoma) of the palate. Review of the recent literature and report of a case. Oral Surg (23): 796–802, 1967.
48. Eneroth C-M, Hertman L, Moberger G. Adenoid cystic carcinoma of the palate. Acta Otolaryngol (66): 248–260, 1968.
49. Spiro RH, Huvos AG, Strong EW. Adenoid cystic carcinoma of salivary origin. A clinicopathologic study of 242 cases. Amer J Surg (128): 512–520, 1974.
50. Shumrick DA. Treatment of malignant tumors of minor salivary glands. Arch Otolaryngol (88): 74–79, 1968.
51. Allen MSA, Marsh WL. Lymph node involvement by direct extension in adenoid cystic carcinoma. Absence of classic embolic lymph node metastasis. Cancer (38): 2017–2021, 1976.
52. Marsh WL, Allen MS. Adenoid cystic carcinoma. Biologic behaviour in 38 patients. Cancer (43): 1463–1473, 1979.

# 4. CLINICAL AND HISTOLOGICAL ASPECTS OF ORAL MALIGNANCIES, EXCLUDING SQUAMOUS CELL CARCINOMAS AND SALIVARY GLAND TUMOURS

MERVYN SHEAR
MARIO ALTINI

## 1. AMELOBLASTOMA

The ameloblastoma is a locally invasive tumour of odontogenic epithelium. There has been extensive discussion on the most appropriate term [1].

### 1.1. Epidemiology

An epidemiological study of ameloblastoma in South Africa has shown that the annual incidence rates, standardized against the standard world population, are 1.96, 1.20, 0.18, and 0.44 per million population for black males, black females, white males, and white females, respectively [2]. The higher incidence of ameloblastoma in blacks than in whites, with a ratio of about 11 to 1, confirms a view that has previously been suggested [3]. In a frequently cited large series of ameloblastoma [4], most cases were diagnosed in the fifth decade and the sex distribution was almost equal.

### 1.2. Etiology

Information about the etiology of ameloblastoma is scant. Lesions resembling ameloblastoma have been induced in animals [5,6]. The concept that the dentigerous cyst has ameloblastomatous potential has little foundation. Occasionally, dentigerous cysts exhibit mural nodules consisting of tissue very similar to that of plexiform ameloblastoma without evidence of infiltration of

*I. van der Waal and G.B. Snow (eds), ORAL ONCOLOGY.* 

epithelium into the cyst wall. Such lesions have been described as "mural ameloblastomas" [7]. They are clearly not infiltrating lesions and do not behave like ameloblastomas [8]. The term *odontogenic papilloma* would probably be more appropriate. Furthermore, the clinical and radiological features of a unicystic or unilocular ameloblastoma that involves a related unerupted tooth are indistinguishable from those of dentigerous cysts [9]. This phenomenon is also partly responsible for the view that dentigerous cysts predispose to ameloblastoma.

### 1.3. Histogenesis

Much has been written about the origin of the odontogenic epithelium that comprises the ameloblastoma. The enamel organ, dental lamina or its remnants, the cell rests of Serres, the cell rests of Malassez, the basal layer of the oral epithelium, and the epithelial lining of odontogenic cysts—all have been suggested as possibilities [10]. Although the solution to the problem may be regarded largely as an academic exercise, it is nevertheless an intriguing one, one that may well be resolved with the development of basic studies on odontogenesis and related oncogenesis [11,12].

### 1.4. Clinical features

Figures approximating 15% have been cited for the frequency of ameloblastoma in the maxilla [4]. However, of approximately 200 ameloblastomas accessioned in our files, only 3 occurred in the maxilla. The molar-angle-ascending ramus regions are most frequently involved.

Ameloblastoma is a slowly growing tumour. It is remarkable how frequently we see patients who have delayed seeking medical attention until their tumours have produced extremely large swellings both intra- and extraorally. The swellings are at first firm when covered by a fairly thick layer of bone. Gradually, the overlying bone is thinned and the tumour may exhibit "springiness." At a later stage, with no overlying bone, fluctuation may be elicited. The ameloblastoma may grow to a fairly large size without producing pain. Other signs and symptoms may be loosening of teeth, ill-fitting dentures, nasal obstruction, bleeding, trismus, or unhealed extraction sockets [13]. Ameloblastoma grows by expansion and local invasion. Its infiltrative nature demands that it be treated by wide excision, and the high frequency of recurrences reported in the literature, such as 33% in the large series of Small and Waldron [4], results from failure to observe this method of treatment. Metastasis to distant sites is a controversial matter. Well-documented cases of pulmonary deposits in patients with ameloblastoma of the jaws have probably resulted from inhalation of tumour cells rather than from blood or lymphatic spread. Cases of ameloblastoma with metastases to regional lymph nodes or to bone have been reported [10]. They may actually be rare examples of malignant ameloblastoma or odontogenic carcinoma, as is discussed later in the chapter.

### 1.5. Radiological features

The radiological features of ameloblastoma vary. There may be a unilocular radiolucent area with a smooth, well-demarcated margin, with or without bony trabeculations. Alternatively, the margins of an unilocular ameloblastoma may be irregular and not sharply demarcated. Unilocular lesions may involve unerupted teeth and must be differentiated from dentigerous [9] and primordial cysts (keratocysts). Ameloblastoma very frequently produces resorption of roots of adjacent teeth, but so do dentigerous cysts, so that root resorption alone cannot distinguish the two. Primordial cysts, however, have a lesser tendency to produce root resorption [14]. Larger lesions are frequently multilocular, the locules being of different shape and size and separated usually by fine bony septa. Multilocular radiolucencies are also found in central giant granuloma and in myxofibroma of the jaws.

### 1.6. Biopsy procedure

An important precaution in taking the biopsy is to remove a solid portion of the tumour. Frequently, the most prominent and readily accessible part of an ameloblastoma is the wall of a large expanded cystic portion of the tumour. Such an expanded cyst may be lined by a thin layer of stratified squamous epithelium, which appears deceptively innocent, and thus a diagnosis of simple jaw cyst may erroneously be made.

### 1.7. Histopathology

There are two main histological patterns of ameloblastoma: the follicular and plexiform. Within these two groups are a number of histological variants, none of which has been shown to influence the prognosis.

The follicular variety consists of variable numbers of epithelial islands of different shapes and sizes lying in a fibrous stroma (figure 4–1). The peripheral cells of each follicle are palisaded, and their nuclei lie toward the centre of the follicles away from the basement membrane. The central cells of the follicles are separated by intercellular oedema, and this zone thus resembles the stellate reticulum of the enamel organ. Coalescence of foci of intercellular oedema leads to the formation of microcysts. Further coalescence and then expansion and dilatation of these intrafollicular cysts lead to the clinically and radiologically overt cysts that are a characteristic of the ameloblastoma.

In the plexiform variety a more or less continuous plexiform network of odontogenic epithelial strands occurs (figure 4–2). The peripheral cells of these narrow strands are also palisaded, but not as conspicuously as in the follicular variety. The central areas of the plexiform strands are not as oedematous as in the follicles, and cysts do not usually form within the epithelium. In the plexiform variety the cysts tend to form in the stroma, which, as a result of oedema, is often looser than the stroma of the follicular variety. The breakdown of connective tissue in the plexiform variety, which leads to stromal cyst

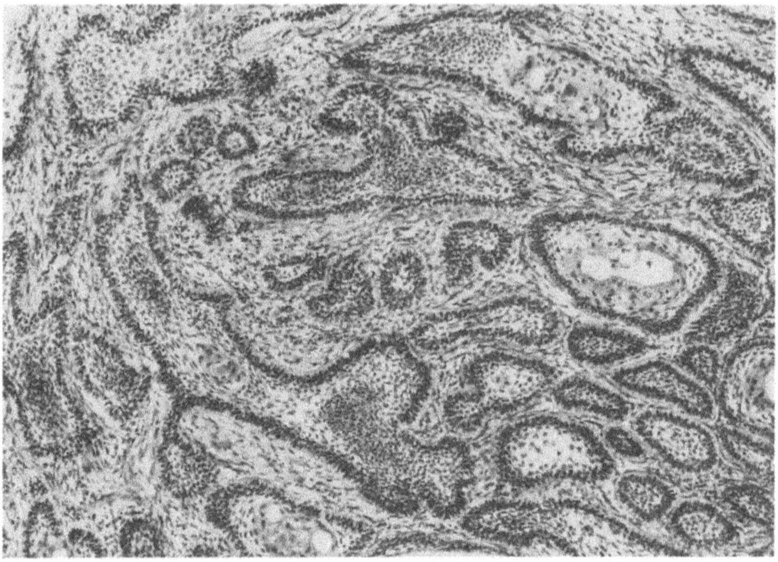

**Figure 4–1.** Follicular variety of ameloblastoma.

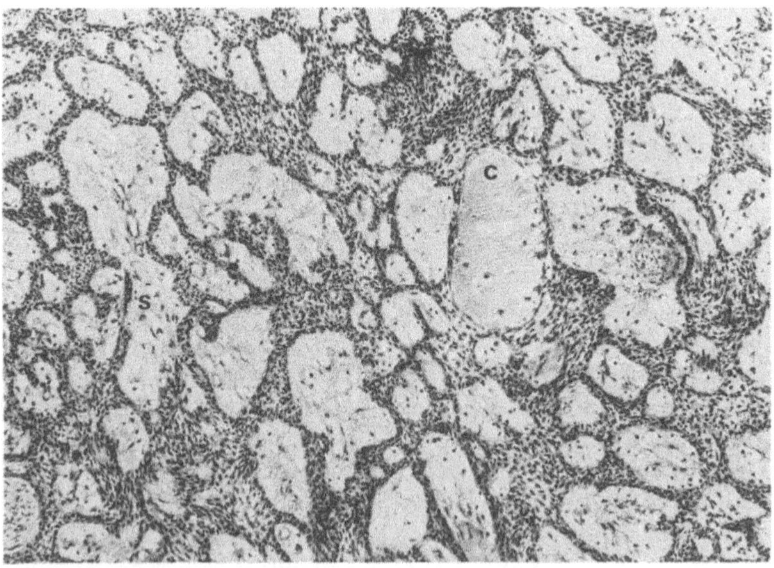


**Figure 4–2.** Plexiform variety of ameloblastoma showing oedematous stroma (S) and formation of stromal microcysts (C).

formation, also affects the blood vessel walls so that they sometimes lose their support, dilate widely, and rupture, giving the tumour a markedly vascular or haemorrhagic appearance.

Histological variants of the above two main patterns are described as the acanthomatous, the granular cell, and the basal cell varieties.

Ameloblastoma does not usually induce the formation of dentine and enamel. When this condition occurs very occasionally, it is termed *odontoameloblastoma* [15].

## 2. MALIGNANT ODONTOGENIC TUMOURS

The World Health Organization classifies the odontogenic tumours into two major groups, benign and malignant [16]. The malignant group is classified further, as follows:

1. Odontogenic carcinomas
   a. Malignant ameloblastoma
   b. Primary intraosseous carcinoma
   c. Other carcinomas arising from odontogenic epithelium, including those arising from odontogenic cysts
2. Odontogenic sarcomas
   a. Ameloblastic fibrosarcoma (ameloblastic sarcoma)
   b. Ameloblastic odontosarcoma

In this section we shall refer also to a third histological variant of odontogenic sarcoma, the ameloblastic dentinosarcoma [17].

### 2.1. Odontogenic carcinoma

Primary carcinoma of the jaws, sometimes referred to as intra-alveolar epidermoid carcinoma, arises from epithelial remnants within the jaws. As these epithelial residues are predominantly odontogenic, it is likely that most primary intra-alveolar carcinomas, and certainly those in the mandible, are of odontogenic origin and are therefore referred to as odontogenic carcinomas [16]. Odontogenic carcinomas may develop by malignant transformation of an ameloblastoma, the so-called malignant ameloblastoma; from residues of odontogenic epithelium, the so-called primary intraosseous carcinoma; and from the epithelial lining of odontogenic cysts. Subclassification of odontogenic carcinomas into these three categories is probably of academic and research interest only. From a clinicopathological point of view, they are best lumped together.

Odontogenic carcinomas are rare lesions. A recent study [18] has shown incidence rates of 0.65, 0.41, 0.22, and 0.17 per million per year for white males, black males, white females and black females, respectively. The incidence may be somewhat higher, but unless the diagnosis is established early it may be difficult to differentiate it from a tumour of surface oral mucosa that has invaded the jaws [19].

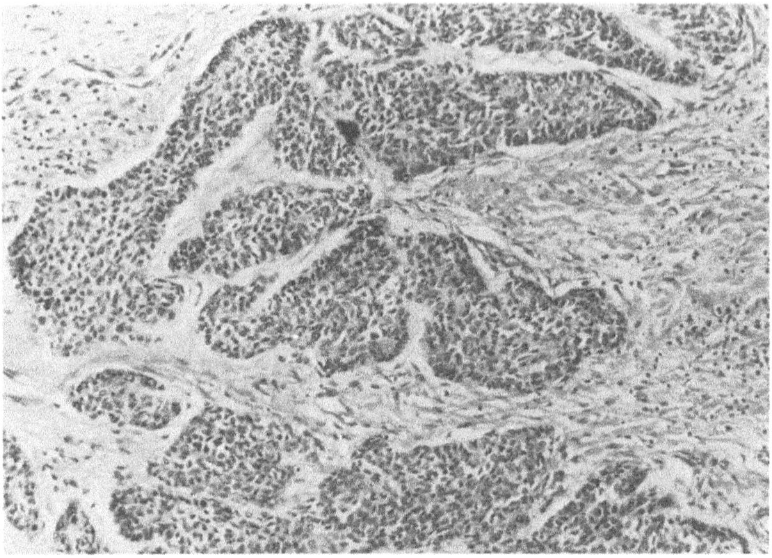

**Figure 4–3.** Odontogenic carcinoma.

Metastases occur to regional lymph nodes and to distant sites. The five-year survival rate of all patients with odontogenic carcinoma appears to be about 30%, but the prognosis is very much worse when there are metastases at the time of treatment [19].

Some of the reported cases of odontogenic carcinoma show histological features of squamous carcinoma that are indistinguishable from squamous carcinoma of the oral mucosa. In others, however, the tumours have a distinctly odontogenic pattern with basal-type cells forming alveoli or arranged in a plexiform pattern with palisading of the peripheral cells [19] (figure 4–3). To make a specific diagnosis of malignant ameloblastoma, rather than the less specific odontogenic carcinoma, would require evidence that the neoplasm was preceded by a conventional ameloblastoma that developed into or recurred as a malignant tumour. Similarly, before the diagnosis of carcinoma arising from a cyst lining can be established, one must exclude the possibilities that the cyst and neoplasm may have developed independently adjacent to one another and ultimately fused in some parts and that the lesion was initially an epithelial neoplasm that underwent secondary cystic change [20].

### 2.2. Odontogenic sarcomas

The ameloblastic fibrosarcoma is a "neoplasm with a similar structure to the ameloblastic fibroma but in which the mesodermal component shows the features of a sarcoma" [16]. It has been stated that the presence of induced dentine and enamel does not alter the basic nature of this neoplasm and that further subclassification into those lesions containing dentine only and those containing both enamel and dentine is unnecessary [21]. A survey of the literature on ameloblastic fibrosarcoma included ten cases and added six new examples [21]. Other individual cases have recently been reported [22,23]. Only one case of ameloblastic dentinosarcoma has been reported [17]. Ameloblastic odontosarcoma is also extremely rare, and very few cases have been reported in the literature [24,25].

A review of the malignant ameloblastic lesions reported in the literature [26] showed that they occur most commonly in the second, third, and fourth decades of life, show no sex predilection, and are found more commonly in the mandible. Paraesthesia of the lip is usually present. This is a very useful diagnostic symptom, as ameloblastomas do not produce lip paraesthesia.

Undoubtedly, many of the malignant ameloblastic lesions result from the malignant transformation of benign counterparts [17,21,25,26]. Of equal interest is the fact that in many instances the epithelial component seems to disappear as malignant transformation progresses, so that eventually all traces of the odontogenic origin may be lost and the histological features become those of a central fibrosarcoma of bone [21,22,27]. This has led to the postulate that many fibrosarcomas of the jaws may be odontogenic in origin [21,26,27]. The high recurrence rate of ameloblastic fibromas [28], together with the occurrence of malignant transformation in some cases, has resulted in the ameloblastic fibroma being regarded in an increasingly suspicious light by clinician and pathologist alike.

Histologically, the malignant lesions show similar features to their benign counterparts, with the exception that the connective tissue is clearly sarcomatous (figure 4–4). The odontogenic epithelial component is present in the form of follicles and strands. The epithelium does not show malignant features. The malignant mesodermal component surrounds the epithelium and consists of spindle cells, which may show whorling and streaming. Areas in which the connective tissue is histologically benign are interspersed with the malignant areas, supporting the concept of transition from a previously benign to a malignant lesion. In the ameloblastic dentinosarcoma, the epithelium appears to induce deposition of dentinoid that in parts is dysplastic. In the ameloblastic odontosarcoma both induced dentine and enamel are present adjacent to each other.

### 3. MALIGNANT MELANOTIC NEUROECTODERMAL TUMOUR OF INFANCY

The melanotic neuroectodermal tumour of infancy is an uncommon tumour of neural crest origin. It occurs in infants, usually in the first year. The maxilla is involved more frequently than any other site in the body. The lesion may appear clinically as a nodular pigmented or nonpigmented mass on the gingiva. The rate of growth varies. Radiologically, the adjacent bone is involved, often irregularly. Recurrences after surgery are rare, and the tumour has been

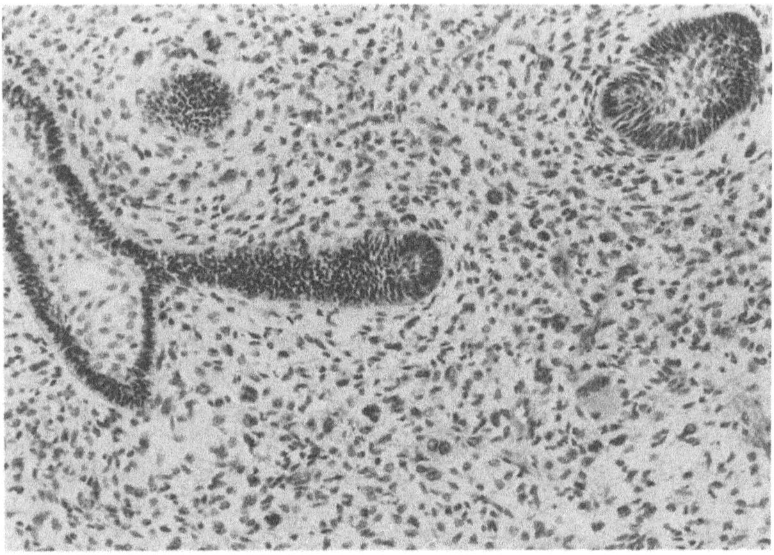

**Figure 4–4.** Odontogenic sarcoma. This variety is an ameloblastic fibrosarcoma. The odontogenic epithelium is not malignant, but the connective tissue component is sarcomatous.

generally regarded as benign [10,15,29]. Two exceptions, however, have been reported: a case in a stillborn infant which had metastasized to lymph nodes, liver, and adrenal [30] and another recent well-documented description of a malignant melanotic neuroectodermal tumour of infancy [31]. In the latter case, histological features of the original tumour and its recurrences were no different from the classical description of the usual benign type.

## 4. FIBROSARCOMA AND RELATED LESIONS

No discussion of fibrosarcoma would be complete without a brief consideration of the fibromatoses and of the locally aggressive and malignant histiocytic tumours of the oral regions, because they provide so many problems in the differential diagnosis of fibrosarcoma.

### 4.1. Fibromatosis

The fibromatoses are a heterogeneous group of lesions that may be described as diffuse, ill-defined overgrowths of fibrous tissues that infiltrate adjacent normal tissues, are difficult to eradicate surgically, and recur but do not metastasize [32]. The fibromatoses generally have their origin in the musculoaponeuroses. On clinical and histological grounds, distinguishing the fibromatoses from fibrosarcoma is often difficult. Fibromatoses of the jaws and oral soft tissues are rare. When they do occur, they are found mostly in children and young adults and more often in females than males, in common with other fibromatoses of the head and neck region.

The terms *desmoplastic fibroma* or *desmoid tumour* have been used to refer to primary aggressive fibromatoses of bone. A recent comprehensive literature review on the subject of desmoplastic fibroma (fibromatosis) of the jaw bones [33] consisted of 26 acceptable cases. The mean age at presentation was 15.7 years. There was no sex predilection. Twenty-four of the tumours were located in the mandible. Swelling of the jaw was the most common presenting complaint. Sixteen of the 22 cases appeared radiographically as well-delineated radiolucencies. Most lesions do not have a uniform histologic appearance. The degree of cellularity varies from case to case and in different areas of the same lesion. The nuclei of the fibroblasts may be either small, elongated and pyknotic, or larger and oval. They are always uniform and lack anaplastic features and significant numbers of mitoses [33].

Most cases of fibromatosis of the soft tissues occur in young individuals. Cases of congenital fibromatosis have been reported in the tongue [34] and in the floor of the mouth [35]. The lesions present as painless, poorly defined grey-white firm masses with a propensity to infiltrate surrounding soft tissue or to erode or actually invade bone [36].

The histological appearance of the fibromatoses is deceptively harmless when one considers the ability of these lesions to attain a large size, to recur, and to infiltrate adjacent structures. This appearance varies from relatively acellular, often hyalinized fibrous tissue, to extremely cellular fibrous tissue often with a "herringbone" pattern. The cells are uniform, there is no anaplasia, and mitoses are infrequent [36].

Both the desmoplastic fibroma and soft tissue fibromatosis, although histologically benign, show considerable local aggressive behaviour. Metastases do not occur. The lesions will recur if treated conservatively. Treatment is aimed at complete removal and consists of surgical excision.

Nodular fasciitis (pseudosarcomatous fibromatosis, pseudosarcomatous fasciitis), previously regarded as a fibromatosis, is most likely a reactive and non-neoplastic lesion occurring in response to injury [37]. It differs from fibromatoses in that it is clinically innocuous but histologically aggressive. It should therefore not be regarded as a fibromatosis [32].

### 4.2. Locally aggressive and malignant histiocytic tumours

The generic term *fibrous histiocytoma* is used to include a heterogeneous group of tumours proposed to have a common origin from the tissue histiocyte. Of the locally aggressive or malignant fibrous histiocytic lesions, only the malignant fibrous histiocytoma (fibroxanthosarcoma) has been documented occasionally in the oral soft tissues [38,39,40] and jaws [41–44].

In many examples of this family of lesions, the "fibroblasts," which may vary in the degree of pleomorphism they exhibit, tend to be arranged spirally,

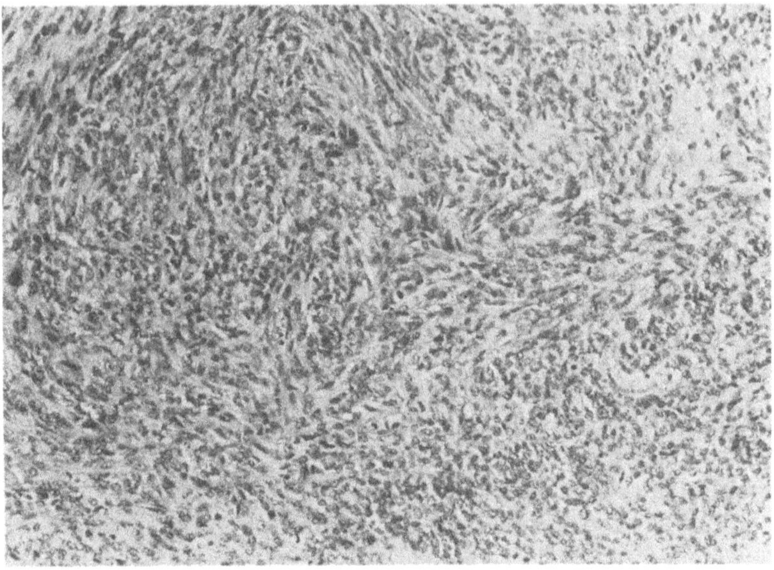

**Figure 4–5.** Malignant fibrous histiocytoma of mandible. The tumour has a "storiform" pattern. There is considerable cellular pleomorphism, and numerous mitoses are present.

usually described by the term *storiform* (figure 4–5). This storiform pattern is by no means pathognomonic of tumours of histiocytic origin, nor is its presence essential to such a diagnosis. Varying numbers of histiocytes as well as bizarre multilobulated and multinucleated giant cells are often present. Histological assessment as to the potential malignancy of a particular lesion is, however, unreliable.

### 4.3. Fibrosarcoma

Fibrosarcoma of the jaws and of the oral soft tissues is not common. An accurate assessment of the frequency of this tumour would be difficult to make from the literature, for a better understanding of fibrous tumours has resulted in a change in the emphasis and outlook of the diagnostic histopathologist to such an extent that many of the lesions previously reported as fibrosarcomas would, if reviewed today, not survive such a diagnosis [10]. The distinction of fibrosarcoma from some of the tumours derived from tissue histiocytes remains a problem [45–47]. Some authors believe the fibrosarcoma may merely be a nonosseous matrix-producing variant of osteosarcoma arising from the same stem cell line [48].

*Fibrosarcoma of bone* may be associated with Paget's disease of bone or giant cell tumor of bone and may seemingly also be induced by chronic osteomyelitis or irradiation [49]. Origin of jaw fibrosarcomas from preexisting ameloblastic fibromas and ameloblastic sarcomas have been reported [21,22,27]. For this reason, the question has arisen as to whether at least some fibrosarcomas of the jaws may be odontogenic in origin [21,26,27]. In a series of 114 cases of fibrosarcoma of bone [27], the mandible was involved in 11.4% and the maxilla in 1.7% of cases. In an extensive review of the literature, 40 reported cases were regarded as acceptable examples of fibrosarcoma of the jaws [26]. Periosteal, antral, and soft tissue fibrosarcomas were excluded. Twenty-five cases were in males and 15 in females. The mandible was involved in 37 cases and the maxilla in 3. Ten cases occurred in the fourth decade, and the remainder were distributed evenly among the first, second, third, and fifth decades. Pain and swelling are the two most frequent complaints. No radiological features distinguish fibrosarcomas of the jaws from other malignant osteolytic tumours.

Less-differentiated fibrosarcomas are more cellular and have less collagen than the well-differentiated ones and they may lack the herringbone pattern of the fibroblasts. Features of anaplasia are prominent. Both low- and high-grade fibrosarcomas may contain variable numbers of benign multinucleated giant cells resembling osteoclasts [48].

Death is reported to have occurred in 13 of the 40 jaw cases in the review referred to above [26].

*Fibrosarcoma of the oral soft tissues* may at first resemble the common reactive fibrous overgrowths of the oral mucosa since at the outset they may be relatively well circumscribed [45]. They grow more rapidly, however, are prone to ulceration, and will soon infiltrate adjacent tissues and spread, thus revealing their malignant nature [10]. Oral soft tissue fibrosarcomas appear to have a better prognosis than either extraoral soft tissue fibrosarcomas or central fibrosarcomas of the jaws.

The histological pattern of soft tissue and jaw fibrosarcomas is similar. The well-differentiated fibrosarcoma has abundant collagen in elongated spindly fibroblasts arranged in interlacing bundles, sometimes having a herringbone pattern (figure 4–6). Mitoses are common, but anaplastic features are slight. Less-differentiated fibrosarcomas are more cellular, have less collagen, and may lack the herringbone pattern. Features of anaplasia may be prominent.

## 5. MALIGNANT TUMOURS OF THE PERIPHERAL NERVES (NEUROGENOUS SARCOMA)

The normal nerve fiber is ensheathed by Schwann cells and is also surrounded by more loosely distributed endoneural fibroblasts. The exact cells of origin of the two principal tumours of peripheral nerves, namely, Schwannoma and neurofibroma, are still in doubt. Perhaps the view that all elements of normal peripheral nerves are involved in the formation of neurofibromas, while Schwann cells are indeed the cells of origin of Schwannomas, is closest to the truth [32,50]. In view of this uncertainty, as well as the difficulty of distinguishing malignant Schwannoma from neurofibrosarcoma, the term *neuroge-*

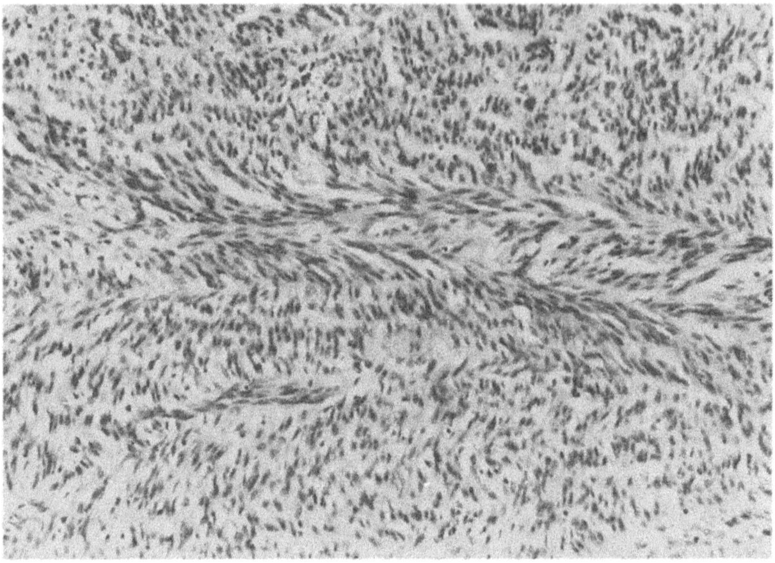

**Figure 4–6.** Well-differentiated fibrosarcoma of tongue. The herringbone pattern is prominent, mitoses are common, but anaplastic features are slight.

*nous* or *neurogenic sarcoma* is preferred by some authors when referring to malignant peripheral nerve sheath tumours [32,45,50].

It has been stated that the only feature distinguishing a neurogenous sarcoma from a fibrosarcoma is its origin from a nerve trunk [32], which tends to support the view that it to classify a tumour as a neurogenous sarcoma solely from its histological pattern is unwise. With this in mind, recent criteria applied [50] to simplify classification of neurogenous sarcomas might be useful. According to this classification neurogenous sarcomas fall into two categories:

1. Malignant change in lesions of neurofibromatosis, designated as neurofibrosarcoma, which occurs in 5.5 to 16% of cases.
2. In the absence of neurofibromatosis, malignant nerve sheath tumours diagnosed on the basis of surgery or, in cases involving the mandible, radiography, with origin from nerve trunk; or those neoplasms that on histologic examination show one of the recognized neural patterns such as Antoni type A tissue in malignant Schwannoma. These lesions may be designated as malignant Schwannoma, or neurogenous sarcoma.

Neurogenous sarcomas of the oral cavity and jaws are rare [45,50]. One literature review [45] included seven peripheral, six both central and peripheral, and six central neurogenous sarcomas. Enlargement of the mental fora-

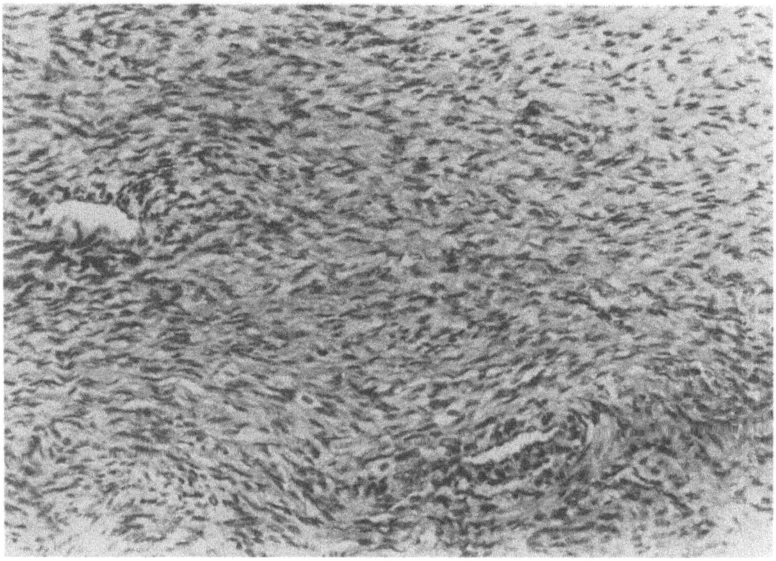

**Figure 4–7.** Neurogenous sarcoma in facial tissues.

men and widening and loss of delineation of the mandibular canal are indicative of origin from the inferior alveolar nerve [50]. No other radiographic features distinguish central neurogenic sarcomas from other malignant central lesions of the jaws. Too few cases of intraoral neurogenous sarcoma are reported for meaningful judgments on the likely prognosis. The propensity for neurogenous sarcomas to extend longitudinally along nerve trunks may well contribute to a high rate of local recurrence because of inadequate removal.

Histologically, neurogenous sarcoma consists of spindle cells showing varying degrees of pleomorphism, often with numerous mitoses. The intercellular fibres may exhibit considerable waviness (figure 4–7). Palisading of nuclei is present in some tumours.

### 6. RHABDOMYOSARCOMA

Rhabdomyosarcomas are among the more common malignant mesenchymal tumours of soft parts, being exceeded in frequency only by liposarcoma and possibly by fibrosarcoma [51]. Several types of rhabdomyosarcoma have been described. Pleomorphic, embryonal, and alveolar rhabdomyosarcomas have been distinguished histologically. Botryoid rhabdomyosarcoma is not a distinct entity but describes a macroscopic form of any embryonic sarcoma involving the mucosal surface of a hollow structure. Whether the alveolar type is a separate entity is also of considerable doubt. Rhabdomyosarcoma is the most common malignant soft tissue neoplasm of the head and neck in children.

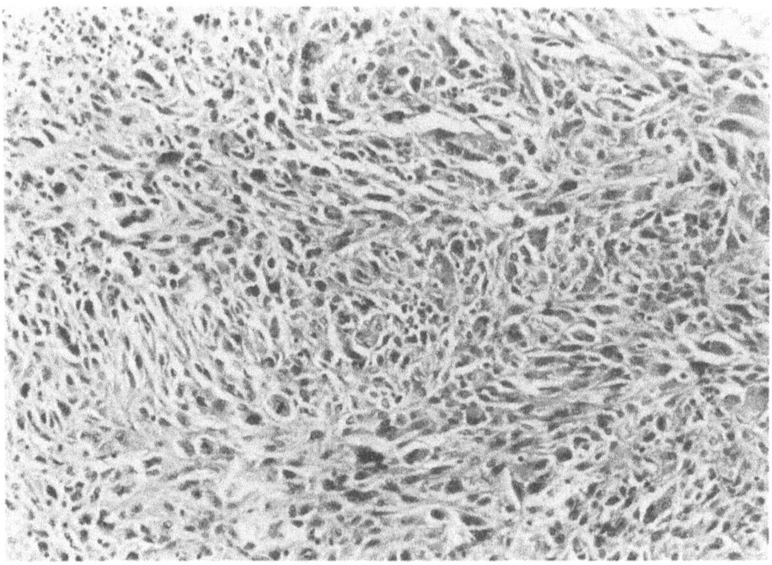

**Figure 4–8.** Pleomorphic rhabdomyosarcoma in the neck.

Twenty-nine percent of rhabdomyosarcomas in the head and neck region have their origin in intraoral and pharyngeal structures [42,52]. Within the oral cavity the palate and the tongue are the sites most frequently affected. Origin from within the jaws is possible [53]. An excellent review of the literature together with the presentation of 11 new cases of embryonal rhabdomyosarcoma of the oral soft tissues has been published [54]. The chief complaint of patients with oral rhabdomyosarcoma is a painless swelling. Generally, the lesions enlarge rapidly, and the size of reported lesions varies from 1 to 7 cm [54,55].

*Pleomorphic* rhabdomyosarcoma is the best differentiated of the group and the most readily recognized, for it resembles adult striated muscle more than does the embryonal variety. Most are characterized by a high degree of cellular pleomorphism (figure 4–8). There are also elongated "strap" cells, often with several nuclei. These cells almost invariably show longitudinal fibrils, but distinct cross striations can rarely be demonstrated [51]. Numerous giant cells of various types with one or more bizarre hyperchromatic nuclei are present in varying numbers. Some of these cells have been referred to as "tadpole" or "raquet" cells. Many of the cells have strongly acidophilic cytoplasm. *Embryonal* rhabdomyosarcoma closely resembles developing muscle in the 7- to ten-week foetus. It consists of sheets of round and spindle cells with scanty cytoplasm. Cross striations were found in only 6 of the 11 cases in one series [54]. It is worth emphasizing that the demonstration of cross striations is not necessary for the diagnosis of embryonal rhabdomyosarcoma. *Alveolar* rhabdomyosarcoma, in which the tumour cells are arranged in an alveolar pattern, is the least common of the subtypes and may not warrant separate classification since it is probably a variant of embryonal rhabdomyosarcoma.

There is a little difference in prognosis between the various histological types of rhabdomyosarcoma of childhood or in the head and neck. In this region orbital rhabdomyosarcomas appear to have the best prognosis. Although capable of local recurrence and local invasion, they are less likely to metastasize. Metastases are generally very common and usually blood borne to lungs, bone marrow, and brain. In addition peripheral rhabdomyosarcomas often metastasize to regional lymph nodes [32]. The addition of adjuvant chemotherapy in combination with wide-field high-dosage radiation and surgery has substantially improved survival. Two-year survival rates as high as 74% have been reported [52].

### 7. LEIOMYOSARCOMA

Smooth muscle tumours are rare in the oral cavity and upper respiratory tract because smooth muscle in these areas is limited [32]. They probably originate from the smooth muscles of the circumvallate papillae and blood vessel walls [56], but origin from undifferentiated mesenchymal cells must also be considered. Literature reviews of oral and jaw leiomyosarcomas and additional new case reports have been published in recent years [56,57,58]. Of 25 reported cases 8 occurred in the jaws and 17 in the soft tissues. The age distribution is wide, with most patients older than 50 years. No notable difference is found in sex distribution. No special clinical or radiological features could assist in distinguishing leiomyosarcoma from other connective tissue malignancies of the oral cavity.

Histologically, leiomyosarcomas (figure 4–9) resemble leiomyomas very closely. The nuclei are elongated and have blunt rounded ends. Mitotic activity is considered to be the major distinguishing factor between leiomyomas and their malignant counterpart [59]. Definite malignancy is present when there is one or more mitosis per high-power field. Other criteria useful for differentiating leiomyosarcoma from leiomyoma are anaplasia, bizarre cell forms, less obvious nuclear palisading, and conspicuous myofibrils. It has been emphasized, however, that the potential of smooth muscle tumours to metastasize cannot always be ascertained histologically and that the histologic degree of differentiation may be misleading as far as behaviour is concerned [32].

Of 19 reported cases of intraoral leiomyosarcoma in which follow-up was available, there were metastases to the cervical lymph nodes in 5 and in 4 cases there were lung metastases. Eight of the patients had died of their disease [57]. Metastases often occurred after repeated local recurrences.

### 8. LIPOSARCOMA

Liposarcoma is thought to be the most common connective tissue malignancy in adults. The occurrence in the head and neck is less than 4% of all sites [60,

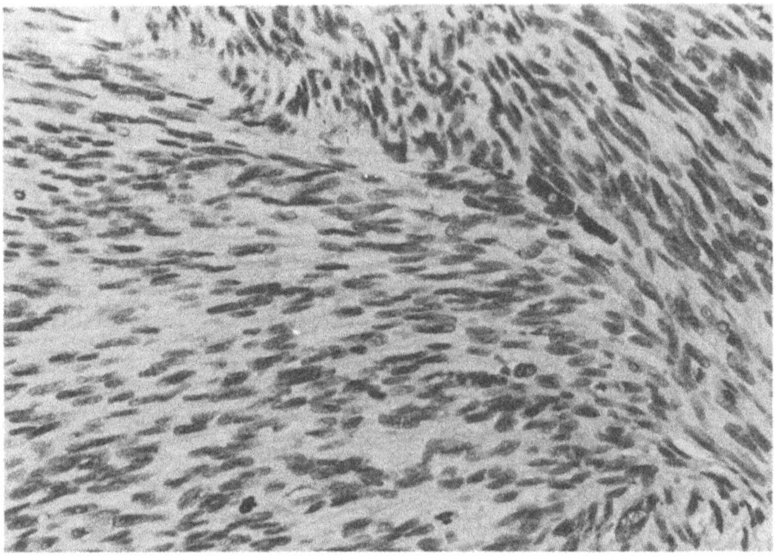

**Figure 4–9.** Leiomyosarcoma of mandible. The nuclei are elongated and have blunt rounded ends.

61,62]. The vast majority of liposarcomas arise spontaneously and not in preexisting lipomas [51]. Comprehensive reviews of liposarcoma of the head and neck region, including intraoral cases, have been published [60,61]. They begin as inconspicuous swellings and usually have attained an appreciable size before being diagnosed. The colour is usually yellowish. The consistency varies from soft mucoid to firm. Pain is not a feature [51]. Tumours arising intraosseously are exceedingly rare [63]. In view of the paucity of documented intraoral cases, drawing definite conclusions regarding their age, sex, and site distribution is not feasible.

Histologically, *well-differentiated* liposarcoma has a lobular architecture and is composed mostly of mature fat in which variable amounts of mucoid and myxomatous tissue are accompanied by fusiform and stellate cells and occasional bizarre lipoblasts. It is usually well circumscribed [51]. *Myxoid* liposarcoma is the most common form of this neoplasm. The appearance of embryonal adipose tissue is reproduced. Occasionally, signet ring cells with a single larger vacuole may be present. Giant cells with pyknotic nuclei may be intermingled. Less-differentiated areas resembling fibrosarcoma may be present. The *round* cell liposarcoma has many features of the myxoid variety but is characterized by a marked proliferation of uniform rounded cells in which lipid formation is not very prominent [61]. *Pleomorphic* liposarcoma is generally highly anaplastic and may be difficult to distinguish from other highly undifferentiated tumours.

It has been pointed out [64] that the diagnosis merely of liposarcoma is of little value since the histological subdivisions mentioned before bear greatly on the clinical outcome. All lesions infiltrate, and more than half of them recur locally. Regional lymph node involvement is rare, but distant metastases occur in about one-third of patients with round cell and pleomorphic variants. The five-year survival rate for patients with the well-differentiated and myxoid varieties is considerably better than for those with the round cell and pleomorphic variants.

## 9. MALIGNANT VASCULAR TUMOURS

Considerable confusion exists regarding the correct terminology and classification of malignant vascular tumours. In order to obviate this confusion, the approach adopted by Batsakis [32] seems a practical one. He believes that usage of the term *haemangioendothelioma* should be restricted to the rare hepatic vascular lesions. Those lesions previously referred as to haemangioendothelioma, sometimes with the adjectives "juvenile, cellular or aggressive," and which are benign, are better classified as proliferative haemangiomas. They are probably hamartomas and will mature in time to typical capillary haemangiomas. Lesions previously termed *malignant haemangioendothelioma* or *haemangioendotheliosarcoma* should be classified as angiosarcoma. The terms *malignant haemangiopericytoma* and *Kaposi's sarcoma* refer to distinctive clinicopathological entities and complete the classification of malignant vascular lesions.

### 9.1. Angiosarcoma

Angiosarcoma is a malignant tumour of the vascular endothelial cell and includes lymphangiosarcoma. Since the level of differentiation is so poor, consideration of lymphangiosarcoma as a separate entity is inadvisable [32]. The most common site for angiosarcoma in the head and neck is the scalp. Primary origin from bone has been well documented [65]. A recent extensive review [66] reported 46 cases of angiosarcoma of the oral regions. Of the 35 intraoral cases in which the age had been recorded, 14 occurred in the first two decades. Females were affected twice as often as males. Three cases were multifocal. The mandible itself was involved in 17 cases. Radiographically, these lesions are radiolucent with poorly defined margins [66]. Approximately 50% of angiosarcomas are cured by primary surgical excision. The remaining patients die within three years [67], with regional lymph node involvement or distant metastases.

There is considerable variation in the histological appearance of this lesion. It is characterized by the formation of irregular anastomosing vascular channels lined by one or more layers of atypical endothelial cells often of immature appearance [54] (figure 4–10). The vascular pattern is seen to its best advantage with silver reticulin stains. The tumour cells are inside the delicate reticulin sheath that encloses each vessel; this characteristic serves to distinguish the

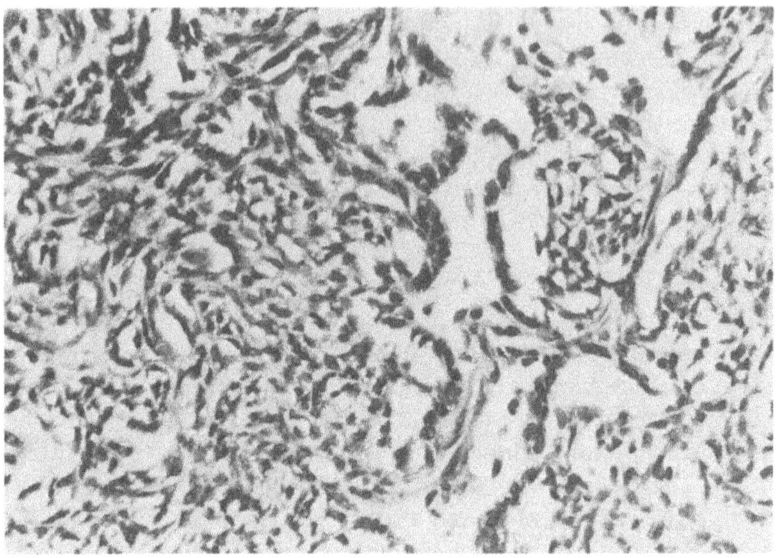

**Figure 4–10.** Angiosarcoma of body of mandible.

neoplasm from the haemangiopericytoma, where the vessels have a normal endothelial lining and the tumour cells are outside the reticulin sheath.

### 9.2. Malignant haemangiopericytoma

The haemangiopericytoma is a complex neoplasm derived from the pericytes and shows great variability in anatomical distribution, histological appearance, pattern of growth, and biological behaviour. Approximately 25% of all cases occur in the region of the head and neck [32]. It has been stated that attempts to classify haemangiopericytomas into benign and malignant forms based on histological criteria are futile [68]. In one study [68], 52% of the cases either recurred locally or metastasized. Another study [69] of 106 haemangiopericytomas from various soft tissue sites suggested, in contradistinction to the view expressed above [68], that a high mitotic count, marked cellularity, the presence of foci of necrosis and haemorrhage, and recurrence of the primary tumour might be indications that the lesion is likely to metastasize. The infantile or congenital haemangiopericytoma is a distinct entity. In contrast to the adult form, these tumours are all biologically benign [69].

A detailed description of the histology [69] has emphasized the continuously ramifying vascular pattern, with large channels extending from the pericapsular tissue into the tumour and branching into dilated sinusoidal spaces or capillaries. All the vessels, regardless of size, lack a muscular coat.

### 9.3. Kaposi's sarcoma (idiopathic multiple haemorrhagic sarcoma)

Kaposi's sarcoma is a multifocal neoplastic disease of the vascular system which rarely metastasizes. It usually occurs on the skin of the extremities but may involve the viscera. It is predominantly a disease of males, with the greatest frequency in the fifth to seventh decades of life. It is found most frequently in patients of Mediterranean extraction as well as in blacks in equatorial Africa and Africa south of the Sahara. In the oral mucosa Kaposi's sarcoma may occur as a solitary lesion or as multiple lesions. Both clinically and histologically, early oral lesions greatly resemble pyogenic granulomas [70]. They may manifest as flat nonpalpable haemorrhagic areas or as definite tumour masses which are occasionally ulcerated. In a literature review of cases in which there was oral involvement [71], the oral lesions were the first manifestation of the disease in nine.

Histologically, the lesion is composed of a network of capillaries in between which are spindle cells and reticulin fibres resembling well-differentiated fibrosarcoma. The relative proportions of the two tissues vary but both must always be present [72]. Mitoses are not present in great numbers. The vascular spaces may not be well formed when they consist of poorly differentiated endothelial cells. Although cutaneous Kaposi's sarcoma is said to be fatal in only 10 to 20% of cases, the mortality rate is much higher for the visceral form of the disease. The cause of death is usually haemorrhage from a visceral lesion. There does not appear to be any significant difference in prognosis or response to therapy between oral lesions and lesions involving other organs.

## 10. OSTEOSARCOMA

Thus far all definitions of osteosarcoma have stressed the importance of the presence of direct formation of osteoid by tumour osteoblasts. Recently, however, [73] it has been proposed that too much emphasis has been placed on the presence of tumour osteoid, which may be absent in some examples of osteosarcoma. The tumour cells in osteosarcoma contain abundant alkaline phosphatase, whereas this enzyme is scanty in chondrosarcoma and fibrosarcoma. The suggestion was made that osteosarcomas be defined as malignant tumours of osteoblasts in which the tumour cells contain abundant alkaline phosphatase, irrespective of whether tumour osteoid is present or not [73]. Whether such an approach will be widely adopted remains to be seen.

Most osteosarcomas are of unknown etiology and pathogenesis. More than half that arise after the age of 40 years, however, do so secondarily to another lesion. The two most common antecedent lesions are Paget's disease of bone and that which follows irradiation. The frequency of malignant transformation in Paget's disease appears to be between 9 and 15% [74].

The jaws are involved in approximately 7% of all cases [66,76]. The age at which jaw lesions are diagnosed is one to two decades later than for osteosarcomas of other bones [75,76,77]. An extensive literature review [76] accumulated 167 cases of jaw osteosarcoma. In this review 70 cases occurred in the maxilla and 90 in the mandible. There was a slight predilection for males.

### 10.1. Clinical features

By far the majority of patients complain of a rapidly enlarging swelling causing facial asymmetry. Less frequently, pain, paraesthesia, and looseness of teeth may be present. The overlying mucosa is usually normal. Jaw lesions are often well differentiated. Distant metastases are less frequent in osteosarcoma of the jaws than in osteosarcomas arising in long bones. With radical resection of the tumour, patients with osteosarcoma of the jaws do significantly better than those with osteosarcoma in general [77]. Two varieties regarded as distinct clinicopathological entities are the well-differentiated intramedullary osteosarcoma and parosteal osteosarcoma. Well-differentiated intramedullary osteosarcomas [78] create diagnostic problems because they are difficult to differentiate from benign lesions. They are of low-grade malignancy, do not frequently metastasize, and have a particularly good prognosis following resection or amputation. Parosteal osteosarcoma (juxtacortical osteosarcoma) is an infrequently encountered variant, accounting for less than 4% of all osteosarcomas [79]. Few cases have been reported in the jaws [80,81]. The prognosis for parosteal osteosarcoma is comparatively good.

Survival rates for osteosarcoma of the jaws, especially of the mandible, appear to be somewhat better than for extrafacial lesions [77]. In a series of 30 cases [82], the five-year survival rate was 50% for maxillary lesions and 71% for mandibular lesions. Local recurrences were the major problem. Distant metastases occurred in less than one-third of the cases.

### 10.2. Radiological features

The radiographic appearance of osteosarcoma of the jaws, as of other bones, is variable. The lesion appears very poorly defined and destructive. It may be sclerotic, lytic, or mixed. Some 25% of osteosarcomas present a "sunray" effect [75]. This occurs only if the neoplasm breaks through the cortex leading to a soft tissue mass. With elevation of the periosteum, reactive new bone may be deposited. Symmetrical widening of the periodontal ligament space is said to be an important early diagnostic feature and is almost peculiar to osteosarcoma [75].

### 10.3. Histopathology

Beyond the production of osteoid, or bone, no single factor can be regarded as being histologically characteristic [75] (figure 4–11). Generally, three histological patterns have been recognized: osteoblastic, chondroblastic, and fibroblastic osteosarcoma. Most lesions consist of plump spindle cells that cytologically appear highly malignant. Many abnormal mitoses are found.

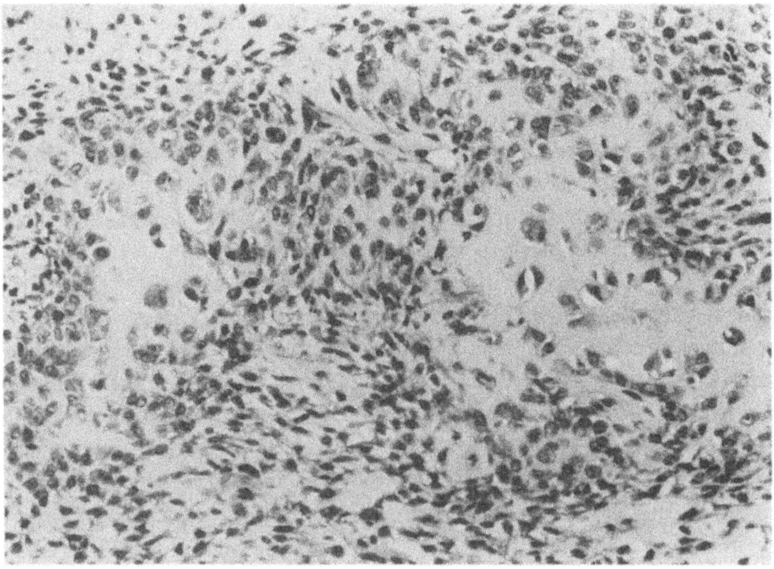

**Figure 4–11.** Osteosarcoma of maxilla. Osteoid is deposited by malignant osteoblasts.

About 50% of lesions produce osteoid in sufficiently large amounts to be called osteoblastic osteosarcoma. In about 25% of cases, the predominant differentiation is toward cartilage. Such lesions are termed *chondroblastic osteosarcoma.* Some of these cases have been erroneously regarded as chondrosarcomas. The remaining 25% of cases show bundles of spindle cells arranged in a herringbone pattern similar to that seen in fibrosarcoma. Osteoid is present in minimal amounts as fine eosinophilic material between tumour cells. Such tumours are classified as fibroblastic osteosarcoma [77].

In this context the question of *malignant giant cell tumour* of the jaws deserves brief mention. Malignant giant cell tumours do undoubtedly occur in bones other than the jaws. It has been stated that "all giant-cell tumours are potentially malignant" as "there is today no agreement on specific histological features that dependably indicate the likelihood of malignant behaviour" [83]. Well-documented examples of malignant giant cell tumours of the jaw are exceptionally rare, and it has been suggested that the diagnosis of osteosarcoma, giant cell variant, may be more appropriate [84].

## 11. CHONDROSARCOMA

Chondrosarcoma is often misdiagnosed as a benign neoplasm, and there may be considerable problems in differentiating benign enchondromas from well-differentiated (grade I) chondrosarcomas.

### 11.1. Clinical features

Chondrosarcomas of the jaws account for approximately 2% of all chondrosarcomas; most of these jaw cases occur in the maxilla [10]. In the mandible there is a predilection for the premolar and molar regions. The temporomandibular joint is a rare site for primary chondrosarcoma [85]. A number of literature reviews and reports of individual cases have been published [86,87,88]. The patients tend to be younger than those with lesions outside of the jaws. They are usually in the third, fourth, or fifth decades, and there is a slight male predominance. In the early stages the tumour is nearly always painless. Patients complain of a mass causing facial asymmetry. The rate of growth is variable. Loosening and drifting of teeth may occur.

Chondrosarcomas have been grouped into three grades, based on histological criteria [88]. The five-year survival rates for grades I, II, and III chondrosarcoma are 90%, 81%, and 43%, respectively [88]. In contrast to the situation in other bones, the five-year survival rate as well as the overall long-term survival is worse for chondrosarcoma of the jaws than it is for osteosarcoma of the jaws. Death is usually related to aggressive local infiltration. Metastases occur in only a small number of cases. Recurrences are common [32,86].

### 11.2. Radiological features

The radiological features of an unequivocal chondrosarcoma are considered classical [48]. The lesions are ill defined and cause expansion of the bone. Some cases show focal or extensive erosion of the cortex, whereas others may show extensive cortical thickening. The lesions are generally radiolucent and contain calcifications of varying size. Large lobules of cartilage may impart a "soap bubble" appearance to the radiolucency, and the calcifications have a characteristic granular appearance. There is often an associated soft tissue mass and a periosteal reaction. Resorption of roots of teeth is a common feature in jaw cases.

### 11.3. Histopathology

The greatest difficulty in the histopathological diagnosis of chondrosarcoma lies in distinguishing the well-differentiated lesions from enchondroma or other benign tumours of cartilage. In contrast to enchondromas—in which the lobules are small to moderate in size, are usually distinct form one another, and are separated by a variable amount of normal bone—the lobules in chondrosarcoma increase progressively in size, become confluent, and may totally replace the normal bone [48]. The degree of nuclear anaplasia varies considerably and depends on the degree of malignancy. Malignant cartilage nuclei are most often large, plump, and round to oval (figure 4–12). An important aid in the diagnosis of nuclear malignancy is the presence of pink to red nucleoli. The presence of two or three nucleoli per cell is regarded as virtually diagnostic of

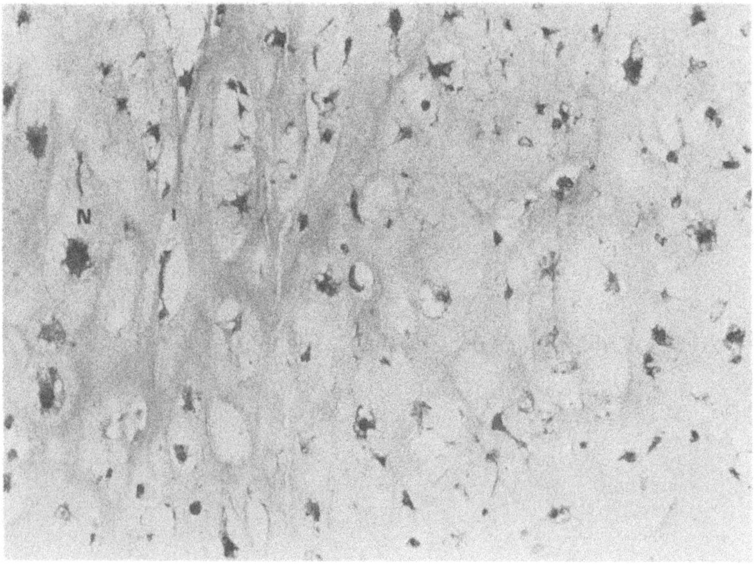


**Figure 4–12.** Chondrosarcoma. The cartilage cells are large. One cell (N) has three nucleoli.

malignancy. Double or triple nuclei within a single cell are important signs of malignancy. One mitotic figure per one or two high-power fields is virtually diagnostic of chondrosarcoma [48].

Two histological variants of chondrosarcoma warrant separate consideration: clear cell chondrosarcoma and mesenchymal chondrosarcoma. Clear cell chondrosarcoma is characterized by the presence of benign giant cells, clear cells, and areas of pleomorphic cells in a cartilagenous matrix [89]. Some have suggested [89,90] that clear cell chondrosarcomas could be chondroblastomas that have undergone malignant change. The prognosis is good. The tumour enlarges slowly and does not often metastasize. Treatment by resection is therefore advocated. Mesenchymal chondrosarcoma is a highly characteristic malignant tumour. The ribs and jaws are the bones most commonly involved [91,92]. There is a wide age distribution and a slight female predominance. The prognosis is generally poor, with multiple recurrences and metastases to lungs and bones occurring in more than half of the cases up to 10 years or more following primary treatment. Histologically, sheets of highly undifferentiated small oval or round cells alternating with zones of easily identifiable cartilagenous material are characteristic (figure 4–13). The amount of chondroid material varies. Pleomorphism and mitoses are not a feature within the undifferentiated cellular component. Metaplastic bone within the islets of well-differentiated cartilage is often found [91].

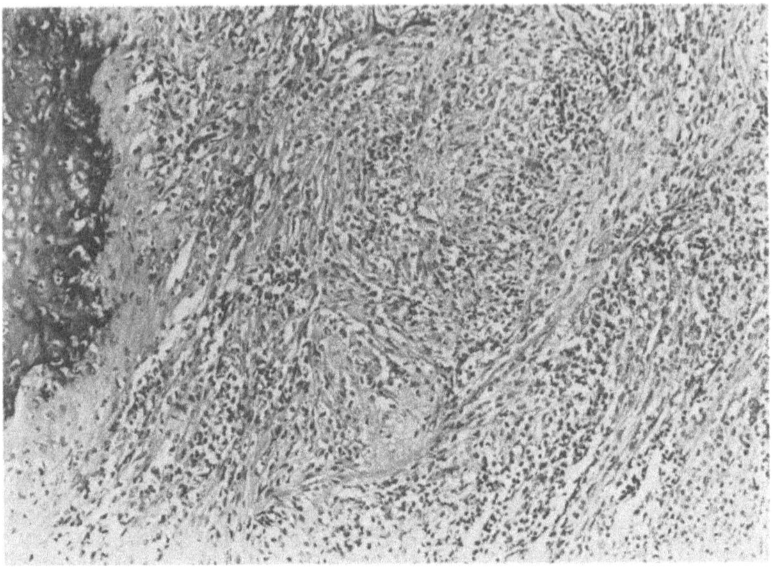

**Figure 4–13.** Mesenchymal chondrosarcoma. There are sheets of small round and oval cells associated with the cartilagenous material.

## 12. EWING'S SARCOMA

Ewing's sarcoma is a highly malignant neoplasm of bone. Its nature and origin have been controversial since its original description by Ewing. It is a tumour occurring predominantly in the second decade and it affects males more frequently than females and may involve almost any bone [93]. The jaw cases are found in young individuals in the first and second decades, and in males more frequently than in females [94]. The mandible is involved far more often than the maxilla [94]. Patients with Ewing's sarcoma have rapidly growing, painful swellings [94], which are usually hard but occasionally are soft and fluctuant. Ulceration into the mouth may occur. Tumours of the maxilla may produce exophthalmos. Abnormal tooth mobility and lip paraesthesia may be encountered. Local recurrences and metastases to other bones, lungs, brain, peritoneum, and liver have been documented. The tendency to involve other bones has suggested a multicentric origin [83]. The prognosis is poor. The majority of documented cases with primary jaw involvement have been dead with the disease within a few years of diagnosis.

The radiological features of Ewing's sarcoma of the jaws are not diagnostic [95]. There may be expansion of bone, increased density of the cortex, and irregular mottled destruction [94], the mottling being the result of patchy reactive bone formation. In the early lesion small punched-out radiolucent areas may be found.

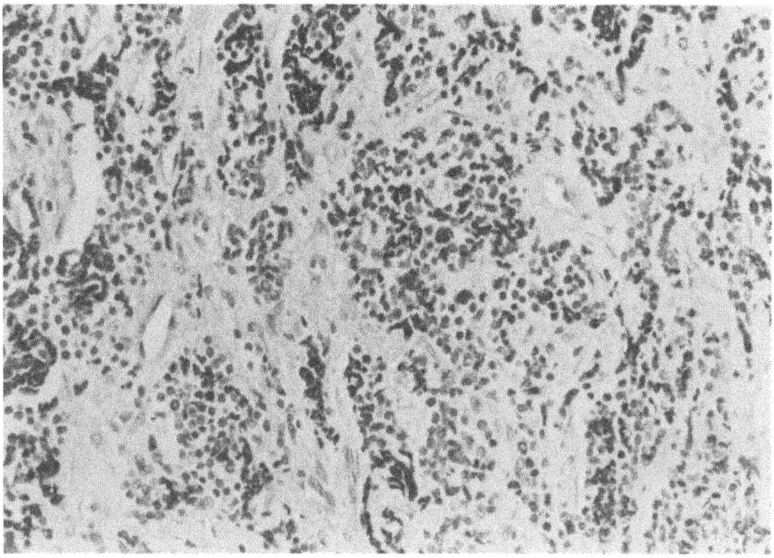

**Figure 4–14.** Ewing's sarcoma.

Microscopically, Ewing's sarcoma consists of closely packed strands or sheets of cells with indistinct borders and small round nuclei without prominent nucleoli (figure 4–14). The tumour cells are separated by fibrous septa. Few mitotic figures are seen. There may be "rosette" formation of tumour cells. Differential diagnosis from reticulosarcoma of bone and metastatic neuroblastoma may be difficult. The demonstration of glycogen granules in the cytoplasm of Ewing's sarcoma cells is a valuable diagnostic aid [96].

### 13. MYELOMA

Myeloma is a common primary malignant tumour of the skeleton. Over 90% of patients are over 40 years of age [48]. Although any bone may be involved, the skull, vertebrae, ribs, sternum, pelvic bones, and jaws are affected most commonly. The tumour occurs in males approximately four times more often than in females.

Myeloma may take various clinical forms. It is usually multiple but may be solitary. Extramedullary forms are also possible. The relationship between the various clinical forms of this disease have long been a subject of contention. A practical approach [97] is that the extramedullary and solitary myelomas (both of which are often referred to as plasmacytoma) are best considered as components of a continuous spectrum of plasma cell disorders, each capable of rendering a variety of clinical expressions. The literature contains numerous reports of lesions in the jaws or oral soft tissues in multiple myeloma. These

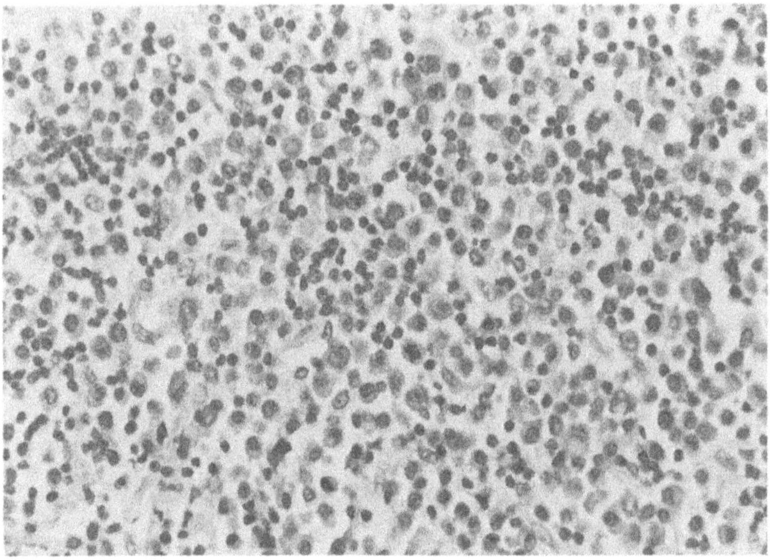

**Figure 4–15.** Myeloma, involving maxilla.

have either been initial lesions in what was soon to become a generalized process or were part of a widespread disease. This mode of presentation is well documented [98]. A recent literature review on solitary plasmacytoma of the mandible included 20 cases [99]. Most cases occurred in the body and ramus of the mandible. Solitary plasmacytoma of the maxilla is much less common [100]. In the jaws in both the multiple and solitary forms of the disease, pain is a common early symptom. Numbness of the lip or chin may be present. Occasionally, macroglossia as a result of amyloidosis may be the earliest manifestation of the disease [10]. In most cases with solitary medullary or extramedullary lesions, no abnormal haematological and biochemical changes occur.

Radiologically, the lesions appear as multiple punched-out cystic or trabeculated radiolucencies. They vary in size, but seldom exceed 1 cm in diameter. Confluence of lesions of the jaws is rarely seen [100].

Myeloma is a malignant neoplasm of plasma cells arising from the bone marrow and is characterized microscopically by nodular aggregates and sheets of plasma cells that vary in their degree of differentiation (figure 4–15). Plasmacytomas are virtually monomorphic, replace tissue, and do not contain other inflammatory cells except if ulcerated. Russell bodies are generally few or absent in plasmacytomas.

Several cases have been reported in which oral amyloidosis was the initial symptom of multiple myeloma [101,102]. The Bence-Jones protein test is positive in only 9% of patients with solitary lesions, as opposed to 65% of patients with multiple lesions [103].

The prognosis for patients with multiple myeloma is very poor. Death results within a very short period of time in virtually all cases. Although the immediate prognosis of solitary and extramedullary myeloma is good, disseminated myelomatosis ultimately develops in approximately 30 to 50% of these patients [99]. Vigorous treatment aimed at eliminating the solitary lesions is mandatory in all cases since it is impossible to predict with certainty which cases will progress to multiple myeloma.

## 14. NON-HODGKIN'S LYMPHOMA

Involvement of extranodal sites in the head and neck by Hodgkin's disease is, in contrast to non-Hodgkin's lymphoma, rare. It has been described in Waldeyer's ring as well as in the oral soft tissue [97,104] and will not be discussed here.

At least six different classifications of non-Hodgkin's lymphoma are in common usage. The Rappaport classification [105] is largely descriptive, whereas some others are functional in nature and are based on the relationships of the various lymphomas to the T and B systems of lymphocytes and on the alterations observed in lymphocyte transformation. In these classifications the lymphomas are identified on the basis of immunological markers. The most widely used classification seems to be that of Rappaport [105,106] or of modifications thereof. This classification is based on the cytological and histological patterns observed. Immunological and functional studies appear to indicate that the Rappaport classification and the concepts associated with it might be erroneous. However, because of the wide usage of this classification by pathologists and clinicians alike as well as the established clinical and prognostic value this classification possesses, it continues to be widely used [97]. Rappaport's classification of non-Hodgkin's lymphomas [10] is as follows:

1. Lymphocytic, well differentiated.
2. Lymphocytic, poorly differentiated (may be diffuse or nodular).
3. Histiocytic (reticulum cell sarcoma) (may be diffuse or nodular).
4. Mixed lymphocytic—histiocytic (may be diffuse or nodular).
5. Undifferentiated non-Burkitt's type.
6. Undifferentiated Burkitt's type (see later discussion).

This basic classification has recently been modified by the addition of a lymphoblastic and an immunoblastic variety as well as by the recognition of mycosis fungoides as a distinct entity [106].

Nodularity in the histological pattern is indicative of a better prognosis. Transition from nodular to a diffuse pattern indicates a worsening of the prognosis.

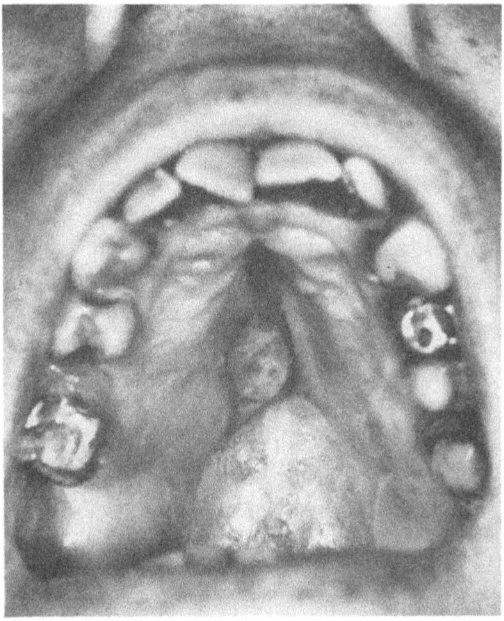

**Figure 4–16.** Malignant lymphoma involving hard palate. (Courtesy Professor J.J. Pindborg, Copenhagen)

### 14.1. Distribution in the oral cavity

Most lymphomas first present in lymph nodes, most often in lymph nodes of the neck. Some lymphomas, however, especially those of the diffuse type, may present initially in other lymphoreticular organs. The most common site of origin of primary extranodal lymphoma in the head and neck is Waldeyer's ring. Less frequent sites of involvement include the soft palate, oropharynx, larynx, salivary glands, and jaws.

Lymphoma in the oral cavity can occur at any site, but there seems to be some predilection for the mucosa of the hard palate (figure 4–16). Lesions can arise in areas usually totally devoid of normal lymphoid tissue. In 1975 Tomich and Shafer [107] described 21 cases of primary lymphoma of the hard palate. Both unilateral and bilateral involvement of the palate occurred. All cases were classified as lymphocytic lymphomas. An additional 8 new cases of lymphoma of the hard palate have recently been reported [108]. In considering primary lymphoma of the palate, the subjects of follicular lymphoid hyperplasia of the hard palate [109,110] and midline nonhealing "granuloma" [111] are extremely important. Extreme caution in distinguishing these lesions from malignant lymphoma is urged. Several reports of lymphoma of the other oral soft tissues and jaws have appeared in the literature [112,113].

Involvement of the oral mucosa has even been reported in *mycosis fungoides* [114,115]. *Primary reticulum cell sarcoma* (histiocytic lymphoma) of the jaws warrants special attention. The majority of cases have been reported in the posterior body and angle of the mandible. An extensive literature review [116] included 22 cases from the mandible and reported a new case. The prognosis seems to be considerably better than for histiocytic lymphoma of soft tissue. Microscopic differentiation from Ewing's sarcoma creates considerable difficulty. The differences have been referred to earlier in this chapter.

### 14.2. Mode or spread and prognosis

The prognosis for extranodal lymphoma of the oral soft tissues depends on the nature of the lesion, the histological pattern, and the clinical stage of the disease. The stage I lesion, that is, the lesion confined to a single site, has the best prognosis, with treatment directed at eliminating the lesion entirely in the hope that involvement of other sites will not occur. Depending on the stage of the disease, radiotherapy and/or chemotherapy is the treatment of choice. Attempts to remove a lymphoma of the palate or other soft tissue by surgical excision do not seem justified [108]. Reticulum cell sarcoma of the mandible is more often a solitary lesion with less tendency to spread than its soft tissue counterpart. A five-year survival rate of up to 70% has been reported for this site [117].

### 14.3. Histopathology

The distinction between neoplastic lymphoid proliferation and various non-neoplastic reactive lymphoid hyperplasias is always a perplexing problem. Dorfman and Warnke [118] have provided an excellent description of the spectrum of morphologic changes produced by a wide variety of antigenic stimuli upon normal lymphoid tissue. The salient features of the various histological types of non-Hodgkin's lymphomas can be summarized as follows [97].

The well-differentiated lymphocytic lymphoma is comparatively rare. The lymphocytes are cytologically indistinguishable from normal lymphocytes, and the diagnosis of lymphoma must be made on the obliteration of the normal nodal architecture by a proliferation of uniform, mature-appearing lymphocytes that do not aggregate into nodules. There is a close relationship between well-differentiated lymphocytic lymphoma and chronic lymphocytic leukaemia.

The poorly differentiated lymphocytic lymphoma is the most common of all lymphocytic lymphomas. The cells are larger than those of the well-differentiated form; the nuclei are pleomorphic, irregular, and commonly have nuclear clefts and indentations. In childhood poorly differentiated lymphocytic lymphomas progress to leukaemia and in the leukaemic phase become indistinguishable from acute lymphocytic leukaemia.

The derivation of histiocytic lymphomas (reticulum cell sarcoma) from his-

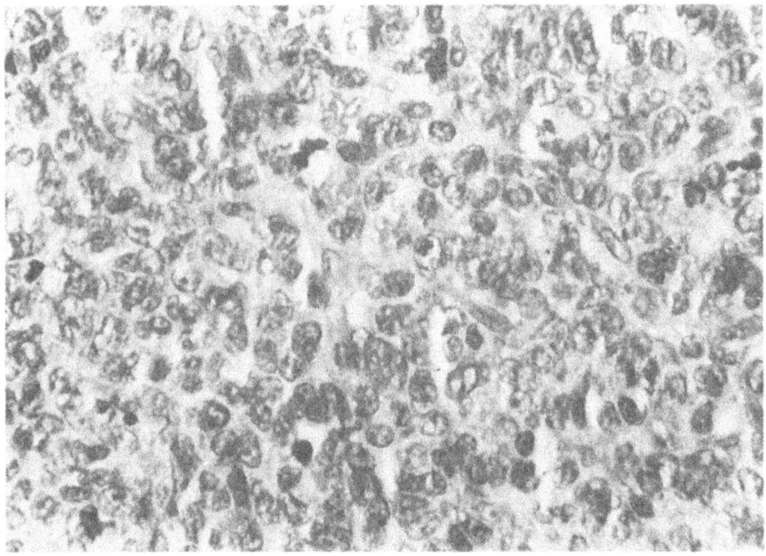

**Figure 4–17.** Histiocytic lymphoma (reticulum cell sarcoma) involving the palate, maxillary alveolus, and cheek.

tiocytes is doubtful. In many instances these cells are derived from B lymphocytes. The cells are larger than those of the lymphocytic lymphomas (figure 4–17). Some of these neoplasms may have very pleomorphic bizarre and multinucleated giant tumour cells.

The mixed (lymphocytic-histiocytic) lymphoma is not common. It is composed of approximately equal numbers of poorly differentiated lymphocytes and histiocytes. A nodular growth pattern is more common than a diffuse one.

The undifferentiated lymphoma—non-Burkitt type—is rare. The cells show considerable pleomorphism. Nucleoli are larger than those in Burkitt's lymphoma. This lymphoma is seen only in the diffuse form, mostly in adults with nodal disease, and has an unfavourable prognosis.

#### 15. BURKITT'S LYMPHOMA

Burkitt's lymphoma is a distinctive clinicopathological entity [119] occurring mainly in African children between the ages of 2 and 14 years. It is the most common malignant tumour of childhood in central Africa, accounting for up to 50% of cases. The disease is usually multifocal and predominantly extranodal. It remains aleukaemic, even at a late stage. In over half the African cases, a jaw tumour is the presenting symptom. The second most frequent presenting symptom is an abdominal mass as a result of kidney, liver, adrenal, and gonadal involvement. Several important differences have been observed between the African and the so-called American cases of Burkitt's lymphoma

[120]. The American cases occur in older individuals, do not commonly show jaw lesions, do not have the same association with the Epstein-Barr virus, and patients do not suffer late relapse after treatment.

The occurrence and significance of jaw lesions in Burkitt's lymphoma has been reviewed [121]. Up to the age of three years, jaw lesions occur in almost 100% of cases. Thereafter, the frequency of jaw lesions gradually decreases. The concept that odontogenesis creates suitable environmental conditions for colonization by circulating Burkitt's lymphoma cells is an interesting one [121].

### 15.1. Etiology

The geographic distribution of endemic cases within a wide belt of equatorial Africa led to the recognition of the possibility that the disease might be related to climatic conditions and therefore that it might be borne by arthropods, particularly mosquitoes [122]. The endemic distribution of Burkitt's lymphoma in Africa and in New Guinea corresponds to the areas of hyperendemic malaria. While malaria alone is not the cause of Burkitt's lymphoma, it might act with a cofactor—a virus for instance—to cause the disease. Various viruses have come under consideration as possible causes of Burkitt's lymphoma. The most likely one is the Epstein-Barr virus (EBV), a member of the Herpes group. The importance of the EBV in relation to Burkitt's lymphoma seems unquestionable, although the nature of the relationship is not clear [123].

### 15.2. Clinical and radiological features

Jaw lesions occur mainly in the posterior regions of the maxilla and mandible. More than one quadrant may be involved, and, frequently, deposits are found in all four quadrants of the jaws. The effect of Burkitt's lymphoma on the teeth and jaws has been reviewed [124]. The presenting symptoms often consist of loosening of the deciduous molar teeth, followed by expansion of the gingiva and displacement and exfoliation of the teeth. Pain is minimal, and tenderness, anaesthesia, or paraesthesia are usually absent.

Initially, small discrete radiolucencies may be seen. These soon coalesce to produce larger radiolucent areas. One of the earliest radiological signs is a loss of or break in the lamina dura. Subperiosteal new bone formation may occur resulting in a "sunray" appearance [124,125].

If untreated, most of the children die within four to six months. Older children may survive up to one year. Dramatic remissions occur in over 90% of patients following high-dose alkylating-agent therapy. Relapse occurs in two-thirds of these patients, most often in those with advanced disease [97].

### 15.3. Histopathology

The tumour consists of sheets of undifferentiated lymphoid cells larger than lymphocytes that do not show cytological or cytochemical evidence of differentiation toward either lymphocytes or histiocytes. A so-called "starry sky"

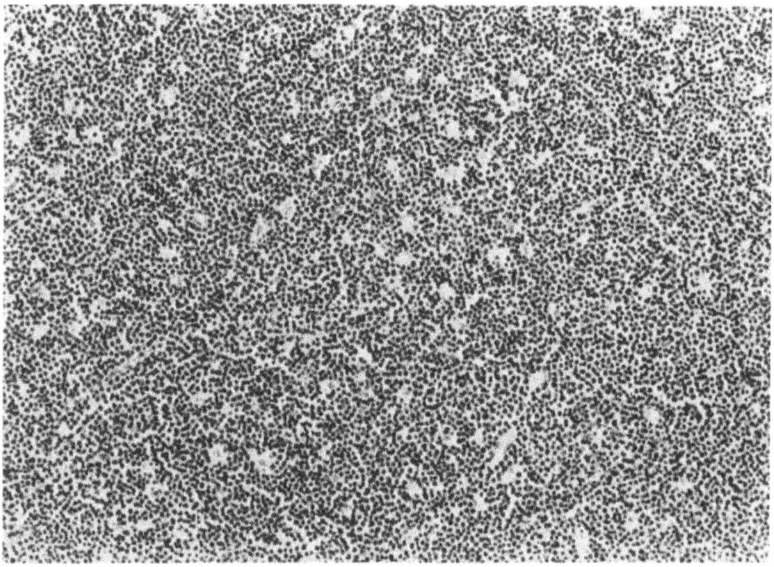

**Figure 4–18.** Burkitt's lymphoma.

pattern because of the presence of benign macrophages scattered among the malignant cells is characteristic of Burkitt's lymphoma (figure 4–18). The starry-sky pattern is not essential to the diagnosis nor is it specific to Burkitt's lymphoma. Mitoses are numerous. The cytoplasm of the cells is markedly pyroninophilic.

### 16. WEGENER'S GRANULOMATOSIS AND MIDLINE (NONHEALING) "GRANULOMA"

The conditions described as Wegener's granulomatosis and midline (nonhealing) "granuloma" were previously regarded as synonymous. It is now clear, however, that although they may share some clinical characteristics, such as necrosis and granulomatous inflammation of the upper respiratory tract and mouth, they have their own spectra of clinical manifestations, they may be distinguished histologically, and they require different forms of treatment.

#### 16.1. Wegener's granulomatosis

Wegener's granulomatosis is characterized by a triad consisting of necrotizing granulomas of the respiratory tract, both upper and lower; focal necrotizing glomerulitis; and a systemic small vessel vasculitis. These different sites may be involved to a varying extent, and limited forms of the disease with a more benign course may occur [126]. In the latter forms, there may be pulmonary or extrapulmonary lesions without glomerulitis. Skin involvement occurs in be-

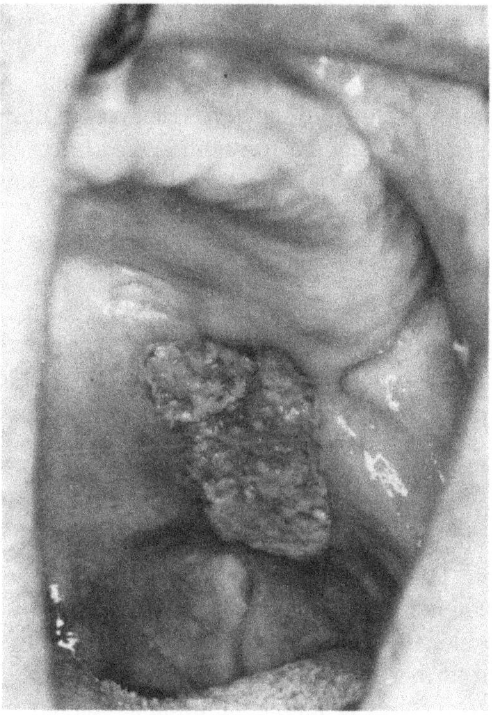

**Figure 4–19.** Wegener's granulomatosis involving the soft palate. (Courtesy Professor J.J. Pindborg, Copenhagen)

tween 40 to 50% of cases. As far as oral involvement is concerned, an extensive literature review [127] indicates that this is fairly common. It may take the form of palatal ulceration independent of nasal lesions; oropharyngeal granulomas involving the fauces, uvula, and soft palate (figure 4–19); inflammation of other oral mucosal surfaces; or failure of extraction sockets to heal. Destruction of the hard palate by extension of a lesion from the nose or sinuses is not a feature of Wegener's granulomatosis although it is of midline (nonhealing) "granuloma" [111,127].

Renal involvement, with focal necrotizing glomerulitis, is the most serious complication, but almost any organ may be involved, especially, in addition to those already mentioned, the eyes, ears, joints, and nervous system. Vasculitis of the coronary vasculature, valvulitis, and pericarditis are the cardiac manifestations [111].

The etiology and pathogenesis of Wegener's granulomatosis are far from clear. No specific causative organism has been demonstrated, nor is there evidence of an autoimmune mechanism [128].

Histologically, Wegener's granulomatosis is similar to polyarteritis nodosa, but Wegener's is more commonly granulomatous. The predominant microscopic features [111] are epithelioid granulomas, fibrinoid necrosis in blood vessel walls, focal vasculitis, and healing vasculitis with thrombosis and fibrous obliteration. There is a subacute to chronic inflammatory cell infiltration with numbers of multinucleate giant cells. Eosinophils are often found. Areas of necrosis including fibrinoid necrosis may be present.

The effective response of Wegener's granulomatosis to immunosuppressive drugs is well established.

### 16.2. Midline (non-healing) "granuloma"

The separation of Wegener's granulomatosis from those disorders previously described as "lethal midline granuloma" leaves a group that, as stated by Batsakis [111], share clinical signs and symptoms referable to the nasal cavity and midfacial tissues, which are not all lethal and not all granulomatous. The term *midline (non-healing) granuloma* has been used to embrace this group, which comprises at least three histologically definable lesions [111]. The first, which has been referred to as idiopathic midline granuloma, is a localized destructive lesion of the upper respiratory tract characterized by a nonspecific acute and chronic inflammatory reaction with necrosis. The second is a pseudolymphomatous reaction called polymorphic reticulosis by others. The third form is extranodal lymphoma, discussed earlier in this chapter, and will not be considered further here.

This histological features of idiopathic midline granuloma are surprisingly nonspecific, in view of this destructive process, being characterized by an acute and chronic inflammatory reaction with necrosis. Vasculitis, granulomas, and giant cells are found only rarely [111]. Long-term remissions have been achieved with radiotherapy.

As indicated earlier, Batsakis [111] separates polymorphic reticulosis as a histologically definable form of the group of midline (non-healing) "granuloma." He also distinguishes this form from the so-called "idiopathic midline granuloma," in that in the latter there is no systemic involvement.

## 17. MALIGNANT MELANOMA

Malignant melanoma is rare in the mouth. Age standardized incidence rates for oral lesions are not available, but the incidence of cutaneous malignant melanoma varies in different populations [129]. The frequency of oral melanoma as a percentage of all recorded melanomas also varies in different reports, from 1.7% [130] to 8% [131]. Oral lesions accounted for 7.5% (22 cases) of a series of 295 autopsied cases of malignant melanoma in a nationwide survey conducted in Japan [132]. Patients with oral melanoma range in age from the third to the tenth decades, with the peak frequency in the fifth and sixth decades [130,132,133]. Some review articles on oral melanoma indicate an equal sex frequency, but in one report males were involved almost twice as often as females [134]. There is general agreement that the majority of oral melanomas involve the mucosa of the maxilla, particularly the hard palate and gingiva.

### 17.1. Special etiologic factors

An association between oral melanoma and a previous pigmented lesion has frequently been reported [132–134]. While excessive exposure to solar radiation is important in the development of cutaneous melanoma, this is clearly not a significant factor with intraoral melanoma. However, repeated trauma to a pigmented lesion, which has also been implicated as a factor in skin melanoma [135], cannot be disregarded as a possible etiologic factor in the genesis of oral melanoma. It has been suggested [123] that several factors support a policy of prophylactic excisional biopsy of any focal pigmented lesion of the oral mucosa that does not have an indisputably innocuous etiology. These are the difficulty in clinical differentiation between focal melanocytic lesions and a number of other pigmentations, particularly as a significant number of melanomas are preceded by asymptomatic pigmentations. Furthermore, a considerable number of malignant melanomas appear innocent clinically.

### 17.2. Clinical features

Patients may complain of long-standing enlargement of a pigmented area or of a mass development in such an area (figure 4–20). These changes may have occurred rapidly [132]. Symptoms noted in published case reports are swelling, bleeding following minimal trauma, ulceration, or delayed healing of extraction sockets.

The presence of dark brown or black pigmentation is obviously very important in making a clinical diagnosis, but this feature is not always found. The lesions may be pink or colourless, and some have been described as vascular or red and fleshy. Ulceration is frequently present, but the lesions are not as indurated as squamous carcinomas and the lesions may bleed [136]. The neoplasm extends to involve bone, and this may lead to loosening of teeth. As in skin lesions, satellite foci may develop in the environment of the primary. In a series of 94 cases of oral melanomas [132], a preexisting melanosis was present in 34 (36%) and a concurrent melanosis in 28 (30%).

There is now some degree of international unanimity [137] that two basic patterns are involved in the development of primary malignant melanoma of the skin. In the first antecedent spreading pigmentation occurs that is characterized histologically by intraepidermal proliferation of melanocytes prior to the appearance of an invasive nodule (figures 4–21, 4–22). In the other the tumour invades the dermis from the beginning, with no such antecedent area of pigmentation. The first pattern is seen with two similar but clinically and histologically distinctive entities [137]: Hutchinson's melanotic freckle (figure 4–21) and noninvasive superficial spreading melanoma (figure 4–22). These two lesions are frequently confused, not least because of the numerous syn-

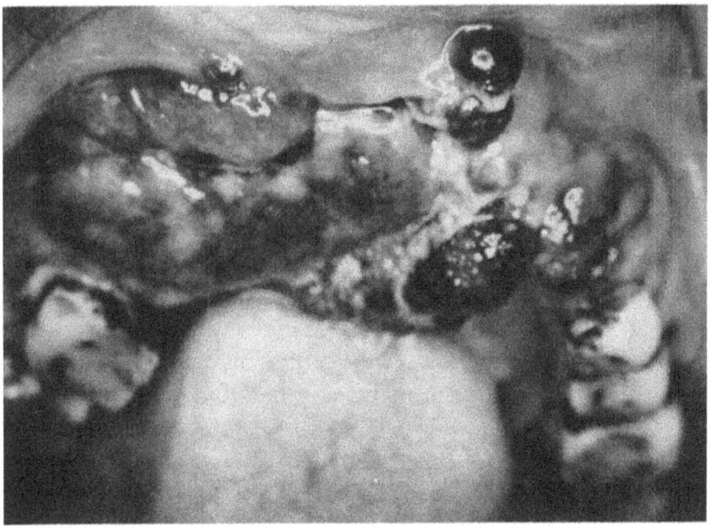

**Figure 4–20.** Malignant melanoma of oral mucosa. (Courtesy Professor J.J. Pindborg, Copenhagen)

onyms that have been applied to each. This confusion has been compounded in discussions on oral melanoma because of the controversy as to whether Hutchinson's melanotic freckle, usually found on areas of skin particularly exposed to the sun, could occur in the mouth. The available evidence indicates that both Hutchinson's melanotic freckle and noninvasive superficial spreading melanoma occur in the mouth [130,137,138].

Hutchinson's melanotic freckle has a number of synonyms in common use: Hutchinson's freckle, sessile freckle, lentigo maligna, melanose circonscrite precancereuse, and Dubreuihl's melanosis circumscripta praecancerosa [137]. Oral lesions of Hutchinson's melanotic freckle with histological confirmation have been described on the buccal mucosa, labial mucosa, floor of mouth, and palate and may extend from one area to another. The lesion is flat and varies in intensity of pigmentation from brown to black with greyish foci. It has an irregular outline. In time nodules of invasive melanoma develop in the oral lesions.

The synonyms for noninvasive superficial spreading melanoma are pagetoid

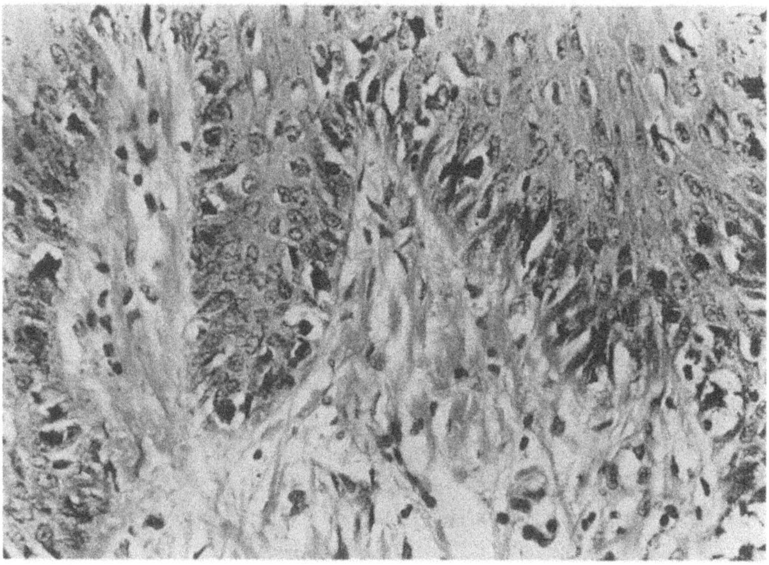

**Figure 4–21.** Hutchinson's melanotic freckle (lentigo maligna) showing proliferation of atypical melanocytes.

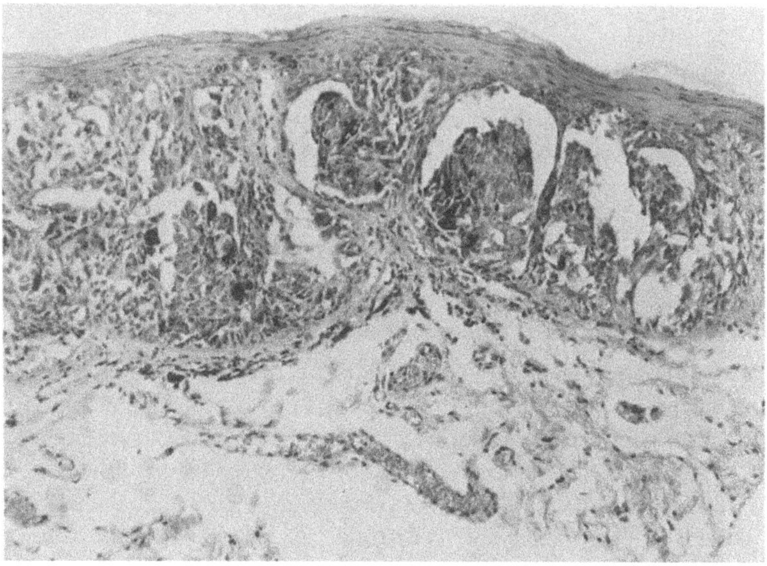

**Figure 4–22.** Superficial spreading melanoma involving vermilion border of lower lip, showing nests of naevus cells invading the epidermis in pagetoid fashion. (Section by courtesy Dr. J.A. Regezi, Ann Arbor)

melanoma, premalignant melanosis, melanose circonscrite precancereuse, Dubreuihl's melanosis circumscripta praecancerose, and in situ melanoma [137]. The term *acral-lentiginous melanoma* has also been used for both forms of superficial melanoma [138]. The overlap of synonyms with those for Hutchinson's melanotic freckle is an indication of the confusion of these two entities. Large series of oral mucosal melanosis associated with melanoma [132] have unfortunately not differentiated the two forms, and distinction between them may, for the time being, have to depend on histological examination. Clearly, a need exists for well-documented publications of oral lesions of the two forms with clinical and supportive histological descriptions.

### 17.3. Mode of spread, biopsy, and prognosis

Local extension of tumour from oral mucosa to underlying bone of maxilla and mandible leads to bone destruction. In a series of 65 cases involving the oral mucosa, metastases were present in the regional nodes of 24 patients on presentation, and general metastases in 5 [130].

Adequate biopsy should, where possible, excise the entire lesion with a rim of normal tissue [137]. This is examined by frozen section or by rapid paraffin section, after which the surgeon decides whether further excision of the area is necessary. No evidence has been found that incisional biopsy, if it must be done, causes spread of malignant melanoma [139].

The prognosis for oral melanoma is worse than for cutaneous melanoma. In a review of 51 patients with oral malignant melanoma [130], the overall five-year survival rate was 19.6%.

### 17.4. Histopathology

Guidelines for the classification of malignant melanoma and its histologic reporting have been published by the group of international authorities already referred to [137]. Although their recommendations are based essentially on the development of primary malignant melanoma of the skin, they may be applied also to the classification and description of melanoma of the oral cavity.

#### *17.4.1. Malignant melanoma, invasive, with adjacent intraepidermal or intraepithelial component of Hutchinson's melanotic freckle type*

Initially, Hutchinson's melanotic freckle is characterized by a linear proliferation of atypical melanocytes in the basal layer (figure 4–21). The proliferating melanocytes produce a considerable amount of melanin pigment which is released and phagocytosed by melanophores. A lymphocytic infiltrate is present in the superficial dermis or lamina propria. At a later stage the melanocytes are palisaded. Then clusters of cells form, usually spindle cells, and foci of invasion are often present. The cells of the invasive areas show considerable pleomorphism. In the noninvasive regions the relative absence of epidermal or epithelial invasion is a distinctive histologic feature [137].

### *17.4.2. Malignant melanoma, invasive, with adjacent intraepidermal or intraepithelial component of superficial type*

Here the proliferating melanocytes are not confined to the junction between epidermis and dermis or epithelium and lamina propria as in Hutchinson's melanotic freckle but invade the epidermis or epithelium in pagetoid fashion. This is not the result of centrifugal spread, but rather an enlarging field effect. The cells are uniform and do not show the pleomorphism seen in Hutchinson's melanotic freckle. When they invade they are either epithelioid, spindle, naevus cell-like, or a mixture. The spread of melanocytes between as well as on rete pegs distinguishes this lesion from the junctional naevus, where the nests are mainly on the rete ridges [137] (figure 4–22).

### *17.4.3. Malignant melanoma, invasive, without any adjacent intraepidermal or intraepithelial component*

Here malignant melanocytes invade from the beginning. The tumours consist of polygonal cells, fusiform cells, or mixtures of the two [133]. There appears to be no correlation between tumour morphology and clinical findings [132,137]. Metastatic foci show a more pleomorphic pattern than in the primary sites and may contain amelanotic nodules [132]. Other histologic points to be sought and recorded are vascular invasion, mitotic activity, and levels of invasion [137]. To assess mitotic activity at least 10 high-power (×300) fields should be examined and the tumours graded as follows:

*Grade 1:* low mitotic activity, less than 1 mitosis per 5 high-power fields. This grade is associated with an 80% five-year survival rate for cutaneous melanomas.

*Grade 2:* medium mitotic activity, 1 to 4 mitoses per 5 high-power fields. This grade is associated with a five-year survival rate of 51 to 69% for cutaneous melanomas.

*Grade 3:* high mitotic activity, 1 or more mitoses per high-power field. This grade is associated with a 40% five-year survival rate for cutaneous melanomas.

Levels of invasion are assessed according to Clark's classification [140], modified slightly for use with oral melanomas:

*Level 1:* Tumour confined to epidermis or epithelium.

*Level 2:* Tumour invading papillary layer, but not into reticular layer of the dermis or lamina propria.

*Level 3:* Tumour extends to and impinges on the interface between the papillary and reticular layers, but does not penetrate reticular layer.

*Level 4:* Tumour penetrates reticular layer.

*Level 5:* Tumour invades subcutaneous or submucosal fat.

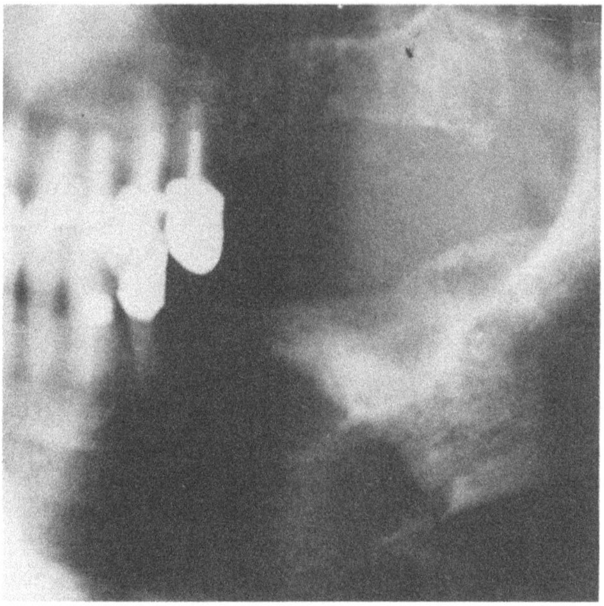

**Figure 4–23.** Radiograph of metastatic deposit of thyroid carcinoma. (Courtesy Professor J.J. Pindborg, Copenhagen)

Regardless of the clinical presentation, the mortality rate for cutaneous melanoma increases in proportion to the depth of invasion at the time of excision [140]. Microstage measurement may also be attempted with division of the lesions into three categories: those less than 3 mm deep, those 3 to 5 mm deep, and those more than 5 mm deep [136].

## 18. METASTATIC TUMOURS TO THE ORAL REGIONS

Malignant tumours may metastasize to the jaws and soft tissues of the mouth from primary sites in many parts of the body and constitute between 1 and 8% of malignant tumours of the oral regions [141]. Metastases have been documented much more frequently in the jaws, especially in the mandible, than in the oral soft tissues (figure 4–23). It is likely, however, that the actual incidence of metastatic deposits in the jaws is higher than that observed since the jaws are not routinely examined at autopsy [142]. Sometimes, the histological diagnosis of an oral lesion may be the first indication of an occult malignant tumour elsewhere [143,144]. As carcinoma of the breast is the commonest source of metastases to the jaws, females preponderate in most large series [141,143]. Although all parts of the mandible may be involved, more cases are found posterior to the canines than in the anterior region [143].

The primary sites of the metastatic deposits based on a review of 391 cases

**Table 4–1.** Primary sites of metastases to oral regions

| Site | Males | Females |
|---|---|---|
| | % | % |
| Carcinomas | | |
| Breast | 1.0 | 44.5 |
| Lung | 27.7 | 4.0 |
| Kidney | 18.8 | 12.5 |
| Prostate | 10.5 | — |
| Colon & rectum | 5.2 | 8.0 |
| Uterus | — | 7.0 |
| Thyroid | 2.1 | 6.0 |
| Testis | 5.2 | — |
| Liver | 4.2 | — |
| Stomach & oesophagus | 5.2 | 1.0 |
| Ovary | — | 2.0 |
| Pancreas | 1.1 | — |
| Gall bladder | — | 0.5 |
| Urinary bladder | 1.1 | — |
| Penis | 0.5 | — |
| | 82.6(n = 158) | 85.5(n = 171) |
| Other tumours | | |
| Neuroblastoma | 9.4 | 7.5 |
| Sarcomas | 6.8 | 6.0 |
| Melanoma | 1.0 | 1.0 |
| | 99.8(n = 191) | 100.0(n = 200) |

From reference 141.

[141] are shown in table 4–1. As in other series, tumours of the breast, lung, and kidney are those most frequently found. As stated previously the oral manifestations were the first evidence of the disease in a substantial proportion of cases, and in most instances where the primary tumour was diagnosed first, the time taken for the oral metastasis to appear was between one to five years [141]. Swelling and pain are the most frequent symptoms, while loosening of teeth, anaesthesia or paraesthesia, fracture of the jaw, and problems with dentures also occur [143].

The prognosis is poor. In the majority of recorded cases, death has occurred shortly after development of the metastasis, but some patients survived for a few years [142]. In some instances, particularly in cases of hypernephroma and thyroid carcinoma, the jaw lesion may be a solitary metastasis, and treatment of this as well as the primary tumour may cure the patient [142]. In most, however, other skeletal metastases coexist, and pulmonary deposits may also be present [143]. Radiological features of metastatic tumours are not characteristic [143], except that they share with other malignant tumours of the jaws the same evidence of irregular bone destruction (figure 4–23). Metastatic prostatic carcinoma and some breast tumours may, however, manifest as radiopaque deposits [142].

The diagnosis of a metastatic neoplasm depends on histological examination, but this is by no means always a simple procedure if the primary is still occult and the biopsied lesion poorly differentiated.

## REFERENCES


1. Baden E. Terminology of the ameloblastoma: History and current usage. J Oral Surg (23): 40–49, 1965.
2. Shear M, Singh S. Age-standardized incidence rates of ameloblastoma and dentigerous cyst on the Witwatersrand, South Africa. Community Dent Oral Epidemiol (6): 195–199, 1978.
3. Adekeye EO. Ameloblastoma of the jaws: A survey of 109 Nigerian patients. J Oral Surg (38): 36–41, 1980.
4. Small IA, Waldron CA. Ameloblastomas of the jaws. Oral Surg (8): 281–297, 1955.
5. Lucas RB. Odontogenic tumours on polyoma virus-infected mice. 4th Proc Int Acad Oral Path, 1969, New York.
6. Herrold KMcD: Odontogenic tumours and epidermoid carcinomas of the oral cavity. Oral Surg (25): 262–272, 1968.
7. Shteyer A, Lustman J, Lewin-Epstein J. The mural ameloblastoma: A review of the literature. J Oral Surg (36): 866–872, 1978.
8. Shear M. Cysts of the Oral Regions. Bristol: John Wright & Sons, 2nd ed. 1983.
9. Robinson L, Martinez MG. Unicystic ameloblastoma. A prognostically distinct entity. Cancer (40): 2278–2285, 1977.
10. Lucas RB. Pathology of Tumours of the Oral Tissues, 3rd ed. Edinburgh, London, and New York: Churchill Livingstone, 1976.
11. Shear M, Altini M. The possible inductive role of ectomesenchyme in the pathogenesis of some odontogenic lesions. J Dent Ass S Afr (31): 649–654, 1976.
12. Lucas RB, Pindborg JJ. Odontogenic tumours and tumour-like lesions. In Scientific Foundations of Dentistry, Cohen B, Kramer IRH (eds). London: Heinemann, 1976, pp. 240–250.
13. Mehlisch DR, Dahlin DC, Masson JK. Ameloblastoma: A clinicopathologic report. J Oral Surg (30): 9–22, 1972.
14. Struthers P, Shear M. Root resorption by ameloblastomas and cysts of the jaws. Int J Oral Surg (5): 128–132, 1976.
15. LaBriola JD, Steiner M, Bernstein ML, Verdi GD, Stannard PF. Odontoameloblastoma. J Oral Surg (38): 139–143, 1980.
16. Pindborg JJ, Kramer IRH, Torloni H. Histological typing of odontogenic tumours, jaw cysts and allied lesions. Geneva, World Health Organization, 1971.
17. Altini M, Smith I. Ameloblastic dentinosarcoma (a case report). Int J Oral Surg (5): 142–147, 1976.
18. Shear M, Rachanis CC. Epidemiology of odontogenic lesions in South Africa. J Dent Ass S Afr (34): 685–688, 1979.
19. Shear, M. Primary intra-alveolar epidermoid carcinoma of the jaw. J Path Bact (97): 645–651, 1969.
20. Kay LW, Kramer IRH. Squamous cell carcinoma arising in a dental cyst. Oral Surg (15): 970–979, 1962.
21. Leider AS, Nelson JF, Trodahl JN. Ameloblastic fibrosarcoma of the jaws. Oral Surg (33): 559–569, 1972.
22. Reichart PA, Zobl H. Transformation of ameloblastic fibroma to fibrosarcoma. Report of a case. Int J Oral Surg (7): 503–507, 1978.
23. Daramola JO, Ajagbe HA, Oluwasanmi JO, Akinyemi OO, Samuel I. Ameloblastic sarcoma of the mandible (report of case). J Oral Surg (37): 432–435, 1979.
24. Forman G, Garrett J. Ameloblastic sarcoma: Report of a case. J Oral Surg (30): 50–54, 1972.
25. Howell RM, Burkes EJ. Malignant transformation of ameloblastic fibro-odontoma to ameloblastic fibrosarcoma. Oral Surg (43): 391–401, 1977.
26. Altini M. The ameloblastic fibroma and related lesions. M Dent dissertation, University of the Witwatersrand, Johannesburg, 1977.
27. Dahlin DC, Irvins JC. Fibrosarcoma of bone. A study of 114 cases. Cancer (23): 35–41, 1969.
28. Trodahl JN. Ameloblastic fibroma. A survey of cases from the Armed Forces Institute of Pathology. Oral Surg (33): 547–558, 1972.

29. Cutler LS, Chaudry AP, Topazian R. Melanotic neuroectodermal tumor of infancy: An ultrastructural study, literature review and reevaluation. Cancer (48): 257–270, 1981.
30. Lindahl F. Malignant melanotic progonoma. One case. Acta Pathol Microbiol Scand (Sect A) (78): 532–536, 1970.
31. Dehner LP, Sibley RK, Sauk JJ, Vickers RA, Nesbit ME, Leonard AS, Waite DE, Neeley JE, Ophoven J. Malignant melanotic neuroectodermal tumor of infancy. A clinical, pathologic, ultrastructural and tissue culture study. Cancer (43): 1389–1410, 1979.
32. Batsakis, JG. Tumors of the Head and Neck, 2nd ed. Baltimore: Williams & Wilkins, 1979.
33. Freedman PD, Cardo VA, Kerpel SM, Lumerman H. Desmoplastic fibroma (fibromatosis) of the jawbones. Report of a case and review of the literature. Oral Surg (46): 386–395, 1978.
34. Kauffman SL, Stout AP. Congenital mesenchymal tumors. Cancer (18): 460–476, 1965.
35. Takagi M, Ishikawa G. Fibrous tumor of infancy—Report of a case originating in the oral cavity. J Oral Path (2): 293–300, 1973.
36. Wilkins SA Jr, Waldron CA, Mathews WH, Droulias CA. Aggressive fibromatosis of the head and neck. Am J Surg (130): 412–415, 1975.
37. Miller R, Cheris L, Stratigos GT. Nodular fasciitis. Oral Surg (40): 399–403, 1975.
38. Kriakos M, Kempson RL. Inflammatory fibrous histiocytoma. Cancer (37): 1584–1606, 1976.
39. Brandenburg JH, Frank TW. Malignant fibrous xanthoma of the lip. Otolaryngol Head & Neck Surg (88): 154–156, 1980.
40. Hoffman S, Martinez MG. Fibrous histiocytomas of the oral mucosa. Oral Surg (52): 277–283, 1981.
41. Spector GT, Ogura JH. Malignant fibrous histiocytoma of the maxilla. Arch Otolaryngol (99): 385–387, 1974.
42. Slootweg PJ, Müller H. Malignant fibrous histiocytoma of the maxilla. Report of a case. Oral Surg (44): 560–566, 1977.
43. Dahlin DC, Unni KK, Matsuno T. Malignant (fibrous) histiocytoma of bone—Fact or fancy? Cancer (39): 1508–1516, 1977.
44. Yoshimura Y, Kawano T, Takada K, Sakai SI, Honda M, Hyo Y, Hoshiya, T. Malignant fibrous histiocytoma of the temporomandibular joint. Report of a case. Int J Oral Surg (7): 573–579, 1978.
45. Eversole LR, Schwartz WD, Sabes WR. Central and peripheral fibrogenic and neurogenic sarcoma of the oral regions. Oral Surg (36): 49–62, 1973.
46. Mackenzie DH. Fibroma: A dangerous diagnosis. A review of 205 cases of fibrosarcoma of soft tissues. Brit J Surg (51): 607–612, 1964.
47. Pritchard DJ, Soule EH, Taylor WF, Ivins JC. Fibrosarcoma—A clinicopathologic and statistical study of 199 tumors of the soft tissues of the extremities and trunk. Cancer (33): 888–897, 1974.
48. Mirra JH. Bone Tumors. Diagnosis and Treatment. Philadelphia: J.B. Lippincott, 1980.
49. Larsson SE, Lorentzon R, Boquist L. Fibrosarcoma of bone. J Bone Joint Surg (58B): 412–417, 1976.
50. Wright BA, Jackson D: Neural tumors of the oral cavity. Oral Surg (49): 509–522, 1980.
51. Shuman R. Mesenchymal tumors of soft tissues. In Pathology, 6th ed., Anderson WAD (ed). St. Louis: C.V. Mosby, 1971.
52. Healey GB, Jaffe N, Cassady JR. Rhabdomyosarcoma of the head and neck: Diagnosis and management. Head & Neck Surg (1): 334–339, 1979.
53. Horn RC, Enterline HT. Rhabdomyosarcoma: A clinicopathologic study and classification of 39 cases. Cancer (11): 181–199, 1958.
54. O'Day RA, Soule EH, Gores RJ. Embryonal rhabdomyosarcoma of the oral soft tissue. Oral Surg (20): 85–93, 1965.
55. Vogel C, Reichart PA, Holgado S, Ostertag H. Rhabdomyosarcoma of the oral cavity in children: Report of five cases with ultrastructural study. Int J Oral Surg (10): suppl. 1: 27–31, 1981.
56. Brandjord RM, Reaume CE, Wesley RK. Leiomyosarcoma of the floor of the mouth. Review of the literature and report of case. J Oral Surg (35): 590–594, 1977.
57. Weitzner S. Leiomyosarcoma of the anterior maxillary ridge. Oral Surg (50): 62–64, 1980.
58. Kratochvil FJ, MacGregor SD, Budnick SD, et al. Leiomyosarcoma of the maxilla. Report of a case and review of the literature. Oral Surg (54): 647–655, 1982.

59. Enzinger FM, Lattes R, Torloni H. Histological typing of soft tissue tumours. World Health Organization, Geneva, 1969.
60. Baden E, Newman R: Liposarcoma of the oropharyngeal region: Review of the literature and report of two cases. Oral Surg (44): 889–902, 1977.
61. Saunders JR, Jaques DA, Casterline PF, Percarpio B, Goodloe S. Liposarcomas of the head and neck: A review of the literature and addition of four cases. Cancer (43): 162–168, 1979.
62. Dahl EC, Hammond HL, Sequeira E. Liposarcomas of the head and neck. J Oral Maxillofac Surg (40): 674–677, 1982.
63. Amarjit S, Bhardivaj DN, Nagpal BL. Intraosseous liposarcoma of the maxilla and mandible (report of two cases). J Oral Surg (37): 593–596, 1979.
64. Enzinger FM. Recent trends in soft tissue pathology. In Tumors of Bone and Soft Tissue. Chicago: Year Book, p. 315, 1965.
65. Campanacci M, Boriani S, Giunti A. Hemangioendothelioma of bone: A study of 29 cases. Cancer (46): 804–814, 1980.
66. Zachariades N, Papadakou A, Koundouris J, Constantinidis J, Angelopoulos, AP. Primary hemangioendotheliosarcoma of the mandible—Review of the literature and report of case. J Oral Surg (38): 288–296, 1980.
67. Farr HW, Carandang CM, Huvos AG. Malignant vascular tumors of the head and neck. Am J Surg (120): 501–504, 1970.
68. Backwinkel KD, Diddams JA. Hemangiopericytoma—Report of a case and comprehensive review of the literature. Cancer (25): 896–901, 1970.
69. Enzinger FM, Smith BH. Hemangiopericytoma. An analysis of 106 cases. Hum Pathol (7): 61–82, 1976.
70. Brauer MK, Gates PE, Doyle JL. Visceral Kaposi's sarcoma presenting with gingival lesions. Oral Surg (50): 151–155, 1980.
71. Farman AG, Uys PB. Oral Kaposi's sarcoma. Oral Surg (39): 288–296, 1975.
72. Stout AP, Lattes R. Tumors of the soft tissues. In Atlas of Tumour Pathology, Second Series, Fascicle 1. Washington D.C.: Armed Forces Institute of Pathology, 1967.
73. Sanerkin NG. Definitions of osteosarcoma, chondrosarcoma and fibrosarcoma of bone. Cancer (46): 178–185, 1980.
74. Rosenmertz SK, Schare HJ. Osteogenic sarcoma arising in Paget's disease of the mandible. Review of the literature and report of a case. Oral Surg (28): 304–309, 1969.
75. Garrington GE, Scofield HH, Cornyn J, Hooker SP. Osteosarcoma of the jaws. Analysis of 56 cases. Cancer (20): 377–391, 1967.
76. Curtis ML, Elmore JS, Sotereanos C. Osteosarcoma of the jaws: Report of case and review of the literature. J Oral Surg (32): 125–130, 1974.
77. Dahlin DC, Unni KK. Osteosarcoma of bone and its important recognizable varieties. Am J Surg Pathol (1): 61–72, 1977.
78. Unni KK, Dahlin DC, McLeod RA, Pritchard DJ. Intraosseous well-differentiated osteosarcoma. Cancer (40): 1337–1347, 1977.
79. Unni KK, Dahlin DC, Beabout JW, Ivins JC. Parosteal osteogenic sarcoma. Cancer (37): 2466–2475, 1976.
80. Newland JR, Ayala AG. Parosteal osteosarcoma of the maxilla. Oral Surg (43): 727–734, 1977.
81. Bras JM, Donner R, van der Kwast WAM, Snow GB, van der Waal I. Juxtacortical osteogenic sarcoma of the jaws. Review of the literature and report of a case. Oral Surg (50): 535–544, 1980.
82. Russ JE, Jesse RH. Management of osteosarcoma of the maxilla and mandible. Am J Surg (140): 572–576, 1980.
83. Schajowicz F, Ackerman LV, Sissons HA. Histological typing of bone and tumours. Geneva, World Health Organization, 1972.
84. Waldron CA, Shafer WG. The central giant cell granuloma of the jaws. An analysis of 38 cases. Am J Clin Path (45): 437–447, 1966.
85. Richter KJ, Freeman NS, Quick CA. Chondrosarcoma of the temporomandibular joint: Report of a case. J Oral Surg (32): 777–781, 1974.
86. Chaudhry AP, Robinovitch MR, Mitchell DF, Vickers RA. Chondrogenic tumours of the jaws. Am J Surg (102): 403–411, 1961.

87. Sato K, Nukaga H, Horikoshi T. Chondrosarcoma of the jaws and facial skeleton: A review of the Japanese literature. J Oral Surg (35): 892–897, 1977.
88. Evans HL, Ayala AG, Romsdahl MM. Prognostic factors in chondrosarcoma of bone. A clinicopathologic analysis with emphasis on histologic grading. Cancer (40): 818–831, 1977.
89. Unni KK, Dahlin DC, Beabout JW, Sim FH. Chondrosarcoma: Clear-cell variant. A report of sixteen cases. J Bone Joint Surg (58A): 676–683, 1976.
90. Slootweg PJ. Clear-cell chondrosarcoma of the maxilla: Report of a case. Oral Surg (50): 233–237, 1980.
91. Salvador AH, Beabout JW, Dahlin DC. Mesenchymal chondrosarcoma—Observations on 30 new cases. Cancer (28): 605–615, 1971.
92. Dabska M, Huvos AG. Mesenchymal chondrosarcoma in the young. Virchows Arch (Path Anat) (399): 89–104, 1983.
93. Dahlin DC, Coventry MB, Scanlon PW. Ewing's sarcoma. A critical analysis of 165 cases. J Bone Joint Surg (43A): 185–192, 1961.
94. Roca AN, Smith JL, MacComb WS, Bao-Shan J. Ewing's sarcoma of the maxilla and mandible. Study of six cases. Oral Surg (25): 194–203, 1968.
95. de Santos LA, Jing B-S. Radiographic findings of Ewing's sarcoma of the jaw. Br J Radiol (51): 682–687, 1978.
96. Schajowicz F. Ewing's sarcoma and reticulum-cell sarcoma of bone. With special reference to the histochemical demonstration of glycogen as an aid to differential diagnosis. J Bone Joint Surg (41A): 349–356, 1959.
97. Schnitzer B, Weaver DK. Lymphoreticular disorders. In Tumors of the Head and Neck, 2nd ed, Batsakis JG (ed). Baltimore: Williams & Wilkins, 1979.
98. Tabachnick TT, Levine B. Multiple myeloma involving the jaws and oral soft tissues. J Oral Surg (34): 931–933, 1976.
99. Christensen RE, Sanders B, Mudd B. Local recurrence of solitary plasmacytoma of the mandible. J Oral Surg (36): 311–313, 1978.
100. Raley LL, Granite EL. Plasmacytoma of the maxilla: Report of case. Oral Surg (35): 497–500, 1977.
101. Kraut RA, Buhler JE, La Rue JR, Acevedo A. Amyloidosis associated with multiple myeloma. Oral Surg (43): 63–68, 1977.
102. Flick WG, Lawrence FR. Oral amyloidosis as initial symptom of multiple myeloma. Oral Surg (49): 18–20, 1980.
103. Christopherson WM, Miller AJ. A re-evaluation of solitary plasma-cell myeloma of bone. Cancer (3): 240–252, 1950.
104. Peters RA, Beltaos E, Greenlaw RH, Schloesser LL. Intraoral extranodal Hodgkin's disease. J Oral Surg (35): 311–312, 1977.
105. Rappaport H. Tumors of hematopoietic system. In Atlas of Tumor Pathology, Section III, Fascicle 8. Washington, D.C.: Armed Forces Institute of Pathology, 1966.
106. Rappaport H. Discussion II: Round table discussion of histopathologic classification. Cancer Treat Rep (61): 1037–1048, 1977.
107. Tomich CE, Shafer WG. Lymphoproliferative disease of the hard palate. A clinicopathologic entity. A study of twenty-one cases. Oral Surg (39): 754–768, 1975.
108. Blok P. van Delden L, van der Waal I. Non-Hodgkin's lymphoma of the hard palate. Oral Surg (47): 445–452, 1979.
109. Harsany DL, Ross J, Fee WE. Follicular lymphoid hyperplasia of the hard palate simulating lymphoma. Otolaryngol Head Neck Surg (88): 349–356, 1980.
110. Wright JM, Dunsworth AR. Follicular lymphoid hyperplasia of the hard palate: A benign lymphoproliferative process. Oral Surg (55): 162–168, 1983.
111. Batsakis JG. Wegener's granulomatosis and midline (nonhealing) "granuloma." Head and Neck Surg (1): 213–222, 1979.
112. Mittelman D, Kaban LB. Recurrent non-Hodgkin's lymphoma presenting with gingival enlargement (report of a case). Oral Surg (42): 792–800, 1976.
113. Fritz GW, Petti NA, Abitbol A, Thelmo WL. Extranodal malignant histiocytic lymphoma of the cheek: report of case. J Oral Surg (38): 200–202, 1980.
114. Laskaris GC, Nicolis GD, Capetanakis JB. Mycosis fungoides with oral manifestations. Oral Surg (46): 40–42, 1978.

115. Wright JM, Balciunas BA, Muus JH. Mycosis fungoides with oral manifestations; report of a case and review of the literature. Oral Surg (51): 24–31, 1981.
116. Campbell RL, Kelly DE, Burkes EJ. Primary reticulum cell sarcoma of the mandible. Review of the literature and report of a case. Oral Surg (39): 918–928, 1975.
117. Lian SL, Nagai T, Kawasaki H, Sakaizumi K, Nakamura Y. Reticulum cell sarcoma of the jaws. Report of two cases and comparison of incidence in Japan and other countries. Oral Surg (50): 110–115, 1980.
118. Dorfman RF, Warnke R. Lymphadenopathy simulating the malignant lymphomas. Hum Pathol (5): 519–550, 1974.
119. Burkitt D. A sarcoma involving the jaws in African children. Brit J Surg (46): 218–223, 1958.
120. Terrill DG, Lee A, Le Donne MA, Nusbaum TG. American Burkitt's lymphoma in Pittsburgh, Pennsylvania. Oral Surg (44): 411–418, 1977.
121. Adatia AK. Significance of jaw lesions in Burkitt's lymphoma. Br Dent J (145): 263–266, 1978.
122. Haddow AJ. In Burkitt's Lymphoma, Burkitt DP and Wright DH (eds). Edinburgh and London: Livingstone, 1970.
123. Epstein MA, Achong BG. In Burkitt's Lymphoma. Burkitt DP and Wright DH (eds). Edinburgh and London: Livingstone, 1970.
124. Adatia AK. Dental tissues and Burkitt's tumor. Oral Surg (25): 221–234, 1968.
125. Hupp JR, Collins FJV, Ross A, Myall RWT. A review of Burkitt's lymphoma. Importance of radiographic diagnosis. J max-fac Surg (10): 240–245, 1982.
126. Carrington CB, Liebow AA. Limited forms of angiitis and granulomatosis of Wegener's type. Am J Med (41): 497–527, 1966.
127. Scott J, Finch LD. Wegener's granulomatosis presenting as gingivitis. Oral Surg (34): 920–933, 1972.
128. Shillitoe EJ, Lehner T, Lessof MH, Harrison DFN. Immunological features of Wegener's granulomatosis. Lancet (1): 281–284, 1974.
129. Waterhouse J, Muir C, Powell J (eds). Cancer Incidence in Five Continents. vol. IV. Int. Lyon: Agency for Research on Cancer, 1982.
130. Liversedge RL. Oral malignant melanoma. Brit J Oral Surg (13): 40–45, 1975.
131. Broomhall C, Lewis MG. Malignant melanoma of the oral cavity in Ugandan Africans. Brit J Surg (54): 581–584, 1967.
132. Takagi M, Ishikawa G, Mori W. Primary malignant melanoma of the oral cavity in Japan. With special reference to mucosal melanosis. Cancer (34): 358–370, 1964.
133. Trodahl JN, Sprague WG. Benign and malignant melanocytic lesions of the oral mucosa. An analysis of 135 cases. Cancer (25): 812–823, 1970.
134. Chaudhry AP, Hampel A, Gorlin RJ. Primary malignant melanoma of the oral cavity. A review of 105 cases. Cancer (11): 923–928, 1958.
135. Lea AJ. Malignant melanoma of the skin: The relationship to trauma. Ann Roy Coll Surg Eng (37): 169–176, 1965.
136. Snow GB, van der Esch EP, van Slooten EA. Mucosal melanomas of the head and neck. Head and Neck Surg (1): 24–30, 1978.
137. McGovern VJ, Mihm MC, Bailly C, Booth JC, Clark WH, Cochran AJ, Hardy EG, Hicks JD, Levene A, Lewis MG, Little JH, Milton GW. The classification of malignant melanoma and its histologic reporting. Cancer (32): 1446–1457, 1973.
138. Regezi JA, Hayward JR, Pickens TN. Superficial melanomas of oral mucous membranes. Oral Surg (45): 730–740, 1978.
139. Ackerman LV, del Regato JA. Cancer, Diagnosis, Treatment and Prognosis, 4th ed. St. Louis: C.V. Mosby, 1970.
140. Clark WH Jr, From L, Bernadino EA, Mihm MC. The histogenesis and biologic behavior of primary human malignant melanomas of the skin. Cancer Res (29): 705–727, 1969.
141. Oikarinen VJ, Calonius PEB, Sainio P. Metastatic tumours to the oral region. I. An analysis of cases in the literature. Proc Finn Dent Soc (71): 58–65, 1975.
142. Cohen B. Secondary tumours of the mandible. Ann Roy Coll Surg Eng (23): 118–130, 1958.
143. Clausen F, Poulsen H. Metastastic carcinoma to the jaws. Acta Path Microbiol Scand (57): 361–374, 1963.
144. Stypulkowska J, Bartkowski S, Panas M, Zaleska M. Metastatic tumors to the jaws and oral cavity. J Oral Surg (37): 805–808, 1979.

# II. TREATMENT

Oral Oncology brings the subject of neoplasia, its diagnosis, and management up to date and presents in a very inclusive manner the state-of-the-art as it is practiced today. The functions of the oral cavity include the intake of food and fluid, mastication and transport of these substances to the pharynx, and, in addition to these physiological functions, participates in sound articulation and breathing and is both directly and indirectly associated with the esthetics of the mid- and lower-third of the face. This combination of factors adds a special importance to this region that demands specific understanding and management. Any treatment directed against benign or malignant neoplasia in this area must detail the nuances of options and complications of an ever-changing variety of surgical techniques, great advances in radiotherapy, and the introduction of chemotherapeutic agents. This treatment program must be coordinated to comply with the gravity of the tumor, either as a single therapeutic force or in combination.

There has been an increase in the recognition of the value of reconstruction of the large defects that are natural consequences of aggressive treatment in this area of a malignant neoplasm. In addition to the technique of rehabilitative surgery, it is necessary to include the use of certain prosthetic devices.

Chapter 5's discussion of treatment has been handled admirably by Professor Snow, who reviews surgical treatment. Professor Cummings elucidates the radiotherapeutic aspects, and Professors Pitman and Bertino cover the chemotherapeutic advances. Professor Tiwari reviews the reconstructive aspects, and Professor Engels covers the prosthetic rehabilitation and dental care. This interdisciplinary team of authors has created a superb collection of papers that describe the best possible chances not only for patient survival, but also for a meaningful life.

The detail of the writing is so complete and complemented by extensive bibliographies in such a way that the book not only has immediate value to specialists in this field, but also can be used profitably by physicians in training as a textbook. No therapeutic modality is omitted, yet proper emphasis is placed on the most essential and most effective types of procedures under accurate classification and criteria. The reconstructive procedures described incorporate both the well-tested and tried standard methods, as well as the new myocutaneous and microvascular techniques.

The value of the oral prosthesis is appreciated most by the individuals who are best rehabilitated in this manner. There are certain situations in radical head and neck surgery where a prosthesis rehabilitates the patient better than any series of protracted and complicated surgical endeavors. This recognition is important in the management of these problems.

JOHN CONLEY

# 5. SURGICAL TREATMENT OF MALIGNANT TUMORS OF THE ORAL CAVITY

G.B. SNOW

## 1. INTRODUCTION

Squamous cell carcinomas make up the great majority of malignant tumors of the oral cavity. There is no unanimity as to the preferred method of treatment of oral cavity carcinoma. Depending on the policy of the institution, the primary cancer is treated either surgically or by radiotherapy. In locally advanced tumors the common practice is to apply radiation therapy as a pre- or postoperative adjuvant to surgical resection. Solid evidence to support the validity of this combined approach, however, is lacking. Although chemotherapy and to a minor degree immunotherapy have received much interest over the last decade, their role in the management of oral cancer has yet to be defined. Treatment of metastatic neck nodes has traditionally been by surgery, although elective irradiation of the neck has been recommended for the management of occult metastasis.

In this chapter the surgical management of oral cavity carcinoma will be reviewed. Certain basic principles of surgical treatment of oral cancer will be discussed. A number of controversies surrounding surgical procedures will be highlighted. As many excellent textbooks and atlases are available on surgical techniques, these will not be dealt with in detail. The role of combined therapy will be analysed. The results of surgical management of cancer of the

*I. van der Waal and G.B. Snow (eds), ORAL ONCOLOGY.* 

various sites within the mouth will be reviewed. The complications of surgical treatment will be presented. Cryosurgery and laser surgery will be mentioned briefly.

## 2. GENERAL ASPECTS OF SURGICAL TREATMENT OF ORAL CANCER

### 2.1. Selection of patients

During the past 25 years major advances have been made in the development of surgery for head and neck cancer. Sophisticated techniques of reconstruction allow for repair of almost every defect. At present virtually every structure in the head and neck can be resected and repaired safely. Furthermore, oral cancer is rarely inoperable on account of its local, regional, or distant spread. However, when the magnitude of the resection will be such that the patient will be left with a functional deficit resulting in a poor future quality of life, the question arises whether the patient is better off left untreated by surgery. An example of this problem in surgery for oral cancer is when total removal of the tongue is required to eradicate the disease. No general clues can be given to this problem; the solution should be individualised for each patient, philosophy and psychology of both patient and doctor playing an important role.

Anaplastic carcinomas should not be treated surgically but by radiotherapy. This also holds true for most of the poorly differentiated squamous cell carcinomas. Both histologic types of tumor, however, are rare in the oral cavity. Very rapidly progressing well- or moderately differentiated squamous cell carcinomas—an unusual situation—should probably better not be attacked by surgery as the first modality of treatment.

Finally, of course, are medical contraindications for surgery. In general, patients over 80 years of age should not be subjected to major head and neck surgery (see later discussion on mortality).

### 2.2. Management of the primary tumor

Careful examination of the cancer, including digital palpation, should form the basis for assessing the choice of surgical procedure. Whenever doubtful about the exact extent of the tumor, local examination under general anaesthesia should be performed. This is particularly helpful when the lesion is painful or posteriorly situated. Also important is the appraisal of the defect likely to result after excision in terms of its several components, mucosa, soft tissue, and bone, so that a general outline of the ensuing reconstructive procedure can be made if necessary. Whenever a segmental resection of the mandible or a maxillectomy is envisaged, this appraisal should be carried out with a dental colleague to allow for preparation of necessary appliances.

Premalignant lesions, carcinoma in situ, and small cancers situated anteriorly can be excised readily through the mouth, that is, by transoral approach (figure 5–1). Adequate exposure of larger cancers and more posteriorly situated tumors requires that the lower lip be divided in the midline and a

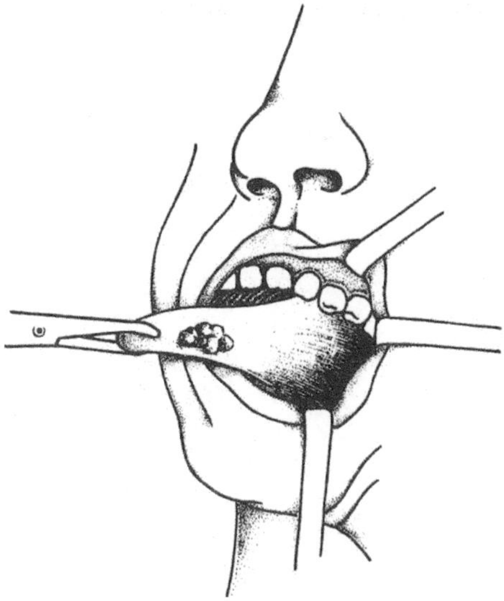

**Figure 5–1.** Small cancers situated anteriorly can be excised through the open mouth.

cheek flap elevated on the side of the lesion (figure 5–2). Division of the lower lip in zigzags results in a less conspicuous scar. On occasion sectioning the mandible stepwise in the midline may be advantageous to obtain adequate access. Subsequently, the mucosa of the floor of the mouth is incised on the side of the lesion, and the anterior belly of the digastric muscle and the mylohyoid muscle are transected. The hemimandible can then be retracted with the cheek flap with a hook (figure 5–3). This mandibular "swing" approach [1,2], which provides wide exposure, is particularly indicated in patients with posteriorly situated tumors and heavy dentate mandibles likely to provide an obstacle to exposure. After the excision of the tumor is completed, the mandible is easily rewired. In large tumors of the anterior floor of the mouth, adequate exposure may be achieved through a visor flap approach, which respects the integrity of the lower lip (figure 5–4). When excision through the open mouth is not possible for cancers in the superior part of the oral cavity, the upper lip is divided and a modified Weber-Fergusson approach is used (figure 5–5).

An important point concerns the adequacy of the extent of surgical margins in oral cancer. Particularly, cancers of the tongue and floor of the mouth may spread easily along submucosal, muscular, and neural planes. It has been brought forward that a margin of 2 cm in all three dimensions is therefore required for all cancers of the tongue [3]. Ballantyne [4] contends that this is necessary for all tongue cancers and advocates determining the extent of the margins in each individual case by clinical evaluation during the surgical pro-

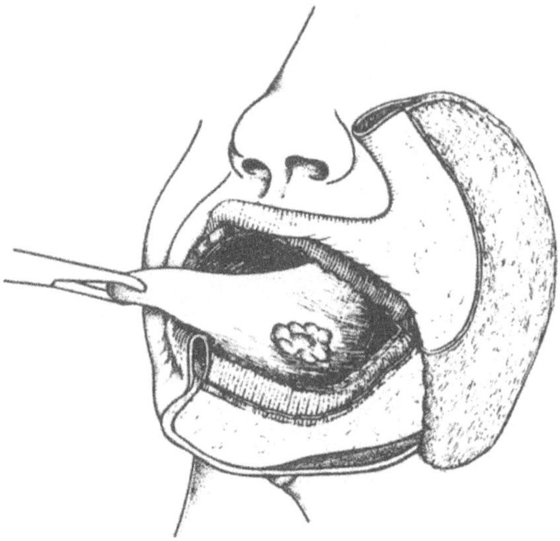

**Figure 5–2.** Adequate exposure of larger and more posteriorly situated tumors often requires that the lower lip is divided and a cheek flap elevated.

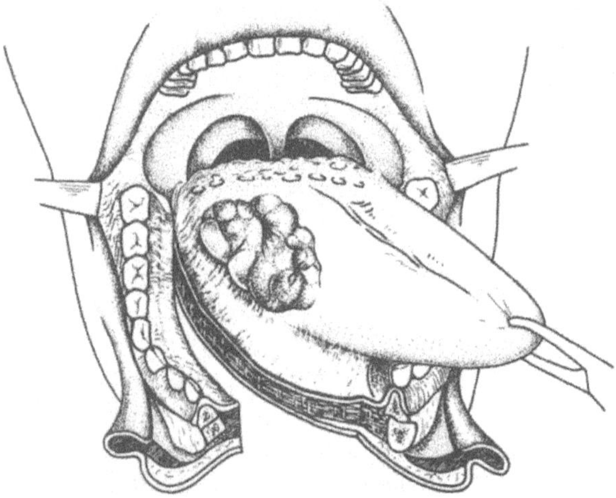

**Figure 5–3.** Exposure of posterior cancers is facilitated by mandibular division and "swing." This is particularly helpful in patients with heavy dentate mandibles.

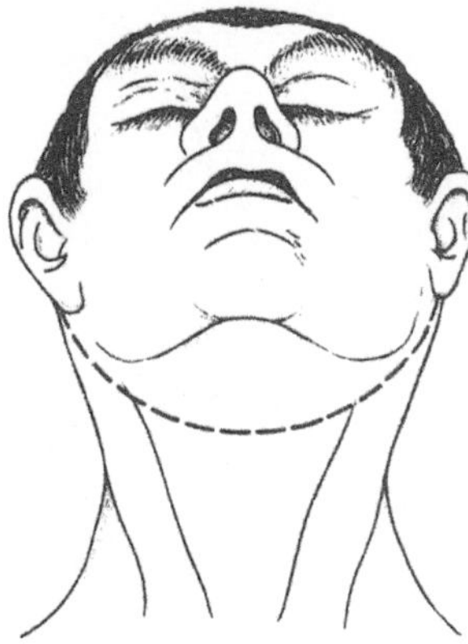

**Figure 5–4.** Visor-flap approach provides adequate exposure of large tumors of the anterior floor of the mouth while respecting the integrity of the lower lip.

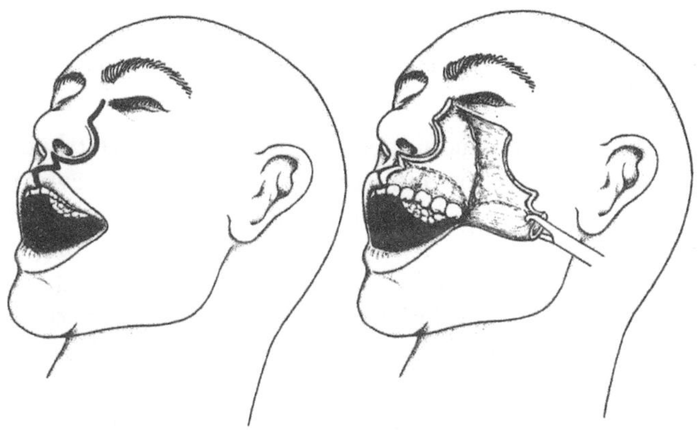

**Figure 5-5.** Upper cheek flap elevated for exposure of larger cancers of the palate or superior alveolar arch.

cedure and with the aid of frozen section microscopic studies. Byers et al. [5] have demonstrated the reliability of the frozen section technique in predicting local control for $T_1$, $T_2$, and $T_3$ tumors. The author of this chapter has found electrocoagulation of the tumor before the excision has begun very helpful in determining the extent of the lesion. Electrocoagulation as the first step of the surgical procedure became routine in our institution some 15 years ago and was primarily aimed at devitalizing the ulcerating surface of the cancer before the excision is carried out so as to minimize the risk of iatrogenic implantation metastasis. Gradually the electrocoagulation procedure has been extended until healthy tissue, at least on macroscopic appearance, is reached. It became apparent

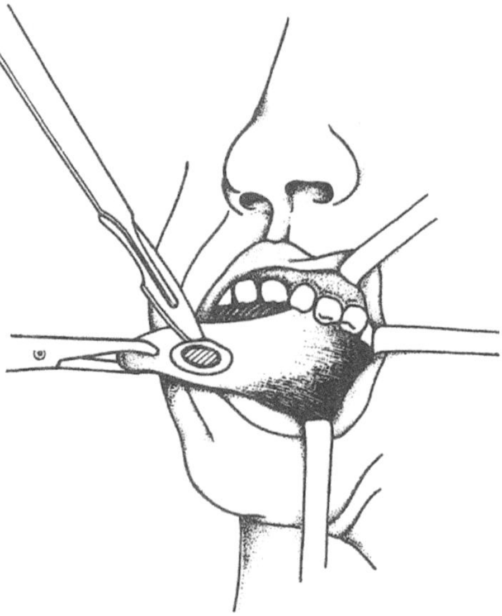

**Figure 5–6.** Excision of tongue cancer after electrocoagulation of the tumor.

that this procedure enables the surgeon to assess more accurately the extent of the tumor than by inspection and palpation alone, because even the smaller offshoots of the tumor can be recognised as they appear as small white points in the underlying red muscle. Another advantage is that during the ensuing phase of excision, the mass of the tumor is no longer in the way. After irrigation with a cell-killing solution of sublimate 1/1,000, the coagulated area is then excised with a clearance of 1 cm (figure 5–6).

Another potential problem in tumors of the inferior complex of the oral cavity consisting of the tongue, the floor of the mouth, and the lower gum, which is closely related both to the aspects of exposure and surgical margins outlined above, is that of management of the mandible. From the point of view of the mandible, patients fall into three categories: those with gross invasion where resection is inevitable, those with a degree of involvement, and those in whom there is still a measurable distance of a few mm of normal mucosa between the gross edge of the lesion and the mandible. It has been held that the mandible, although uninvolved by tumor, should be resected in large tumors of the tongue and the floor of the mouth so as to get better access to the primary tumor and to facilitate primary closure. With the available procedures of exposure outlined above and the methods of reconstruction discussed in chapter 8, this view is certainly obsolete. It has also been stated that the lymphatic channels draining the tongue and the floor of the mouth communicate with the periosteal lymphatics of the mandible and that this necessitates resection of the bone. This view too is to be discarded since Marchetta et al. [6]

and Carter et al. [7] have clearly demonstrated that involvement of the periosteum or the underlying bone is by direct extension of the tumor and not through periosteal lymphatics. In most patients belonging to the two last categories mentioned above, a more conservative management of the mandible, marginal mandibulectomy, is to be considered. Whether this procedure can be carried out safely depends on the relationship between the tumor and the mandible. This is assessed by bimanual palpation, preferably under general anaesthesia, and radiographs (see later in this chapter). In general marginal mandibulectomy is justified when the tumor is superior to the mylohyoid line, unless it concerns an edentulous mandible with major atrophy of the bone [8].

### 2.3. Management of cervical lymph nodes

For any patient who has clinical evidence of cervical node involvement, a radical neck dissection is carried out. When nodal metastasis is present on admission, the neck operation is performed in continuity with the excision of the primary tumor because viable tumor cells may be present in the lymphatics between the primary and the regional nodes. However, Spiro and Strong [9] have demonstrated that the principle of incontinuity neck dissection may be abandoned in selected patients without affecting the cure rate.

Controversy exists regarding the treatment policy of the clinically negative neck ($N_0$). Long-standing, continuing discussion as to the indications for elective radical neck dissection [10] is furthermore complicated by the more recent publications that elective irradiation of the neck might be equally effective in eliminating microscopic nodal disease (see chapter 6). In general, elective treatment of regional neck nodes is considered indicated when there is a high likelihood of occult nodal metastasis, when the status of the cervical nodes cannot be adequately assessed as in patients with short muscular necks, when the patient will not be available for regular follow-up visits, or when the neck must be entered for the resection of the primary tumor.

Until recently, the classical radical neck dissection, as described by Crile [11] in 1906 and reemphasized by Martin et al. [12] and Beahrs et al. (13), has not been challenged. In 1967 Bocca and Pignataro [14] introduced a "conservation" neck dissection, which later became widely known as functional neck dissection, for the control of regional metastasis when disease in the neck is either occult or still confined to mobile lymph nodes. The anatomic rationale of functional neck dissection involves the concept of the neck being a group of aponeurotic compartments, filled with areolar tissue and lymphatics, which are distinct from the muscular, vascular, and neural structures. Accordingly, in this technique the spinal accessory nerve, the sternocleidomastoid muscle, and the internal jugular vein are preserved. Bocca and other advocates [15,16,17, 18,19,20] of this operation state that from the oncological point of view these structures may be saved as long as metastatic tumor has not spread beyond the capsule of the nodes and that in those cases the procedure is oncologically equally effective but less mutilating as standard radical neck dissection. Extranodal spread as demonstrated histologically in neck dissection specimens has indeed been shown by many [21,22,23,24,25,26,27,28] to be strongly correlated with local recurrence in the neck and thus to bear heavily on prognosis. Functional neck dissection would certainly not appear to be an adequate procedure when extranodal spread is present. The question then arises as to how one can assess clinically whether extranodal spread is present. Until recently, it has been held that nodes less than 3 cm in diameter do not have extracapsular spread. Cachin et al. [26], Johnson et al. [27], and Snow et al. [28], however, have demonstrated clearly that nodes less than 3 cm in diameter do show extracapsular spread in a high percentage. In the first and the last of these three studies, evidence of extranodal spread was even present in 14% and 22%, respectively, of nodes that were less than 1 cm in diameter. These findings strongly caution against preservation of a structure like the internal jugular vein which has such a close relationship to the most frequently involved groups of nodes.

The question whether the spinal accessory nerve may be preserved deserves special attention, if only for the fact that the most disabling alteration of function following the classical radical neck dissection is the "shoulder syndrome" resulting from the sacrifice of the spinal accessory nerve. This syndrome is characterized by a weakened, deformed, and often painful shoulder with a considerable decreased range of motion. The degree of discomfort varies considerably, but in general patients feel more handicapped than is commonly believed [29]. Dargent [30] in 1945 was one of the first advocates of preservation of the nerve in selected cases when peripheral nodes were not involved, followed, among others, by Pietrantoni [31]. Recent reports by Clarenfelt et al. [32] and Brandenburg et al. [33] strongly suggest that the spinal accessory nerve may indeed be preserved without jeopardizing the chances of cure in elective neck dissections and selected therapeutic neck dissections. In both reports, however, selection is not furthermore specified. Obviously, patients in whom the site and size of the primary tumor do not favour spread to lymph nodes adjacent to the course of the nerve would be considered candidates for the procedure. Schuller et al. [34], however, caution that preservation of the nerve cannot be justified solely on the basis of an infrequent relationship to cancerous nodes. Although nodal metastases along the spinal accessory nerve in its course through the posterior triangle of the neck are rare [35], Schuller et al. [34] have demonstrated clearly that metastases are not uncommon along the superior portion of the nerve, where it is intimately associated with the proximal end of the internal jugular vein and related lymphatics. The feasibility of preservation of the spinal accessory nerve in each individual case has to be carefully evaluated by the surgeon during the dissection. Nahum [36] rightly states that variations in technique of radical neck dissection, such as preservation of the eleventh cranial nerve, should be performed by surgeons with wide experience with the procedure. The technique of preservation of this nerve has recently been described by Becker et al. [37].

Interestingly, preservation of the nerve does not preclude impaired shoulder function. Clarenfelt and Eliasson [38] found persisting major paresis in 17% of their patients in whom the spinal accessory nerve had been preserved. On the other hand, physical therapy rehabilitation programs can minimize shoulder problems in selective patients in whom the nerve has been sacrificed [39].

Suprahyoid neck dissection is another modification. It is particularly tempting to carry out this procedure in patients with a clinically negative neck when the neck must be entered for the resection of a primary tumor in the oral cavity. Chu et al. [40], however, have demonstrated that this operation is associated with a high recurrence rate in the neck below the level of dissection, even in patients with histologically negative nodes. Its use, therefore, is to be discarded.

It is realised that one may take a different view from the one just expressed at the various types of neck dissection if they are combined with radiation therapy, as is being practised at the M.D. Anderson Hospital [41]. However, one must remember that the surgical and radiotherapeutic expertise needed for such approach is available at a few centres only.

## 3. GENERAL ASPECTS OF COMBINED THERAPY FOR ORAL CANCER

### 3.1. Radiation and surgery

Combined radiation and surgery became popular in the 1960s for advanced head and neck cancers at certain sites, such as in the oral cavity. These advanced lesions pose primarily a locally recurrent or regionally metastatic problem. This multimodality approach attempts to increase the effectiveness of therapy to these problem areas. The philosophy behind this type of treatment is that surgery fails at the periphery and radiotherapy at the poorly oxygenated centre of the tumor and that, hopefully, a combination of the two might do better than either alone.

Radiotherapy can be administered either preoperatively or postoperatively; both methods have their advantages and disadvantages [42]. Preoperative radiation is supposed to sterilize tumor cells at the margin of the tumor and to reduce the risk of implantation of metastasis within the surgical field and of iatrogenic metastasis beyond the head and neck. However, it entails the disadvantage of increasing the complication rate of surgery. Furthermore, it limits the possibility of more directed postoperative radiation when this is desirable. Another disadvantage of preoperative radiotherapy is that it may obscure tumor margins, which may render it very difficult for the surgeon to determine the adequacy of resection margins. Postoperative radiotherapy carries three advantages: on the basis of the histopathological report of the surgical specimen, radiation can be justified and planned more selectively, it has no influence on surgical complication rates, and it is usually better tolerated by the patient than preoperative radiation therapy. However, at least on theoretical grounds, radiotherapy is assumed to be less effective when the vascularisation of the tissues has been disrupted by previous surgery. Furthermore, postoperative irradiation may be delayed by complications in wound healing. Finally, it obviously has no influence on any iatrogenic metastasis to distant sites.

Most experiences have been gained with preoperative radiation therapy. Terz and Lawrence [43] recently have reviewed all literature reporting the results of clinical experience with preoperative radiation for head and neck cancer between 1969 and 1979. Regarding retrospective studies the evidence is conflicting. Initial studies in selected patient populations have reported a beneficial role of radiation therapy as a preoperative adjunct. In contrast, later studies [44,45] could not establish that combined therapy offers improvement over surgery alone. More importantly, all three randomized prospective clinical trials [46,47,48] failed to demonstrate any higher survival for those patients receiving preoperative radiation when compared with control groups treated by surgery alone. The question regarding the role of preoperative radiotherapy in the management of head and neck cancer finally appears to have been answered by the outcome of these randomized trials. To this conclusion the objection might be raised that the low doses of irradiation used in two of these three randomized studies might not be as effective as higher doses given over a longer period of time. The higher incidence of postoperative complications associated with higher doses, however, may well preclude the feasibility of such a preoperative radiation approach.

An increasing number of reports advocate postoperative radiation therapy rather than preoperative irradiation [49,50,51,52,53]. The histopathological information on the resected specimen can be used to select the patients who are most likely to benefit from combined treatment, that is, those patients with a significant probability of local and/or regional failure after surgery only. The value of postoperative irradiation therapy has been demonstrated particularly in regard to failure in the neck. The reported recurrence rate in the neck after radical neck dissection alone varies from 14 to 30% [54,55,56]. Such recurrences depend directly on the extent of metastatic disease present at the time of surgery. Histopathologic examination of the neck dissection specimen has been shown to be far more accurate than nodal palpability in the assessment of the extent of metastatic disease in the neck. Particularly when extranodal spread and multiple histologically positive nodes are present, there is a high risk of recurrence in the neck [23,24,26,27,28]. In these cases surgery should be followed by radiotherapy. Jesse and Fletcher [56] and Bartelink et al. [53] have demonstrated that postoperative radiation therapy is effective in reducing the number of recurrences in the neck. Regarding the primary tumor, indications for postoperative radiotherapy include adverse findings as inadequate margins of surgical resection or perineural invasion. If irradiation is given postoperatively, it must cover the entire operated area that is at risk of having been infested. When there is a substantial risk of contralateral neck node metastasis, postoperative irradiation is given to the opposite side of the neck as well. An important point in postoperative radiotherapy, as stressed by Jesse and Lindberg [49], is that it preferably should be started within three to four weeks after the surgical procedure. Vikram [57] demonstrated in a small series of patients that delay in the start of postoperative radiation therapy might indeed affect the results adversely. The surgical procedure must therefore provide rapid primary healing. Immediate repair is essential. Staged methods of reconstruction should be avoided.

Many studies have observed that decrease of local and regional failures by combined therapy is not reflected in a proportionate increase of the five-years survival rates. As fewer patients die from uncontrolled disease in the head and neck, more are exposed to the risk of disseminated disease below the clavicles. Efforts should be directed toward the development of adjuvant chemotherapy regimens effective in destroying micrometastases.

### 3.2. Chemotherapy and surgery

Several effective chemotherapeutic agents in head and neck cancer are available, such as methotrexate, cis-platinum, and bleomycin. The recognition that surgery and radiotherapy have reached a plateau in their ability to cure head and neck cancer has recently stimulated the integration of chemotherapy into combined modality treatment. The data available at present are still minimal and do not allow for definitive evaluation of the role of chemotherapy as an adjunct to surgery or to combined surgery and radiotherapy. Certain observations, however, can be made.

Chemotherapy can be used either preoperatively or postoperatively. Preoperative chemotherapy aims at initial tumor shrinkage. Chemotherapy ranks first in the order of treatment, based on the experience that chemotherapy is more effective in the untreated case than after surgery (or radiotherapy), when the blood supply to the tumor has been seriously interfered with. Most experiences have been gained with methotrexate as a single agent. There is a continuing controversy over the intra-arterial route of administration versus systemic administration. Response rates to preoperative methotrexate vary from 40 to 70%, depending on the site of the tumor within the head and neck, the histologic degree of differentiation of the squamous cell carcinoma, and the dose schedule of methotrexate [58]. Methotrexate as a single agent is well tolerated by the patient, and surgery following methotrexate is not fraught with any more complications than surgery alone. No randomized clinical trials have been carried out to compare the results of preoperative methotrexate followed by surgery with those of surgery alone. The key question regarding whether good responders to methotrexate will do better in the long run, therefore, cannot be answered. Although multiple drug regimens are likely shown to be superior to methotrexate as a single agent in advanced recurrent head and neck cancer [59], this has yet to be demonstrated for untreated advanced though operable cases. Multiple drug regimens, moreover, are associated with more toxicity and may well preclude their feasibility as a preoperative adjunct.

Postoperative chemotherapy—adjuvant chemotherapy in *sensu strictu*—aims at destruction of micrometastases or microresidual tumors. In patients at high risk for local/regional recurrence or distant metastases, chemotherapy is started shortly after conventional therapy, when the total number of tumor cells is in the chemotherapeutically curable range, and continued on an intermittent maintenance schedule. It is assumed that each treatment kills a fraction of tumor cells, and it is hoped that repeated treatment will result in cure.

It is generally felt that such chemotherapy is not as yet feasible in head and neck cancer. One of the many problems associated with the design of studies of this kind of chemotherapy is the definition of those groups of patients at high risk for recurrence in the head and neck or distant metastases. Usually these groups are defined on the basis of TNM classification, that is, on clinical grounds. In oral cancer neck node metastasis is the single most important prognostic factor. Difficulty in assessing lymph node involvement, however, is generally appreciated. Usually an overall error of 20 to 25% in assessing the presence or absence of cervical lymph node metastases from clinical evaluation alone is reported. Histopathologic examination of neck dissection specimens has been shown to be far more accurate than nodal palpability in the assessment of the extent of metastatic disease in the neck (see earlier discussion). A strong plea is made to include such histologic parameters in the criteria of selection for randomized trials which aim to assess the role of adjuvant chemotherapy.

## 4. SURGICAL TREATMENT OF CANCER AT SPECIFIC SITES WITHIN THE ORAL CAVITY

### 4.1. Carcinoma of the mobile part of the tongue

Small tumors of the oral tongue can be treated either by surgery or radiation therapy with an almost equal cure [60]. As the lesions increase in size and as they become more infiltrative, the results of surgery are considerably better than those obtained by radiation therapy [61]. Furthermore, there are a number of circumstances in which surgery is favoured over radiotherapy [4]. Surgery appears to be the treatment of choice for cancers occurring in patients who have multifocal leukoplakia and who can be expected to develop future cancers in the mouth and for cancer occurring in alcoholic smokers who tolerate radiation therapy poorly. Elderly patients tolerate the minimal morbidity of partial glossectomy better than the prolonged morbidity of radiation therapy. These circumstances naturally pertain to other sites within the oral cavity as well.

In $T_1$ and $T_2$ tumors, which fortunately constitute the great majority of tongue cancers today, partial glossectomy results in a high percentage of control at the primary site, in the order of 90% and 80%, respectively [62,63]. The defect is usually closed primarily; this does not impair tongue mobility to a great extent, because the floor of the mouth mucosa is stretched out. Large superficial defects resulting from excision of carcinoma in situ with extensive areas of leukoplakia are resurfaced with a split skin graft. Successful take of the graft depends on close and immobile contact between the graft and its bed. In a mobile area such as the tongue this can be achieved best with the so-called "quilting technique" [64]. Partial glossectomy requires only a few hospital days, and the effect on speech and swallowing is usually minimal.

In $T_3$ and $T_4$ tumors surgery of the en bloc composite type is needed, usually followed by major reconstruction procedures to restore oral function and cosmetic appearance. The rehabilitation of these patients has improved considerably through the recent advent of myocutaneous flaps, as will be discussed in chapter 8.

Cancer of the tongue is a highly aggressive disease. The single most important prognostic factor is the status of the cervical lymph nodes. This is well demonstrated by the figures from Memorial Hospital as reported by Harrold [65]: for patients who never had metastatic nodes at any time, the five-year survival rate was 75% as compared to 18.5% for those with metastatic nodes on admission. The behaviour of these tumors with regard to their metastases to regional lymph nodes, therefore, is of utmost importance in establishing any plan of therapy. If suspicious nodes are palpable on admission, treatment should encompass both the primary tumor and the regional node areas; usually surgery of the en bloc composite type is indicated. When there is no clinical evidence of cervical node involvement, the problem is far more complex and many factors have to be taken into account.

Vandenbrouck et al. [66] are the only investigators to have carried out a randomized clinical trial to ascertain whether elective treatment of the neck is beneficial for patients with occult nodal metastasis as compared with those presenting later with clinical conversion. Their study concerns 75 patients with a squamous cell carcinoma of the mobile tongue or the floor of the mouth, staged $T_1N_0$, $T_2N_0$, or $T_3N_0$. These patients were divided into two groups. The first group comprised 39 patients who underwent elective radical neck dissection; nodal involvement was present in 49%, with extranodal spread in 13%. In the second group of 36 patients, neck disease appeared during follow-up in 19 cases. Therapeutic radical neck dissection was carried out in 17; the nodes were histologically positive in 15, 9 of which had extranodal spread. Although the second group demonstrated 25% of extranodal spread as compared to 13% in the first group, comparison of the survival curves did not reveal any difference between the two groups. The authors concluded that in cancer of the tongue and the floor of the mouth staged $T_1N_0$, $T_2N_0$, or $T_3N_0$, to delay neck dissection until a node becomes clinically detectable appears to be justified.

It should be realised, however, that in most institutions, based on indirect evidence, a more aggressive management policy as to the clinically negative neck is being carried out [67,68,69]. Cervical nodal metastasis is common throughout the clinical course of carcinoma of the tongue. The nodal conversion rate in $T_2N_0$ and $T_3N_0$ lesions is 25% and 50%, respectively. Treatment of late-onset cervical metastasis carries a poor prognosis: not more than 35% of these patients can be cured. Generally, therefore, elective treatment of the neck is considered indicated for lesions larger than 2 cm. Even 20% of patients who have a $T_1$ lesion and whose nodes are initially disease free will have a metastasis develop in the neck. Johnson et al. [70] have suggested guidelines that may aid in selecting patients with $T_1N_0$ lesions who require elective neck treatment.

If it is decided to treat the clinically negative neck, this can be done by surgery or by radiation therapy. The choice of treatment depends, among other factors, on the choice of treatment for the primary tumor. In lesions crossing or approaching the midline, radiation therapy offers the advantage of treating both sides of the neck.

### 4.2. Carcinoma of the floor of the mouth

In most European countries and in the United States, the floor of the mouth is the second most frequent site of cancer of the oral cavity, surpassed only by carcinoma of the tongue. Cancers of the tongue and floor of the mouth together account for approximately 70% of oral cancer [71]. The floor of the mouth is anatomically defined as the U-shaped groove anterior to the palatine folds, bounded laterally and anteriorly by gingiva, medially by the tongue, and inferiorly by the sublingual salivary glands and the supporting mylohyoid, hyoglossus, and geniohyoid muscles. The floor of the mouth can be arbitrarily divided into an anterior or sublingual area and a lateral or gingivolingual sulcus.

Helfrich et al. [72] in a series of 166 patients with a squamous carcinoma of the floor of the mouth found the following distribution of lesions: 64% were located in the lateral gingivolingual sulcus, in 29% the bulk of the tumor occupied the anterior floor of mouth with extension across the midline to the contralateral side, whereas only 7% of the lesions seemed to arise in the midline. Keim et al. [73] made the observation that lateral lesions usually assume an elongated shape, extending parallel to the axis of the floor of the mouth, while the anterior midline lesions tend to assume an almost circular shape. In a series of 804 patients with squamous cancer of the floor of the mouth, Harrold [74] reported the cancer was localised to the floor of the mouth in 23% of the patients and in the remainder it had invaded gingiva and/or tongue, either alone or in combination with another structure, with bone being involved in 15%. Hardingham et al. [75] found active invasion of the mandible causing radiological signs of bone erosion in only 7% of a series of 189 patients.

Lederman [76], in an illuminating study of the anatomy of cancer of the upper air and food passages, points to the importance of the anatomical relationships of the most posterior part of the lower alveololingual sulcus or retromylohyoid space. In this region the muscular and fascial floor of the oral cavity is absent, the mucous membrane alone forming the barrier between the oral cavity and tissue spaces of the neck. A neoplasm affecting the floor of the mouth in this particular region has, therefore, direct access to the neck. Lederman cautions that a carcinoma affecting this area should never be regarded purely as an intraoral carcinoma and that any treatment method restricting itself to the intraoral part of the disease alone is usually doomed to failure.

The incidence of cervical lymph node metastases at the time of initial treatment is approximately 50% [74,77]. Difficulty in assessing regional lymph node involvement is generally appreciated. In this particular site the fact that Wharton's duct may become involved by tumor and/or inflammation with secondary hypertrophy of the submandibular gland, which may be interpreted as adenopathy, adds to this problem. Harrold [74] reports that histologically proven cervical node metastasis was present on admission in 39%. Of those who had no involvement of nodes at the time of initial treatment, nodal involvement occurred in 17% during follow-up, so that a total of 56% had node metastasis at some time during the course of the disease. The incidence of bilateral cervical node metastasis at some time in the clinical course was 17%. An important observation by Harrold regarding the level of nodal involvement is that 10% of patients demonstrated metastasis in the middle and/or lower neck levels unassociated with metastases in the upper levels; such metastases probably result from tumor cells that have spread through a lymphatic trunk that runs from the floor of the mouth medial to the submandibular gland and lateral to the hyoid and its muscles directly to the lower jugular chain nodes superior to the crossing omohyoid muscle [78]. These findings caution strongly against suprahyoid neck dissection and emphasize the importance of performing complete neck dissection.

Guillamondegui et al. [79] reviewed the final outcome of 104 patients with a cancer of the floor of the mouth according to T stage and modality of therapy. For those with tumors staged $T_1$ and $T_2$ treated with surgery alone, the determinate survival was 89%; those who received radiotherapy had a determinate survival of 64%. In the advanced tumors, staged $T_3$ and $T_4$, the determinate survival was 56% for the patients who had surgical resection and 37% for those treated exclusively with radiotherapy. Taking into account that this report comes from the M.D. Anderson Hospital, where both radiation therapy and surgery are presumably performed by experts, little doubt remains that surgery is superior to radiotherapy in the management of cancer of the floor of the mouth. Patients with associated diseases of other systems such as cardiac and respiratory systems, however, are probably best treated with irradiation to avoid the high risk of postoperative complications [80].

Selection of the type of operation to be performed is based on the site, size, and degree of infiltration of the primary tumor and the status of the cervical lymph nodes. In small, superficially infiltrating lesions—$T_1$ and $T_2$ lesions up to 3 cm in greatest dimension—of the anterior floor of mouth with the neck being clinically negative for metastatic nodes, local excision by transoral route may be carried out. Marginal mandibulectomy plays an important role in access to and control of the disease in the surgical management of carcinoma of the floor of the mouth [73,81]. Primary closure in the anterior floor of the mouth area often leads to severe impairment of tongue mobility. Resurfacing of the defect with a free split skin graft using a pressure dressing for fixation of the graft gives a superior functional end result. Kolson et al. [82] report good results from allowing the wound to heal by secondary intention. In larger, deeper infiltrating and/or posteriorly situated lesions, a combined local and regional operation is usually needed. This often results in major soft tissue loss which may be associated with a segmental defect of the mandible. In most cases flaps must then be used for adequate rehabilitation. Mandibular reconstruction is optimal in lateral arch defects, but mandatory when the continuity of the anterior arch is lost. The problems encountered in reconstruction of this area are still formidable. Their management will be discussed in chapter 8.

The occurrence of multiple primary cancers of the mucous membranes of the upper air and food passages is well recognised. The incidence of secondary primary tumors appears to be particularly high in cancer of the floor of the mouth [77,79,80]. This demands particular attention at follow-up visits.

### 4.3. Oral carcinoma at other sites

#### *4.3.1. Carcinoma of the lower gum*

Radiotherapy is usually not successful in lesions close to bone or invading bone [83]. Surgery, therefore, is to be preferred under these circumstances. The type of operation to be carried out depends on the degree of bone involvement, the size and extension of the tumor, and the status of the neck nodes.

The presence or absence of bone involvement is traditionally assessed by radiology. A routine set of oblique and posteroanterior views, an orthopantomogram, and intraoral radiographs are taken. Whitehouse [84] studied the radiological bone changes produced by carcinoma involving the lower alveolus in a series of 50 patients. There was underlying bone involvement in 56% of primary lower gum carcinomas. The commonest radiological sign of osseous involvement is an ill-defined area of irregular permeative bone destruction, which Whitehouse calls the "invasive" appearance. Less often, there is loss of cortex with a well-defined defect within the bone. This appearance may be termed "erosive." An erosive bone defect probably necessitates less radical therapy than a lesion that is actually invading bone.

In the elderly edentulous patient, the alveolar bone is absorbed and the inferior dental canal is no longer sited deeply in the body of the mandible but lies close to the alveolar mucosa. Consequently, a tumor involving bone may readily spread along the inferior dental nerve [85]; major resection of the mandible is mandatory, and excision must encompass at least the whole length of the inferior dental canal.

Little information, however, is available on the accuracy of the radiograph in determining mandibular invasion. Weisman et al. [86] have compared bone scans with conventional radiographs in correlation with histopathology in patients who underwent some type of mandibulectomy. These authors conclude that the bone scan is more accurate than the roentgenogram in predicting tumor invasion of the mandible. The bone scan, however, has a high false positive rate due to the associated inflammation.

The majority of small lesions staged $T_1$ can be treated by intraoral resection of soft tissue removal with a margin of underlying cortical bone. Larger tumors usually require resection of a complete segment of the mandible. When the neck must be entered for the resection of the primary tumor or when clinically positive nodes are present, an en bloc neck dissection is carried out. The incidence of nodal metastasis does not warrant elective neck dissection. Byers et al. [87] report excellent local/regional control rates from surgical treatment. Cady et al. [88] and Nathansson et al. [89] point to the poor prognosis of patients with clinically positive neck nodes on admission.

*4.3.2. Carcinoma of the cheek mucosa*

Squamous cell cancer of the buccal mucosa most frequently develops along or inferior to the plane of occlusion. Extension to the mandible therefore is more common than to the maxilla. The anteroposterior position in the buccal mucosa area may vary. The majority, however, occur posteriorly, which facilitates their extension into the mandible, the pterygoid region, the parotid gland, and the infratemporal space [90]. In advanced tumors determining whether the tumor originated in the buccal mucosa or in a neighbouring area such as the retromolar trigone can be very difficult at times. The essential lymphatic drainage is to the submaxillary nodes along the facial vein and artery and the deep jugular chain. When the primary tumor is situated posteriorly in the buccal mucosa, parotid and paraglandular lymph nodes may be involved. A routine neck dissection may be of no avail when not combined with parotid dissection in such cases. The incidence of neck node metastasis is high: Vegers et al. [91] and Bloom et al. [92] report an incidence rate on admission of 42% and 38%, respectively, and an overall incidence of 59% and 56%, respectively.

Cheek mucosa cancer in many instances is wrongly considered as a not too difficult surgical problem to handle. In $T_1$ and $T_2$ cases local excision and resurfacing with a free split thickness skin graft poses no problems. In the more advanced lesions, composite resection may result in extensive soft tissue loss and bone defects. Particularly after excision of anterior lesions involving the oral commissure, both internal and external resurfacing may be needed. Bloom et al. [92] report an overall five-year survival after surgery alone of 42%. These authors demonstrated that the presence or absence of nodal involvement is, as for oral cancer in general, the most significant prognostic factor. Treatment of the clinically negative neck may be appropriate in all patients except those with $T_1$ lesions.

Vegers et al. [91] found that surgery proved superior over radiotherapy for each T and N category. However, these authors report good results from combined treatment of intra-arterial chemotherapy followed by radiotherapy in patients with advanced lesions in whom composite resection was not contemplated on general grounds.

*4.3.3. Carcinoma of the hard palate and upper gum*

Squamous cell carcinomas at these sites are rare. These tumors may extend into the soft palate, the cheek, nose and paranasal sinuses, and pterygomaxillary space. Anteroposterior tomography and computerized axial tomography are of great help in the assessment of the extent of the lesion and its potential resectability. Konrad et al. [93] point to the tendency of some of these tumors to follow nerves. Resection therefore must include the greater palatine foramen and pterygoid canal. Defects following maxillary resection are rehabilitated best by a prosthetic appliance. Tumors confined to the hard palate have a low incidence of neck node metastases. The incidence, however, rises when the lesion spreads to neighbouring structures.

A review of the treatment results is impracticable, for most publications on carcinoma of the palate [93,94,95], group together tumors of the hard palate and of the soft palate.

## 5. COMPLICATIONS OF SURGICAL TREATMENT

### 5.1. General aspects

*5.1.1. Introduction*

Operations for cancer of the head and neck in general, and cancer of the oral cavity in particular, can be limited, but often they are major procedures. The anatomy of the region is complex, involving many important structures. Many and serious complications may result. Adequate knowledge concerning possible complications and their avoidance can prevent or reduce the seriousness of complications. Many details require constant and careful attention.

Many patients are of advanced age and have a variety of other diseases, chronic pulmonary problems being most frequent. It is of paramount importance that the general condition of the patient is at its most favourable state before instituting surgical treatment. A majority of patients are heavy smokers and many use alcohol excessively. Some have associated liver disease. Identification of the alcoholic patient is important so that appropriate measures can be taken to lessen the postoperative withdrawal syndrome.

*5.1.2. Nutrition*

Awareness of the necessity of proper nutritional support is critical in the management of patients with oral cancer. Patients with oral cancer often have a history of poor dietary habits, which may be associated with alcoholism, resulting in protein, vitamin, and mineral deficiences. Oral cancer itself can cause an insufficient dietary intake because of pain on swallowing and inability to chew properly. As a result patients with oral cancer are often protein-calorie malnourished at the time their tumor is diagnosed and they are admitted to undergo surgical treatment. Major operative therapy puts a metabolic stress on the patient at a time when food intake is absent, and surgical therapy for oral cancer in particular often results in diminished oral intake for a prolonged period of time. In addition subsequent radiotherapy is often required which produces oral mucositis and diminished salivary secretions and may thus further decrease oral intake. A vicious catabolic cycle may readily result, which greatly enhances the risks of complications of treatment. Every effort, therefore, should be taken to restore the patient's nutritional condition and maintain it at an optimal level.

Prior to the start of appropriate nutritional therapy, the patient's nutritional status must be assessed by clinical observation and the usual laboratory tests. Taking into account the anticipated surgical procedure and the possibility of postoperative radiotherapy, an estimation can be made of the degree and duration of nutritional problems as a result of treatment. Based on this evaluation Copeland et al. [96] have devised a nutritional status score that allows calculation of the amount of nutrition required. As most oral cancer patients have normal gastrointestinal tracts, nasogastric tube feeding is usually appropriate—and also efficacious in the great majority of patients. Nasogastric tube feeding, however, is by no means free of complications [97]. A nasogastric tube can cause intolerable discomfort on rare occasions, and then gastrostomy may be indicated. In certain malnourished patients the gastrointestinal tract may not be available for nutritional support. In others alimentation via the enteral route may not be rapid enough to achieve adequate nutritional repletion prior to surgery. For these patients intravenous hyperalimentation may be indicated [98]. Daly et al. [99] reported on their experiences with intravenous hyperalimentation in 70 malnourished head and neck cancer patients, 53 of whom received this parenteral nutrition perioperatively. These authors found that weight gain, increase in muscle strength, and a significant rise in serum albumin concentration were much easier to accomplish when parenteral nutrition was administered preoperatively rather than postoperatively. They emphasize that nutritional repletion should be undertaken before surgical intervention rather than waiting until postoperative complications have occurred. However, in those patients in whom nutritional support was used postoperatively only, weight gain was achieved, pneumonia resolved, wound infection regressed, and flaps could be used to close fistula openings. In patients with head and neck cancer, however, parenteral nutrition via the subclavian vein poses some problems. Particularly, a high potential exists for catheter site contamination by secretions from stomas or fistulas with the risk of sepsis.

### *5.1.3. Mortality and morbidity*

Over the past 25 years the incidence of serious complications associated with head and neck cancer surgery has steadily declined. Improved general anaesthesia, meticulous surgical technique, careful medical supervision, and intensive nursing care, among other factors, have contributed to this favourable development.

The mortality rate from surgery for oral cancer is low. Removal of the primary lesion is rarely associated with death. The mortality rate—usually defined as death from any cause occurring within 30 days of surgery—for radical neck dissection is 1.5% [54,100]. When the procedure is combined with resection of primary lesions of the upper food and air passages, a mortality rate of 3% [101,102] is reported. When these composite or combined operations are being carried out after previous irradiation, the mortality rate may rise to as high as 23% [103].

Simultaneous bilateral neck dissection and bilateral staged neck dissection have an operative mortality of 10% and 3%, respectively [104]. When one-stage bilateral neck dissection is indicated, preservation of one of the internal jugular veins is recommended.

About half of the deaths are due to local complications such as haemorrhage or airway obstruction, while the other half are related to systemic disease, most often cardiovascular or pulmonary conditions [105]. McGuirt et al. [106] and Williams et al. [107] found a significant increase in mortality in patients over 80 years. Deaths in the older age group were due primarily to pulmonary and cardiovascular complications, whereas the incidence of surgical complications was not different in age groups above and below 70 years. In general, the age of 80 appears to mark the limit for major head and neck surgery.

Regarding morbidity after surgical treatment, one has to distinguish between true complications and sequelae, although, admittedly, a sharp division between the two is not always feasible. The patient should be well informed in advance about the particular deficits associated with the impending surgical procedure. Certain sequelae should be expected and accepted. These patients require knowledgeable nursing care and encouragement to cope with cosmetic and functional disability. For specific sequelae such as shoulder dysfunction after radical neck dissection rehabilitation programs may be beneficial.

Surgical complications are usually divided into major and minor complications; further definition of these two categories, however, is generally not precise, if not lacking at all. Donald [108] gives the following criteria for a major complication: a carotid artery blow out, a fistula that persisted longer than 10 days, a major loss of a neck flap, wound separation greater than 6 cm in length, and osteoradionecrosis. His criteria for a minor complication are (1) a fistula that persisted less than 10 days, (2) wound separation less than 6 cm in length, and (3) a wound infection that did not result in a large fistula or major flap necrosis. Smits et al. [109] define a major loss of a neck flap as a tissue loss greater than 2 × 2 cm. Another often used criterion for a major complication is whether a secondary procedure is required for correction. Obviously, these criteria are arbitrary, but they do provide guidelines. McGuirt et al. [102] and Yarington et al. [100] report a 17% major complication rate from extensive head and neck surgery. Their total complication rate is 38.8% and 25%, respectively. This difference, apparently, is attributable to the former authors' inclusion of even the very minor "complications." McGuirt et al. [102], furthermore, report a 28% incidence for medical complications. Twelve percent of patients had a medical complication alone. The surgical complication rate, particularly that of major complications, rises considerably when the surgery is performed after previous full-dose radiotherapy has failed to cure the lesion or after planned preoperative irradiation [109,103,108].

### 5.2. Specific surgical complications

A discussion of all possible surgical complications is not practicable within the scope of this chapter. Only major complications and those that occur frequently will be reviewed. The two most serious complications, likely to lead to death, are carotid artery haemorrhage and airway obstruction. Wound infection is the most common complication. Methods of preventing these complications will be presented, and their management will be briefly discussed.

#### *5.2.1. Wound infection*

The oral cavity and oropharynx are an ideal incubator for microorganisms. In the variety of species, number of organisms, and potential for virulence, the microbial flora of the human mouth exceed that of any other area of the body [110]. Any surgical procedure in the oral cavity, by disrupting the intact mucous membrane barrier, gives a large inoculum of bacteria access to the depths of the open tissues. All such procedures must therefore be classified as "highly contaminated." Surprisingly, therefore, infection is a rare occurrence after local excision alone by transoral route. Only when the local defense mechanisms against infection have been lowered by previous irradiation, is infection not uncommon after local excision alone. However, infection does become a frequent problem when the surgical procedure is extended to encompass both the primary tumor and the neck nodes. This most often occurs after the completion of the operation because of breakdown of the intraoral closure. Oral secretions with their microflora will accumulate in the neck wound. Major problems of neck flap necrosis, development of fistulas, and carotid artery rupture may then result.

Prevention of infection includes pre-, intra-, and postoperative measures. The importance of an optimal general condition of the patient has already been emphasized. Attention should be paid to oral hygiene. A complete dental evaluation prior to surgery is mandatory, especially if radiation therapy might be required after surgery [111]. Nonrestorable carious teeth are identified for extraction at the time of surgery, after resection of the tumor has been completed. Meticulous intraoral closure avoiding any tension on the suture lines is essential. To achieve this the use of flaps is often indicated, particularly when the continuity of the mandible has been preserved. Haemovac suction drainage is used in all patients undergoing composite resection. The drainage system is carefully monitored and the neck palpated for evidence of haematoma formation, particularly during the first 48 hours. Collection of fluid under the neck flaps in this critical period usually results in wound infection. If a haematoma develops, the neck should be reopened and the haematoma evacuated. Usage of prophylactic antibiotics with a wide spectrum is common practice in composite procedures. The aim of this protection is to achieve an adequate level of antibiotic prior to bacterial penetration and proliferation. The administration of antibiotics should therefore be started shortly before surgery and should be continued for not too long after surgery so as to minimize the risk of the emergence of resistant strains. Despite the use of preventive measures, wound infections do occur. Their treatment consists of adequate drainage, local wound debridement, and administration of culture-specific antibiotics. The majority of fistulas will heal spontaneously with meticulous wound care. Persistent fistulas are closed using regional flaps [112].

*5.2.2. Carotid artery rupture*

The incidence of carotid artery rupture after major head and neck surgery is approximately 3% [113]. Neck dissection alone is rarely associated with a carotid artery complication and then only after previous heavy irradiation to the neck. Once the surgery is extended into a composite resection, a major increase is seen in the incidence of infection, skin flap necrosis, and fistula, which may expose the major vessels in the neck and ultimately give rise to a carotid artery rupture. Usually, a combination of factors leads to this disastrous event. Poor general condition, cardiovascular disease, chronic obstructive pulmonary disease, and particularly diabetes are general high-risk factors for infection and poor healing quality. Previous irradiation is the single most important local adverse factor. The measures to prevent carotid artery rupture include aims to prevent infection (see earlier discussion on wound infection). In addition the choice of incision is most important. The most vulnerable site of the carotid system is the carotid bulb in the region of the bifurcation. Skin flaps, therefore, are designed and positioned in such a way that the carotid bulb area is well protected. A three-point junction of incision lines over the carotid bifurcation as in the classic Y-incision should be avoided at all times. In postirradiation patients or patients in whom poor healing is otherwise expected, carotid coverage with a dermal skin graft or a levator scapulae muscle swing is indicated [113].

A significant clinical sign of impending rupture of the carotid artery is slight bleeding from its wall. Extension of the necrotic slough into the artery itself with erosion of its wall is another such sign. Conley [114] advocates elective ligation of the carotid artery under these circumstances. Elective ligation of these vessels is better tolerated by the patient than emergency ligation after rupture. The two major complications of ligation are serious neurologic deficits such as hemiplegia and death. Unfortunately, no tests are available to predict who will tolerate carotid artery ligation without a complication and who will not.

*5.2.3. Airway obstruction*

Obstruction of the airway can readily result after major head and neck surgery from edema of the larynx or base of tongue area, from posterior displacement of the tongue and epiglottis, and from aspiration of secretions, blood, or vomitus in a situation in which coughing and swallowing are usually a problem. If obstruction of the airway is anticipated, an elective tracheostomy is indicated. An emergency tracheostomy with its attendant increased risks to the patient should be avoided. The indications for elective tracheostomy are well established. Whereas a tracheostomy is not needed in a radical neck dissection alone, bilateral simultaneous or nonsimultaneous radical neck dissection does require a tracheostomy because of the risk of edema of the larynx. In all composite operations a tracheostomy should be carried out because these procedures carry with them a high risk for all the causes of airway obstruction mentioned above. No set rules can be given as to the indications for elective tracheostomy in transoral cancer surgery on its own. Limited resection anteriorly in the oral cavity does not require a tracheostomy. However, when the excision involves a substantial part of the tongue and certainly when it extends posteriorly to the base of the tongue, a tracheostomy is indicated. Not only can upper airway obstruction then occur due to edema, but if bleeding occurs, the patient will be much safer after a tracheostomy.

Within the scope of a composite resection, tracheostomy might easily be looked upon as a minor procedure to be rapidly carried out either before or just after the composite resection. This attitude is to be discarded: tracheostomy has its own complications and mortality [115]. Only meticulous technique and careful attention to detail can keep the complication rate at a very minimum.

## 6. CRYOSURGERY

Freezing kills cells and can be used to destroy tumors. The availability of liquid nitrogen that boils at −196° C, and the development in the early 1960s of suitable instrumentation to utilize this refrigerant, has stimulated the therapeutic use of extreme cold. Liquid nitrogen may be used by either of two methods. In a closed system the liquid nitrogen is passed into and through an appropriate probe, which is placed in contact with the tissues being treated. In an open system the liquid nitrogen is brought into direct contact with the tissues. This may be accomplished by means of a spray. This arrangement is more difficult to monitor and control, also in regard to damage to the normal surrounding tissues. The following variables determine success or failure in cryosurgery: rate of freeze, lowest temperature of freeze, use of repetitive freezing after spontaneous thaw, and adequate freezing of the entire tumor [116]. The usual practice is to cool as rapidly as possible. The rate of freeze depends on the size of the probe. The temperature of the tissue to be destructed must be carried down to at least −20° C and preferably to −30° C. Tissue temperatures can be monitored by means of thermocouples positioned at the periphery of the tumor. Placing of these thermocouples, however, is not always feasible in posteriorly sited tumors in the oral cavity. Repetitive freezing and thawing of tissues is more effective than one freeze-thaw cycle. Each freeze cycle is continued for a minimum of three to a maximum of six minutes after tissue temperatures of −20° C have been established. For tumors in the anterior part of the oral cavity, the procedure does not require general anaesthesia. During treatment haemorrhage is absent.

Following cryosurgery edema of the treated tissues spreads easily to the surroundings and progresses to a maximum after 18 to 24 hours. When treatment involves the posterior part of the oral cavity, a temporary tracheostomy is often required. It usually takes a few days before the edema begins to subside. Subsequently, necrosis becomes evident, and necrotic tissues will slough during the ensuing weeks. This phase is associated with an uncomfortable odor, and there is a risk of secondary bleeding. It takes about six weeks before the treated area is clean and healed.

Cryosurgery has been used in the treatment of oral cancer with palliative and curative aims. In general, results of cryosurgical palliation have been disappointing, as serious complications did occur [117,118]. Recurrence in a maxillectomy cavity is one of the few situations in which cryosurgery might be of palliative benefit to the patient. The experiences with cryosurgery in patients in whom it was used to effect cure are more favourable [117,118,119,120,121]. As cryosurgery lacks precision and has a depth effect of not more than 1 cm, not surprisingly, the best results have been obtained in slow growing, well-delineated, only superficially infiltrative well-differentiated oral cancers. Bekke et al. [121] report particularly good results in small $T_1$ and $T_2$ lesions localised over bone of either the mandible or the maxilla. This finding appears to confirm that tumor infiltration in bone can be destroyed by cryosurgery [122]. Specifically suitable are easily accessible lesions anteriorly in the oral cavity, such as tumors of the buccal mucosa and the gums. At these sites the procedure can be carried out under local anaesthesia and is usually reasonably well tolerated. Cryosurgery for oral cancer is to be considered in elderly patients who are considered unsuitable for conventional resection because of general health and whose cancer meets the criteria mentioned above. Furthermore, cryosurgery appears to be a good alternative to surgical excision in certain extensive or multifocal leukoplakia with dysplasia of the oral mucosa. Healing in general is excellent without loss of function [121].

### 7. CARBON DIOXIDE LASER SURGERY

A laser (light amplification by stimulated emission of radiation) is a device that produces coherent light, a narrow intense beam of pure monochromatic light in which all the light waves are of the same length and travel in phase and in the same direction. The beam can be focused by a lens to a fine point. In the last two decades, a large number of lasers have been developed. The nature of the stimulated lasing medium determines the wave length of the laser light, and the wave length the site of its absorption in the body. The carbon dioxide laser produces infrared coherent light at a wave length of 10.6 microns, which is absorbed by water and therefore by body tissues, which contain 80% water.

The absorption by the tissues is very strong; 200 microns beneath the surface only 5% of the energy is left. That is, at the level of the focus, nearly all of the energy of the laser beam will be absorbed by a very small amount of tissue. As a result intracellular water is boiled and the cells rupture. Cellular particles are released and burned in the beam and deposited as debris around the laser wound. The scattered cellular matter and debris are harmless [123,124]. Thus, tissue destruction by the carbon dioxide laser is by cell vaporization. When the focus of the laser beam is moved over the surface of the tissue, an incision will result. The laser, therefore, may also be used as a scalpel to excise tumors with adequate margins of healthy tissue, and a specimen will be provided for histological examination.

The laser device is attached to the operating microscope, which provides a well-illuminated, magnified operative field. The laser beam is guided by a micromanipulator, which allows for accurate positioning of the beam. The depth of penetration of the beam into the tissues is also under precise control. The absence of an active probe, as needed with diathermy or cryosurgery, enables continuous observation of the target area.

A number of features of the $CO_2$ laser–soft tissue interaction appear to make this instrument particularly feasible for transoral surgery. Dissection is almost bloodless, as vessels up to 0.5 mm in diameter are sealed by the beam. Section of larger vessels is controlled by ligature or diathermy. Damage to normal tissue is minimal, as unwanted heat coagulation adjacent to the wound is not more than 100 to 200 microns. That is, there is no postoperative edema, and healing is rapid. Healing is by migration of the epithelium across the defect. Strong et al. [125,126], reporting on the transoral management of localised carcinoma of the oral cavity in 57 patients using $CO_2$ laser, found only minimal scar contracture, particularly after resection of lesions of the lip, the floor of the mouth, the retromolar area, and the palatine arch. Contracture in these areas would lead to serious functional deficits. Carruth [127] reported a series of 25 tongue resections carried out with the $CO_2$ laser. The defect was left open, and lack of scarring enabled the tongue remnant to retain maximal residual function. Both authors reported no postoperative edema and no airway problems. A tracheostomy is not needed. Lack of pain is one of the most remarkable findings following laser resection. The morbidity is minimal, so that patients can almost always be discharged on the following day.

Despite the reported advantages of carbon dioxide laser surgery, it is to be realised that the experiences with this new tool so far are limited and that follow-up periods are short. Finally, the use of the $CO_2$ laser is not without danger. The safety aspects have been well covered by Carruth et al. [128].

## 8. MINOR SALIVARY GLAND TUMORS

Minor salivary gland tumors are rare. They can occur any where in the upper aerodigestive tracts, but are most frequently seen in the oral cavity. The palate is the site of predilection, followed by cheek, upper lip, and tongue. Tumors of minor salivary glands are similar histologically to those occurring in major salivary glands. However, tumors arising in minor salivary glands are much more likely to be malignant than those arising in major salivary glands. Adenoid cystic carcinoma is the histologic type most frequently encountered, followed by adenocarcinoma and mucoepidermoid tumors [129,130].

The great majority of patients have noticed only an asymptomatic nonulcerative swelling in the mouth. Pain is reported with greater frequency in those with a malignant tumor. However, neither the symptomatology nor the gross appearance of the tumor is of assistance in predicting the true nature of the neoplasm.

Biopsy is recommended prior to institution of definitive therapy. Because of the inherent diagnostic difficulties these tumors present to pathologists, one should not utilise frozen section examination, but rely only on paraffin sections. Small lesions may be excised for biopsy, and this will prove therapeutic in approximately half of the cases. In larger lesions or clinically invasive lesions, an incisional biopsy is indicated. The type of definite operation to be performed depends upon the histologic type and upon the anatomic site and the extent of the tumor. All malignant tumors should have at least a 1 or 2 cm margin of normal healthy tissue included in the specimen. When the lesion is situated on the palate, excision of a portion of the maxilla is involved. When there is clinical evidence of cervical node involvement, a radical neck dissection is carried out. As lymph node metastases are infrequent in malignant salivary gland tumors, elective treatment of the neck is generally not indicated. As in malignant tumors of the major salivary glands, the common practice today is to apply postoperative irradiation to the primary site with the aim of reducing the incidence of local recurrence [131]. This is particularly useful in adenoid cystic carcinoma.

In benign lesions the overlying mucosa and the biopsy incision are always included in the excision. Enucleation techniques must be discarded. The palatal bone can usually be preserved in benign tumors. The bone can be resurfaced with a split skin graft or left bare to heal by secondary intention; mucosal flaps to cover the bone should never be used in these circumstances.

The prognosis depends on histologic type, anatomic site, and extent of the disease. As salivary gland tumors have a prolonged life history, periods of at least 10 to 15 years are necessary to evaluate their course. This is particularly true for adenoid cystic carcinoma. Conley and Dingman [132] report 20% survival with no evidence of disease at 15 years posttreatment for adenoid cystic carcinoma in the head and neck. In the series of these authors, however, adenoid cystic carcinomas of the minor salivary glands proved to have a much poorer prognosis than their counterparts in the major salivary glands.

## 9. MUCOSAL MELANOMAS

Malignant melanoma arising in the mucosa of the upper air and food passages is a rare disease. The great majority occur in the oral cavity and the nasal cavity. The site of predilection for malignant melanomas of the oral cavity, in contrast to squamous carcinoma, is the upper jaw [133]. Particularly, the palate is affected. The actual melanoma is usually surrounded by areas of mucosal pigmentation known as oral melanosis. This makes it at times extremely difficult, if not impossible, to accurately determine the size of the melanoma on clinical examination. These tumors may cause bone destruction, although roentgenographic evidence of this is usually absent.

Surgical treatment offers the best chance for local control [134,135,136]. The excision should encompass all pigmented areas of the mucosa in the surroundings, as well as the underlying bone. For lesions on the upper jaw, this usually entails total removal of the hard palate and the superior alveolar arch.

It has generally been recognized that melanoma of the mucous membranes of the head and neck has a poor prognosis in comparison to melanoma of the skin. Histologic differences have been cited as reasons for this discrepancy [137]. Snow et al. [136] were impressed by the thickness of the lesions in comparison to cutaneous melanoma. Further, anatomic relationships often preclude surgery with generous margins around the visible lesions, as is well reflected by the high percentage of local recurrence [135,136]. Five-year survival rates are in the range of 20 to 25% [135]. One of the most intriguing features of this unusual tumor is the unpredictability of its clinical course. In some cases it is explosive, characterized by rapid, widespread dissemination. At other times, long dormant periods of more than 10 years' duration may be followed by recurrence with a fatal outcome [137]. Patients who survive longer than five years, therefore, are not necessarily cured of their melanoma.

## REFERENCES


1. Shumrick DA. Carcinoma of the supraglottis and tongue treated by supraglottic laryngectomy and mandibular swing. Laryngoscope (79): 1443–1452, 1969.
2. Spiro RH, Gerold FP, Strong EW. Mandibular "swing" approach for oral and oropharyngeal tumors. Head & Neck Surg (3): 371–378, 1981.
3. Westbury G. Carcinoma of the tongue. In Operative Surgery, Head and Neck, Rob C, Smith R (gen. eds), Wilson JSP (cons. ed). London: Butterworths, 1981, 664–671.
4. Ballantyne AJ. Current controversies in the management of cancer of the tongue and floor of the mouth. In Head and Neck Oncology, Controversies in Cancer Treatment, Kagan AR, Miles JW (eds). Boston: GK Hall, 1981, pp. 87–98.
5. Byers RM, Bland KI, Borlase B, Luna M. The prognostic and therapeutic value of frozen section determinations in the surgical treatment of squamous carcinoma of the head and neck. Am J Surg (136): 525–528, 1978.
6. Marchetta FC, Sako K, Murphy J. The periosteum of the mandible and intraoral carcinoma. Am J Surg (122): 711–713, 1971.
7. Carter RL, Tanner NSB, Clifford P, Shaw HJ. Direct bone invasion in squamous carcinomas of the head and neck: Pathological and clinical implications. Clin Otolaryngol (5): 107–116, 1980.
8. McGregor IA. Problems of reconstructive surgery of the oral cavity. J Laryngol Otol (91): 445–465, 1977.
9. Spiro RH, Strong EW. Discontinuous partial glossectomy and radical neck dissection in selected patients with epidermoid carcinoma of the mobile tongue. Amer J Surg (126): 544–546, 1973.
10. Nahum AM, Bone RC, Davidson TM. The case for elective prophylactic neck dissection. Laryngoscope (87): 588–599, 1977.

11. Crile G. Excision of cancer of the head and neck, with special reference to the plan of dissection based upon 132 operations. JAMA (47): 1780–1786, 1906.
12. Martin H, Del Valle B, Ehrlich H, Cahan WG. Neck dissection. Cancer (4): 441–499, 1951.
13. Beahrs OH, Gossel JD, Hollingshead WH. Technique and surgical anatomy of radical neck dissection. Amer J Surg (90): 490–516, 1955.
14. Bocca E, Pignataro O. A conservation technique in radical neck dissection. Ann Otol (76): 975–987, 1967.
15. Bocca E, Pignataro O, Sasaki C. Functional neck dissection. Arch Otolaryngol (106): 524–527, 1980.
16. Dayal VS, Da Silva AJ. Functional and radical neck dissection. Arch Otolaryngol (93): 413–415, 1971.
17. Lingeman RE, Stephens R, Helmus C, Ulm J. Neck dissection: radical or conservative. Ann Otol (86): 737–744, 1977.
18. Chu W, Strawitz JG. Results in suprahyoid, modified radical, and standard radical neck dissections for metastatic squamous cell carcinoma: Recurrence and survival. Amer J Surg (136): 512–515, 1978.
19. Jesse RH, Ballantyne AJ, Larson D. Radical or modified neck dissection: A therapeutic dilemma. Amer J Surg (136): 516–519, 1978.
20. Molinari R, Chiesa F, Cantu G, Grandi C. Retrospective comparison of conservative and radical neck dissection in laryngeal cancer. Ann Otol (89): 578–581, 1980.
21. Noone RB, Bonner H, Raymond S, Brown AS, Graham WP, Lehr HB. Lymph node metastases in oral carcinoma. A correlation of histopathology with survival. Plast Reconstr Surg (53): 158–166, 1974.
22. Pointon RCS, Jelly GO. Block dissection of the neck for squamous cell carcinoma of the mouth and lips. Proc R Soc Med (69): 414–416, 1976.
23. Kalnis IK, Leonard AG, Sako K, Razack MS, Shedd DP. Correlation between prognosis and degree of lymph node involvement in carcinoma of the oral cavity. Amer J Surg (134): 450–454, 1977.
24. Micheau C, Sancho H, Gerard-Marchant R. Prognostic des adenopathies cervicales metastatiques en fonction des facteurs anatomopathologiques. Nuovo Arch Ital Otol VI (1): 5–14, 1978.
25. Zoller M, Goodman ML, Cummings CW. Guidelines for prognosis in head and neck cancer with nodal metastasis. Laryngoscope (88): 135–141, 1978.
26. Cachin Y, Sancho-Garnier H, Micheau C, Marandas P. Nodal metastasis from carcinomas of the oropharynx. Otolaryngol Clin N Am (12): 145–154, 1979.
27. Johnson, JT, Barnes EL, Myers EN, Schramm VL Jr, Borochovitz D, Sigler B. The extracapsular spread of tumors in cervical node metastasis. Arch Otolaryngol (107): 725–729, 1981.
28. Snow GB, Annyas AA, van Slooten EA, Bartelink H, Hart AAM. Prognostic factors of neck node metastasis. Clin Otolaryngol (7): 185–192, 1982.
29. Carenfelt C, Eliasson K. Radical neck dissection and permanent sequelae associated with spinal accessory nerve injuries. Acta Otolaryngol (91): 155–160, 1981.
30. Dargent M, Papillon J. Résultats éloignés de l'évidement ganglionaire du cou avec conservation du filet mentonier et du spinal. Lyon Chir (41): 715–721, 1945.
31. Pietrantoni L, Fior R. Clinical and surgical problems of cancer of larynx and hypopharynx. Acta Otolaryngol, Suppl. 142, 1958.
32. Carenfelt C, Eliasson K. Cervical metastases following radical neck dissection that preserved the spinal accessory nerve. Head & Neck Surg (2): 181–184, 1980.
33. Brandenburg JH, Lee CYS. The eleventh nerve in radical neck dissection. Laryngoscope (91): 1851–1858, 1981.
34. Schuller DE, Platz CE, Krause CJ. Spinal accessory lymph nodes: A prospective study of metastatic involvement. Laryngoscope (88): 439–451, 1978.
35. Skolnik EM, Yee KF, Friedman M, Golden TA. The posterior triangle in radical neck surgery. Arch Otolaryngol (102): 1–4, 1976.
36. Nahum, AM. Radical neck dissection: Theme and variations. Head & Neck Surg (2): 179–180, 1980.
37. Becker GD, Parell GJ. Technique of preserving the spinal accessory nerve during radical neck dissection. Laryngoscope (89): 827–831, 1979.

38. Carenfelt C, Eliasson K. Occurrence, duration and prognosis of unexpected accessory nerve paresis in radical neck dissection. Acta Otolaryngol (90): 470–473, 1980.
39. Saunders WH, Johnson EW. Rehabilitation of the shoulder after radical neck dissection. Ann Otol (84): 812–816, 1975.
40. Chu W, Strawitz JG. Results in suprahyoid, modified radical and standard radical neck dissection for metastatic squamous cell carcinoma: Recurrence and survival. Amer J Surg (136): 512–515, 1978.
41. Jesse RH. Modified neck dissection with and without radiation. In Head and Neck Oncology, Controversies in Cancer Treatment, Kagan AR, Miles JW (eds). Boston: G.K. Hall, 1981, pp. 247–254.
42. Cachin Y, Eschwege F. Combination of radiotherapy and surgery in the treatment of head and neck cancers. Cancer Treatm Rev (2): 177–191, 1975.
43. Terz JJ, Lawrence W Jr. Ineffectiveness of combined radiation and surgery in the management of malignancies of the oral cavity, larynx and pharynx. In Head and Neck Oncology, Controversies in Cancer Treatment, Kagan AR, Miles JW (eds). Boston: G.K. Hall, 1981, pp. 111–123.
44. Carpenter RJ III, De Santo LW, Devine KD et al. Cancer of the hypopharynx: Analysis of treatment and results in 162 patients. Arch Otolaryngol (102): 716–721, 1976.
45. Schuller DE, McGuirt WF, Krause CJ, McGabe BF, Pflug BK. Increased survival with surgery alone vs. combined therapy. Laryngoscope (89): 582–594, 1979.
46. Strong MS, Vaughan CW, Kayne HL, Aral IM, Ucmakli A, Feldman M, Healy GB. A randomized trial of preoperative radiotherapy in cancer of the oropharynx and hypopharynx. Amer J Surg (136): 494–500, 1978.
47. Hintz B, Charynler K, Chandler JR, Sudarsanam A, Garciga C. Randomized study of control of the primary tumor and survival using preoperative radiation, radiation alone, or surgery alone in head and neck carcinomas. J Surg Oncol (12): 75–85, 1979.
48. Terz JJ, King ER, Lawrence W Jr. Preoperative irradiation for head and neck cancer: Results of a prospective study. Surgery (89): 449–453, 1981.
49. Jesse RH, Lindberg RD. The efficacy of combining radiation therapy with a surgical procedure in patients with cervical metastasis from squamous cancer of the oropharynx and hypopharynx. Cancer (35): 1163–1166, 1975.
50. Vandenbrouck C, Sancho H, Le Fut R, Richard JM, Cachin Y. Results of a randomized clinical trial of preoperative irradiation versus postoperative in treatment of tumors of the hypopharynx. Cancer (39): 1445–1449, 1977.
51. Marcus RB Jr, Million RR, Cassissi, NJ. Postoperative irradiation for squamous cell carcinomas of the head and neck: Analysis of time-dose factors related to control above the clavicles. Int J Radiat Oncol Biol Phys (5): 1943–1949, 1979.
52. Snow JB, Gelber RD, Kramer S, Davis LW, Marcial VA, Lowry LD. Comparison of preoperative and postoperative radiation therapy for patients with carcinoma of the head and neck. Acta Otolaryngol (91): 611–626, 1981.
53. Bartelink H, Breur H, Hart G, Annyas AA, van Slooten WA, Snow GB. The value of postoperative radiotherapy as an adjuvant to radical neck dissection. Cancer (52): 1008–1013, 1983.
54. Beahrs OH, Barber KW. The value of radical dissection of structures of the neck in the management of carcinoma of the lip, mouth and larynx. Arch Surg (85): 49–56, 1962.
55. Strong EW, Henschke UK, Nickson JJ, Frazell EL, Tollefsen R, Hilaris BS. Preoperative x-ray therapy as an adjunct to radical neck dissection. Cancer (19): 1509–1516, 1966.
56. Jesse RH, Fletcher GH. Treatment of the neck in patients with squamous cell carcinoma of the head and neck. Cancer (39): 868–872, 1977.
57. Vikram B. Importance of the time interval between surgery and postoperative radiation therapy in the combined management of head and neck cancer. Int J Radiat Oncol Biol Phys (5): 1837–1840, 1979.
58. Versluis RJJ, Snow GB, Waal I van der. Preoperative administration of methotrexate in head and neck cancer. In press.
59. Kish J, Drelichman A, Weaver A, Jacobs J, Bergsman K, Al-sarraf M. Cis-platinum and 5-fluorouracil infusion in patients with recurrent and disseminated epidermoid cancer of the head and neck. Proc Amer Soc Clin Onc 1: 193, 1982.
60. Frazell EL. A review of the treatment of cancer of the mobile portion of the tongue. Cancer (28): 1178–1181, 1971.

61. White D, Byers RM. What is the preferred initial method of treatment for squamous carcinoma of the tongue? Amer J Surg (149): 553–555, 1980.
62. Marks JE, Lee F, Freeman RB, Zivnuska FR, Ogura JH. Carcinoma of the oral tongue: A study of patient selection and treatment results. Laryngoscope (91): 1548–1559, 1981.
63. Spiro RH, Strong EW. Epidermoid carcinoma of the mobile tongue: Treatment by partial glossectomy alone. Amer J Surg (122): 707–710, 1971.
64. McGregor IA, McGrouther DA. Skin-graft reconstruction in carcinoma of the tongue. Head & Neck Surg (1): 47–51, 1978.
65. Harrold CC Jr. Cancer of the tongue: Some comments on surgical treatment. In Symposium on Cancer of the Head and Neck; Total Treatment and Reconstructive Rehabilitation, vol II, Gaisford JC (ed). St. Louis: C.V. Mosby, 1969, pp. 185–190.
66. Vandenbrouck C, Sancho-Garnier H, Chassagne D, Saravane D, Cachin Y, Micheau C. Elective versus therapeutic radical neck dissection in epidermoid carcinoma of the oral cavity, results of a randomized clinical trial. Cancer (46): 386–390, 1980.
67. Spiro RH, Strong EW. Epidermoid carcinoma of the oral cavity and oropharynx. Elective vs. therapeutic radical neck dissection as treatment. Arch Surg (107): 382–384, 1973.
68. Mendelson BC, Woods JE, Beahrs OH. Neck dissection in the treatment of carcinoma of the anterior two-thirds of the tongue. Surg Gyn Obst (143): 75–80, 1976.
69. Whitehurst JO, Droulias CA. Surgical treatment of squamous cell carcinoma of the oral tongue. Arch Otolaryngol (103): 212–215, 1977.
70. Johnson JT, Leipzig B, Cummings CW. Management of $T_1$ carcinoma of the anterior aspect of the tongue. Arch Otolaryngol (106): 249–251, 1980.
71. Moore C, Catlin D. Anatomic origins and locations of oral cancer. Amer J Surg (114): 510–513, 1967.
72. Helfrich GB, Nickels ME, El-Domeiri A, Das Gupta TK. Management of cancer of the floor of the mouth. Amer J Surg (124): 559–562, 1972.
73. Keim WF, Lowenberg S. Marginal mandibulectomy in treatment of carcinoma of the floor of the mouth. Laryngoscope (80): 1566–1579, 1970.
74. Harrold CC. Management of cancers of the floor of the mouth. Amer J Surg (122): 487–493, 1971.
75. Hardingham M, Dalley VM, Shaw HJ. Cancer of the floor of the mouth: Clinical features and results of treatment. Clin Oncology (3): 227–246, 1977.
76. Lederman M. The anatomy of cancer with special reference to tumours of the upper air and food passages. J Laryngol Otol (197): 181–208, 1964.
77. Ballard BR, Suess GR, Pickren JW, Greene GW Jr, Shedd DP. Squamous cell carcinoma of the floor of the mouth. Oral Surg Med Path (45): 568–579, 1978.
78. Feind CR, Cole RM. Cancer of the floor of the mouth and its lymphatic spread. Amer J Surg (116): 482–287, 1968.
79. Guillamondegui OM, Oliver B, Hayden R. Cancer of the anterior floor of the mouth, selective choice of treatment and analysis of failures. Amer J Surg (140): 560–562, 1980.
80. Flynn MB, Mullins FX, Moore C. Selection of treatment in squamous carcinoma of the floor of the mouth. Amer J Surg (126): 477–481, 1973.
81. Guillamondegui OM, Jesse R. Surgical treatment of advanced carcinoma of the floor of the mouth. Am J Roentenol (126): 1256–1259, 1976.
82. Kolson H, Spiro RH, Rosewit B, Lawson W. Epidermoid carcinoma of the floor of the mouth. Arch Otolaryngol (93): 280–283, 1971.
83. Lee ES, Wilson JSP. Carcinoma involving the lower alveolus. Brit J Surg (60): 85–107, 1973.
84. Whitehouse GH. Radiological bone changes produced by intraoral squamous carcinomata involving the lower alveolus. Clin Otolaryng (1): 45–52, 1976.
85. Southam JC. The extension of squamous carcinoma along the inferior dental and neurovascular bundle. Br J Oral Surg (7): 137–145, 1970.
86. Weisman RA, Kimmelman CP. Bone scanning in the assessment of mandibular invasion by oral cavity carcinomas. Laryngoscope (92): 1–4, 1982.
87. Byers RM, Newman R, Russell N, Yue A. Results of treatment for squamous carcinoma of the lower gum. Cancer (47): 2236–2238, 1981.
88. Cady B, Catlin D. Epidermoid carcinoma of the gums. A 20-year survey. Cancer (3): 551–569, 1969.

89. Nathansson A, Jakobsson PA, Wersäll J. Prognosis of squamous cell carcinoma of the gums. Acta Otolaryng (75): 301–303, 1973.
90. Conley J. Squamous cell cancer of the buccal mucosa, a review of 90 cases. Arch Otolaryngol (97): 330–333, 1973.
91. Vegers JWM, Snow GB, v.d. Waal I. Squamous cell carcinoma of the buccal mucosa. A review of 85 cases. Arch Otolaryng (105): 192–195, 1979.
92. Bloom ND, Spiro RH. Carcinoma of the cheek mucosa, a retrospective analysis. Amer J Surg (149): 556–559, 1980.
93. Konrad HR, Canalis RE, Calcaterra TC. Epidermoid carcinoma of the palate. Arch Otolaryngol (104): 208–212, 1978.
94. Eneroth CM, Hjertman L, Moberger G. Squamous cell carcinomas of the palate. Acta Otolaryng (73): 418–427, 1972.
95. Evans JF, Shah JP. Epidermoid carcinoma of the palate. Amer J Surg (142): 451–455, 1981.
96. Copeland EM, Daly JM, Dundrick SJ. Nutritional concepts in the treatment of head and neck malignancies. Head & Neck Surg (1): 350–363, 1979.
97. Sobol SM, Conoyer JM, Zill R, Thawley SE, Ogura JH. Nutritional concepts in the management of the head and neck cancer patient. Laryngoscope (89): 962–979, 1979.
98. Close LG. Indications for hyperalimentation in the treatment of head and neck malignancies. Otolaryngol Head Neck Surg (88): 700–706, 1980.
99. Daly JM, Dudrick SJ, Copeland EM. Parenteral nutrition in patients with head and neck cancer: Techniques and results. Otolaryngol Head Neck Surg (88): 707–713, 1980.
100. Yarington CT Jr, Yonkers AJ, Beddoc GM. Radical neck dissection, mortality and morbidity. Arch Otolaryngol (97): 306–308, 1973.
101. Simons JN, Beahrs OH, Woolner IB. Tumors of the submaxillary gland. Am J Surg (108): 485–494, 1964.
102. McGuirt WF, McCabe BF, Krause CJ. Complications of radical neck dissection: A survey of 788 patients. Head & Neck Surg (1): 481–487, 1979.
103. Joseph DL, Shumrick DL. Risks of head and neck surgery in previously irradiated patients. Arch Otolaryngol (97): 381–384, 1973.
104. Razack MS, Baffi R, Sako K. Bilateral radical neck dissection. Cancer (47): 197–199, 1981.
105. Beahrs OH. Complications of surgery for cancer of the head and neck. In Management of Surgical Complications, Artz CP, Hardy JD (eds). Philadelphia: Saunders, 1975, pp. 277–290.
106. McGuirt WF, Loevy S, McCabe BF, Krause CJ. The risks of major head and neck surgery in the aged population. Laryngoscope (87): 1378–1382, 1977.
107. Williams RG, Murtagh GP. Mortality in surgery for head and neck cancer. J Laryngol Otol (87): 431–440, 1973.
108. Donald PJ. Complications of combined therapy in head and neck carcinomas. Arch Otolaryngol (104): 329–322, 1978.
109. Smits RG, Krause CJ, McCabe BF. Complications associated with combined therapy of oral and pharyngeal neoplasms. Ann Otol (81): 496–500, 1972.
110. Krizek TJ, Ariyan S. Infection. In Complications of Head and Neck Surgery, Conley JJ (ed). Philadelphia: Saunders, 1979, pp. 99–123.
111. Daly TE, Drane JB. Dental care for irradiated patients. In Neoplasia of Head and Neck, Chicago: Year Book, 1974, pp. 225–232.
112. Conley JJ. Oropharyngocutaneous fistula. In Complications of Head and Neck Surgery, Conley JJ (ed). Philadelphia: Saunders, 1979, pp. 92–98.
113. Shumrick DA. Carotid artery rupture. Laryngoscope (83): 1051–1061, 1973.
114. Conley JJ. Carotid artery ligation. In Complications of Head and Neck Surgery, Conley JJ (ed). Philadelphia: Saunders, 1979, pp. 81–91.
115. Conley JJ. Tracheostomy complications. In Complications of Head and Neck Surgery, Conley JJ (ed). Philadelphia: Saunders, 1979, pp. 274–292.
116. Neel HB III, Ketcham AS, Hammond WG. Requisites for successful cryogenic surgery of cancer. Arch Surg (102): 45–48, 1971.
117. De Santo LW. The curative, palliative and adjunctive uses of cryosurgery in the head and neck. Laryngoscope (82): 1282–1291, 1972.
118. Chandler JR. Cryosurgery for recurrent cancer of the head and neck. Otolaryngol Clin N Am (7): 193–204, 1974.

119. Gage AA. Five-year survival following cryosurgery for oral cancer. Arch Surg (111): 990–994, 1976.
120. Smith DB, Weaver AW. Cryosurgery for oral cancer, a six-year retrospective study. J Oral Surg (34): 245–248, 1976.
121. Bekke JPH, Baart JA. Six years' experience with cryosurgery in the oral cavity. Int J Oral Surg (8): 251–270, 1979.
122. Bradley, PF. Modern trends in cryosurgery of bone in the maxillofacial region. Int J Oral Surg (7): 405–415, 1978.
123. Mihashi S, Jako GJ, Incze J, Strong MS, Vaughan CW. Laser surgery in otolaryngology: Interaction of $CO_2$ laser and soft tissues. Bull NY Acad Sci (267): 263–294, 1975.
124. Oosterhuis JW, Verschueren RCJ, Eibergen R, Oldhoff J. The viability of cells in the waste products of $CO_2$-laser evaporation of Cloudman mouse melanomas. Cancer (49): 61–68, 1982.
125. Strong MS, Vaughan CW, Jealy GB, Shapshay SM, Jako GJ. Transoral management of localised carcinoma of the oral cavity using the $CO_2$ laser. Laryngoscope (89): 897–905, 1979.
126. Strong MS, Vaughan CW, Jako GJ, Polanyi T. Transoral resection of cancer of the oral cavity: The role of the $CO_2$ laser. Otolaryngol Clin North Am (12): 207–218, 1979.
127. Carruth JAS. Resection of the tongue with the carbon dioxide laser. J Laryngol Otol (96): 529–543, 1982.
128. Carruth JAS, McKenzie AL, Wainwright AC. The carbon dioxide laser: Safety aspects. J Laryngol Otol (94): 411–417.
129. Chaudhry AP, Vickers RA, Gorlin RJ. Intraoral minor salivary gland tumors. An analysis of 1414 cases. Oral Surg. (14): 1194–1226, 1961.
130. Spiro RH, Koss PG, Hadju S, Strong EW. Tumors of minor salivary origin. A clinicopathologic study of 492 cases. Cancer (31): 117–129, 1973.
131. Snow GB. Tumours of the parotid gland. Clin. Otolaryngol (4): 457–467, 1979.
132. Conley J, Dingman DL. Adenoid cystic carcinoma in the head and neck (cylindroma). Arch Otolaryngol (100): 81–90, 1974.
133. Chaudhry AP, Hampel A, Gorlin RJ. Primary malignant melanoma of the oral cavity. Cancer (11): 923–928, 1958.
134. Conley J, Pack GT. Melanoma of the mucous membranes of the head and neck. Arch Otolaryngol (99): 315–319, 1974.
135. Shah JP, Huvos AG, Stron EW. Mucosal melanoma of the head and neck. Amer J Surg (134): 531–535, 1977.
136. Snow GB, van der Esch EP, van Slooten EA. Mucosal melanoma of the head and neck. Head & Neck Surg (1): 24–30, 1978.
137. Eneroth CM, Lundberg C. Mucosal malignant melanomas of the head and neck. Laryngoscope (87): 760–764, 1976.

# 6. RADIOTHERAPY ASPECTS OF MALIGNANT DISEASES OF THE ORAL CAVITY

B.J. CUMMINGS

## 1. INTRODUCTION

The oral cavity forms the most proximal portion of the alimentary tract and serves as part of the upper airway. It provides the portal of entry to the body for food and fluids and serves as the initial site of digestive function through the mechanisms of mastication and salivation. The structures within the mouth, including the palate, tongue, and buccal regions, are an integral part of the speech apparatus. The oral mucosa is a protective barrier and collects sensory information relating to touch, pain, temperature, and taste. Efforts to treat tumors arising in the oral cavity must be directed not only at preserving the life of the patient, but also at preserving these functions as completely as possible.

Malignant tumors of the oral cavity make up approximately 40% of tumors of the head and neck region. More than 90% are squamous cell carcinomas, with tumors of the minor salivary glands making up most of the remainder. The various sites within the oral cavity, their interrelationships, and the influence of oral anatomy on the local patterns of tumor spread within the mouth have been described by Lederman [1].

The author acknowledges with thanks the secretarial assistance of Miss E. Eisenreich in preparing this manuscript and the assistance of Miss J. Collingwood in compiling the reference list.

The results of the treatment of oral cancer are influenced by both the patient population and the end points of treatment chosen for reference. These end points may include survival, control within the treated area, or response for varying lengths of time. The assessment of tumor stage may differ between physicians, and the reporting of results by stage without including the outcome of treatment for all patients may influence the results obtained in any centre. Patient characteristics, such as age, general health, and the development of second primary tumors, also affect the outcome of treatment. Certain tumor sites within the oral cavity are more accessible to some treatment methods than to others.

Although the two most commonly used staging systems, those of the International Union Against Cancer (UICC) and the American Joint Committee for Cancer Staging (AJC), employ common symbols—primary T(umor), N(ode), and M(etastasis)—they are not identical, and both have been revised on several occasions. It is impossible to reconcile and standardize the staging systems used in papers cited in this review, and the original papers should be consulted for specific details.

The morbidity associated with various methods of treatment is often quite different, and measures of "quality of life" after treatment are either completely lacking or imprecise, although they represent an active area of current research.

The purpose of this review is not to suggest that the results obtained in the management of oral cancer with radiation therapy are "better" or "worse" than those obtained with other modalities of treatment. Rather, it is to present those results that have been obtained with radiation therapy and to highlight both the benefits and the potential morbidity associated with the use of radiation therapy. The treatment of cancer is properly the task of a cooperative group of physicians and is not competitive.

This review will consider first the management of the primary tumor by radiation therapy or planned combined radiation and surgery. This will be followed by a discussion of the treatment of the cervical lymph node areas. A brief overview of treatments presently under investigation in attempts to improve the results of radiation therapy is included. Finally there will be a description of the complications associated with treatment of the oral cavity by irradiation.

## 2. TREATMENT OF THE PRIMARY TUMOR

The importance of successful treatment of the primary tumor is apparent from the inferior results invariably obtained in the treatment of recurring tumors even though they may be of similar size. Failure to control the primary tumor is the most significant problem in the management of oral carcinoma [2]. For convenience, treatment of the primary tumor will be considered first for small tumors less than 4 cm in diameter, and then for more extensive tumors.

### 2.1. Treatment of small lesions

Radiation therapy has produced high rates of control in small lesions in all sites within the oral cavity. If the various determinants of selection for treatment are considered, then either surgery or radiation therapy appear capable of producing control rates of the order of 80% or better in lesions up to 4 cm in size [3,4, 5]. Approximately one-half of those tumors that recur after initial irradiation may be controlled by subsequent surgery [4]. Hintz et al. [6] have reported a randomized trial comparing radiation to primary surgery, but only small numbers of patients were available and within that constraint no differences were seen.

Since the continuing dicussion concerning the relative merits of surgery and radiation cannot be resolved, the information available has been reviewed to determine how the primary tumor and neck nodes may be controlled most effectively by radiation.

The major forms of radiation in use today are external beam megavoltage equipment that delivers photon or electron radiation, and a variety of rigid or flexible interstitial radioactive sources. Kilovoltage equipment may be used occasionally with intraoral applicators. Optimum tumor doses and daily fractionation schemes have not been established, but similar results have been achieved with external beam doses of from 5,000 cGy in three weeks to 7,000 cGy in seven weeks. Daily dosage rates from approximately 180 to 300 cGy have been used, in five fractions each week. Interstitial radiation may be added to external beam therapy or used as the only treatment. Reference should be made to the papers cited for detailed dose prescriptions.

When carcinomas are only 1 to 2 cm in size and easily accessible, surgical excision offers the simplest treatment, provided it can be accomplished without significant risk or morbidity. However, when an "excisional biopsy" rather than a "curative" resection has been performed, the extent of the original lesion is often doubtful, and consideration must be given to the need for further treatment. In one study of patients with only residual scars or induration after biopsy excision, interstitial radium needle implant was used and no local recurrences were seen up to two years later [7]. Doses of 5,500 to 6,000 cGy by implant were considered adequate for subclinical disease, and neither external beam treatment nor elective neck irradiation was recommended unless nodularity of more than 2 cm diameter was present.

Typical results reported for the treatment of primary tumors of the tongue and floor of mouth are shown in table 6–1. Interstitial radiation appears to be effective in increasing local control rates over those achieved by external beam therapy alone. This benefit has been attributed both to the relatively intense local irradiation and to the continuous exposure while the implant is in place. Such factors as the tumor site and jaw configuration which may determine the choice of treatment are not always clear, but the results reported by various

**Table 6–1.** Local control in tumors < 4 cm size external beam (E) ± interstitial treatment (I)

| Site | I | I + E | E | Reference |
|---|---|---|---|---|
| Tongue | 25/33 | 13/17 | — | Fu et al. [8] |
| Tongue | 91/103 | 36/40 | 5/9 | Chu, Fletcher [9] |
| Tongue | 18/27 | 12/18 | 7/25 | Lees [10] |
| Tongue | — | 4/9 | 4/6 | Mendenhall [11] |
| Tongue | 9/10 | 2/3 | 3/6 | Gilbert et al. [12] |
| Tongue | 58/61 | — | — | Pierquin et al. [13] |
| Overall | 201/234 (85%) | 67/87 (77%) | 19/46 (41%) | |
| Floor of mouth | 61/65 | 27/28 | 28/33 | Chu, Fletcher [9] |
| Floor of mouth | — | 6/6 | 0/1 | Mendenhall [11] |
| Floor of mouth | 25/30 | 58/76 | 70/112 | Fitzpatrick [5] |
| Overall | 86/95 (90%) | 91/110 (82%) | 98/146 (67%) | |

authors are consistent. There is no agreement on the appropriate sequence when both external irradiation and interstitial therapy are used, with some authors preferring to apply the implant when the clinical boundaries of the tumor are still distinct and others preferring to implant local residual tumor only.

Several attempts to determine optimum time-dose relationships have been made, but only general conclusions can be drawn. The reported doses delivered by interstitial irradiation are imprecise because of irregular dose distribution within an implant volume and because of different conventions in specifying implant doses. The dose rate from different interstitial sources varies considerably, but similar rates of control have been achieved by implants delivering from 30 to 100 cGy per hour [8]. The incidence of subsequent necrosis shows some relationship to both dose and volume implanted [8] and to proximity of the radioactive sources to bone [14]. The optimal minimum tumor dose for local control of tumors less than 2 cm in diameter is approximately 6,000 cGy, and for tumors 2 to 4 cm diameter 6,500 cGy when interstitial implants alone are used [8]. Control rates of 90% or better have been achieved with such tumors [8,9,13].

When reporting combined treatment techniques, most authors add the radiation dose from interstitial and external sources while recognizing that this is convenient but not strictly in accord with radiobiological principles. Combined external-interstitial doses of 7,500 to 8,500 cGy have been recommended [8,15,16], and higher doses do not appear to be any more effective [17]. Combined treatment is generally used when treatment to the regional nodes is required. If the neck nodes are believed to require 5,000 cGy in five weeks' external beam radiation, then only limited interstitial treatment may be possible. Although the minimum effective interstitial dose has not been established, reduction of this component may be associated with lower primary tumor control rates [11].

Since small carcinomas of the retromolar trigone area, buccal mucosa, and gingiva are usually well lateralized, they can be treated with either a homolateral wedge field arrangement or a homolateral direct beam. This spares the contralateral salivary gland tissues and reduces the amount of mandible irradiated. Undertreatment due to inadequate field size occurred most frequently in one series with retromolar trigone lesions that infiltrated either the soft palate or the anterior buccal mucosa [18]. The initial control rates for small carcinomas in these sites may not be as good as in either the tongue or floor of mouth [4], perhaps because interstitial treatment is often technically impossible. However, surgical salvage is usually good. High local control rates have been obtained with doses equivalent to 7,000 cGy in seven weeks [19], and in the retromolar trigone region, even quite large tumors may remain superficial and be readily controlled by radiation.

Gingival ridge tumors often infiltrate the underlying bone quite early so that even tumors 2 to 3 cm in diameter may show bone involvement radiologically. Primary carcinomas of the upper alveolar ridge and hard palate are relatively uncommon, and many tumors that first present there are extensions of primary tumors of the maxillary antrum. Small superficial tumors are probably treated most readily by excision, although some may be accessible to intraoral cone therapy. The small amounts of bone irradiated can usually tolerate the kilovoltage beams employed, although irradiated mucosa, especially on the gingiva, may be subject to erosion by dental plates. A five-year control rate of 50% has been achieved with supervoltage treatment of primary carcinoma of the hard palate, and this was similar to the control rate following surgery [20].

### 2.2. Treatment of large tumors

The results obtained in the treatment of more advanced oral cavity carcinomas are often unsatisfactory. These tumors are more than 4 cm in diameter and may invade structures in the oral framework or extend to adjacent regions. Many patients with advanced tumors are unable to tolerate radical attempts at cure by any modality. Appropriate case selection may identify those patients most likely to benefit from radiation, surgery or combined treatment, and there is no general agreement on management policies for these complex cases. Local control may be improved if interstitial treatment in addition to external beam therapy is feasible (table 6–2), although tumor bulk and location often make these implants technically impossible. In one report, although three-quarters of patients with carcinoma of the anterior tongue or floor of mouth greater than 4 cm in size were controlled by radiation and surgical resection for recurrence, this control rate fell to one-third in patients with bone involvement or with massive tumors involving the base of tongue. In these patients surgical salvage was rarely possible [9]. Larger tumors are also more likely to be

**Table 6–2.** Local control in tumors > 4 cm size external beam (E) ± interstitial treatment (I)

| Site | I | I + E | E | Reference |
|---|---|---|---|---|
| Tongue | 9/16 | 28/47 | 12/32 | Chu, Fletcher [9] |
| Tongue | — | 3/8 | 3/8 | Fu et al. [8] |
| Tongue | — | 2/3 | 3/19 | Lees [10] |
| Tongue | 1/1 | 4/9 | 7/26 | Gilbert et al. [12] |
| Overall | 10/17 (58%) | 37/67 (55%) | 25/85 (29%) | |
| Floor of mouth | 16/21 | 16/22 | 19/41 | Chu, Fletcher [9] |
| Floor of mouth | — | 7/23 | 25/99 | Fitzpatrick, Tepperman [5] |
| Overall | 16/21 (76%) | 23/45 (51%) | 44/140 (31%) | |

associated with lymph node involvement, which further worsens the prognosis. Fitzpatrick [5] reported control by irradiation in 76% of floor of mouth tumors 4 cm or less in diameter without clinically enlarged lymph nodes; this fell to 40% in those with larger tumors including those with bone involvement, and to 20% when nodes were involved.

Most surgical groups have been equally unsuccessful in controlling advanced tumors with surgery alone [21], and combined radiation-surgery protocols have been explored for these tumors. The general theoretical principles of *combined radiation and surgery*, and many of the studies reported for all head and neck primary tumor sites, were reviewed by Cachin and Eschwege in 1975 [22]. They concluded that the randomized studies reported did not favour the use of preoperative radiation therapy. The major studies to that date used 1,000 cGy single dose 24 hours prior to surgery [23] or 1,400 cGy in 2 fractions prior to surgery [24], and neither regimen produced improvements in local control or survival.

A recently reported randomized trial by the Radiation Therapy Oncology Group (RTOG) comparing preoperative and postoperative irradiation in patients with advanced head and neck cancer has failed to identify any benefit from combined treatment in patients with oral cavity cancer [25]. Patients had carcinomas greater than 2 cm in diameter and were appropriately stratified for site, primary tumor size, and node category. Preoperative radiation consisted of 5,000 cGy in five weeks to the primary and both sides of the neck, followed by surgery four to eight weeks later. Postoperative radiation was commenced within four weeks of surgery, and 6,000 cGy in six weeks were delivered to the primary and 5,000 cGy to the neck. The third randomization was to radical radiation, which prescribed 5,000 cGy in five weeks to the primary and both sides of the neck plus local boost therapy of approximately 1,500 to 3,000 cGy using external beam or interstitial implant. Forty-nine patients with oral cavity primary tumors were included in this trial. The estimated rates of survival at two years for these patients were 53% for preoperative radiation and surgery,

59% for postoperative radiation and surgery, and 42% for radiation only. These differences were not statistically significant, but with the small numbers of patients in the study only very large differences could reach normal levels of statistical significance. The surgical complication rates were similar for planned preoperative and postoperative radiation and slightly greater for those who had salvage surgery after primary radiation treatment. The incidence of distant metastases in each group was similar. Even though undertaken by a large cooperative group, this study illustrates the difficulties in accruing sufficient patients to detect relatively small differences in outcome when appropriate attention is paid to the stratification of known prognostic factors.

In a retrospective review of patients with advanced oral cavity or oropharyngeal carcinoma treated with preoperative or postoperative schedules similar to those used by the RTOG, control in the primary site and neck was achieved for 2 years or longer in 18 of 36 patients. Forty of 49 (81%) had continued control at the primary site until death or last follow-up [26].

Marcus et al. [27] have discussed time-dose factors to achieve tumor control by irradiation following surgery. They concluded that although 5,000 cGy in five weeks will control 90% of patients with subclinical squamous cell carcinoma when surgery has not been performed, postoperative irradiation to that dose results in only about 45% control of subclinical residual tumor. In order to achieve 90% control rates, postoperative treatment apparently requires higher doses of the order of 6,500 to 7,000 cGy in 7 1/2 to 8 weeks [26,27]. This is possibly due to disruption of the vasculature at the time of surgery and to local hypoxia. It has also been suggested that unless radiation is started within seven weeks of surgery, higher failure rates might occur, although the surgery to radiation interval was not correlated with the radiation doses given [28]. Different dose schedules have not been studied in a comparative trial in postoperative patients.

When surgical margins are inadequate, local recurrence has been reported in up to 70% [29]. In one series of patients with inadequate margins who received postoperative irradiation, local recurrence still occurred in 42% [30]. Even so, this was a considerably better result than the 89% failure rate that occurred when gross postsurgical tumor recurrence was present at the time of radiation [30].

For most patients larger radiation fields are necessary postoperatively than preoperatively in order to cover all surgical scars and dissected tissues. There is a risk of significant subcutaneous fibrosis after extensive surgery and radiation. Treatment to the doses recommended by Marcus [27] should be probably be restricted to patients with positive surgical margins with any size primary tumor and to those patients with other poor prognostic features such as large primary tumors, poorly differentiated histological grade, or extensive cervical node involvement. Apparently, the appropriate place of combined radiation and surgery in the management of advanced oral carcinoma has not yet been established.

### 2.3. Contraindications to radiation therapy

Two conditions deserve special mention when radiation therapy for oral carcinoma is considered: verrucous carcinoma and bone involvement.

#### 2.3.1. *Verrucous carcinoma*

Verrucous carcinoma is a clinicopathological variant of squamous cell carcinoma and may occur at any site in the oral cavity but is most commonly found arising from the buccal regions or buccoalveolar grooves. The use of radiation therapy in its management has been disputed. Reported control rates have ranged from 0 to 17 patients [31] to 19 of 32 patients [32]. This latter rate was achieved with doses of 6,000 cGy in six weeks or greater. One series also reported transformation from well-differentiated to undifferentiated histological type following irradiation in 4 of 17 patients [31], but other authors have not found such changes [32,33]. However, the presence of squamous cell carcinoma in association with verrucous carcinoma was noted both at diagnosis and following irradiation [32,33].

Since regional lymph node metastases from verrucous cancers are relatively uncommon, treatment of more than the proximal cervical nodes is probably unnecessary even in the presence of extensive primary tumors. Firm recommendations for the management of verrucous carcinoma cannot be made from review of the literature, and if radiation therapy is chosen as the primary modality of treatment, the same principles of management as those for squamous cell carcinoma generally should be used.

#### 2.3.2. *Bone involvement*

Bone involvement or proximity of a tumor to bone has also been considered a contraindication to radiation therapy. From 3 to 20% of all cases of oral carcinoma may invade bone. Although bone will absorb more radiation than soft tissue because of its increased density (1.8 times that of soft tissue), the radiation absorption gram for gram of tissue will be approximately equivalent when megavoltage equipment is available. In 55 patients with involvement of the mandible who were treated with external cobalt 60 irradiation to doses of 6,500 cGy in six to seven weeks, the five-year survival was 40% [34]. The primary tumor was controlled by radiation in 36%. Only one episode of bone necrosis occurred, and this healed spontaneously; surgical procedures were performed in nine patients without necrosis developing. In a study of 251 patients with carcinoma of the alveolus, 71 (28%) showed bone invasion [35]. This increased the risk of recurrence up to two years after treatment but not thereafter, the cumulative risk of recurrence being 39% for those without bone involvement compared with 58% when bone was invaded. The risk of necrosis, however, was similar in each group.

Some authors have described increased risks of late spontaneous necrosis of bone when the primary tumor lies adjacent to or over bone even where radiological bone invasion is not identified. This is presumably due to relative atrophy of the mucosa after radiation [14]. Tumors adjacent to bone may have to be treated solely by external beam therapy, since the use of interstitial irradiation may not be possible technically and is also associated with an increased risk of bone necrosis. However, a proportion of patients with bone involvement can be cured by irradiation alone. These patients should be evaluated prior to treatment by both surgeon and radiotherapist to determine the management likely to give the best chance of cure with the least functional loss.

### 2.4. Pattern of management: Princess Margaret Hospital

The pattern of management for primary oral carcinoma favored at the Princess Margaret Hospital has been developed from consideration of results such as those already described [5,125]. Superficial tumors less than about 2 cm diameter that can be easily excised without significant interference with oral cavity function are treated surgically. Most other carcinomas are treated with external beam radiation to doses in the range of 5,000 cGy in four weeks to 6,000 cGy in six weeks, with additional interstitial radiation when this is feasible. Patients with verrucous carcinoma are treated in the same way as those with other types of carcinoma. Those patients with only moderate bone involvement are also treated initially with curative doses of radiation, but those with extensive or infected bone involvement are treated by surgical resection.

Patients who have persistent or recurrent carcinoma undergo surgery whenever possible, but planned combined treatment is used infrequently for the primary tumor. This policy results in tumor control rates similar to those reported from other centres, and structural and cosmetic morbidity is kept to as low a level as possible. The major functional morbidity is xerostomia, but whenever practicable some salivary gland tissue is excluded from the radiation beams.

## 3. TREATMENT OF CERVICAL LYMPH NODE METASTASES

No evidence exists that metastatic neck nodes are any more or less sensitive to radiation than is the primary carcinoma [36]. The individual lymph node groups associated developmentally with each site in the oral cavity have been detailed by anatomists, and several points deserve special attention when treatment is being considered [37]:

1. Although some lymphatics from the tip of the tongue and lower gingiva anterior to the incisor teeth may reach the submental nodes, they are seldom of clinical significance.
2. The lymphatics from the lateral and inferior surfaces of the tongue end in either the submandibular or upper deep cervical lymph nodes; those lymphatics that arise more anteriorly end in nodes situated more inferiorly in the upper neck.

3. Lymphatics from the medial tongue and floor of mouth may drain to the contralateral upper deep cervical nodes.
4. Lymphatics from the buccal mucosa follow the course of the facial vessels, and although most reach the submandibular and upper deep cervical nodes, some may terminate in nodes where the facial vessels cross the mandible, or in the lower parotid region.

Lindberg [38] reviewed the incidence and topographical distribution of lymph node metastases at the time of presentation in 2,044 patients with previously untreated squamous cell carcinoma of the head and neck. The nodes most frequently involved by carcinoma of the oral tongue were the upper deep cervical (subdigastric) group, with a lesser proportion in the submandibular region. A few patients had involvement of either submental, midcervical, or contralateral nodes. When the primary tumor arose in the floor of the mouth, the more anteriorly situated submandibular nodes were involved as often as the upper deep cervical nodes. Again, other sites in the neck, and especially contralateral nodes, were infrequently involved. As expected, the more advanced primary tumors were more likely to be associated with clinical node involvement. Less than 15% of patients with primary tumors of 2 cm diameter or less had positive nodes, but 30% had positive nodes when the tumor was between 2 and 4 cm in diameter. Only about one-half of patients with more advanced tumors were free of nodes at presentation.

Clinical assessment of the neck nodes is widely recognized to be less accurate than histological examination. The incidence of histologically positive nodes in necks considered clinically negative has ranged from 4 to 60% [40,41], with most reports in the 30-to-40% region. From 8 to 35% of palpable nodes may be enlarged from causes other than malignancy [40,42]. The accuracy of clinical assessment improves as the number of involved nodes increases and as the distal neck becomes involved [21].

There has been considerable discussion concerning the appropriate terminology for describing treatment of the neck nodes, but in this chapter the term *therapeutic* will be used to describe treatment for clinically enlarged nodes; and the term *elective* for treatment where no nodes can be detected on clinical examination.

### 3.1. Elective treatment

Elective treatment has been advocated because of the high incidence of histologically positive nodes frequently found in patients who did not have palpable nodes [39]. The use of radiation for elective treatment must be conditional, based on several questions.

1. Does elective irradiation produce better control and survival than therapeutic treatment for nodes that later become enlarged?
2. Does elective irradiation give better results than elective neck dissection?

3. If elective irradiation is given, what are the appropriate volume-dose-time factors?
4. What is the morbidity associated with elective irradiation?

Review of most retrospective series shows that of those patients who develop involved neck nodes after initial treatment of the primary tumor, some cannot be salvaged [21,39]. Farr and Arthur [21] reported a 48% five-year survival in those who presented without nodes as compared to only 25% when nodes were clinically enlarged at presentation and 32% when nodes appeared later.

Two randomized trials were conducted in which elective treatment was compared with therapeutic treatment. Vandenbrouck et al. [43] conducted a trial in 80 patients with carcinoma of the tongue in whom the primary tumor was treated by interstitial irradiation. These patients were then randomized to either elective or therapeutic radical neck dissection. The five-year survival and disease-free curves were similar for both groups. At the Christie Hospital, Manchester, 204 patients with oral cancer who did not have enlarged nodes were randomized to receive either elective neck irradiation or therapeutic neck dissection. The radiation dose was 5,000 cGy given dose (4 MeV photons or 10 MeV electrons) to the whole ipsilateral neck in 15 fractions in 3 weeks. Although fewer patients in the irradiated group developed enlarged nodes and required neck dissection, survival was approximately the same in each group [44].

While one could argue that in these two trials the study patients were under close observation so that adverse effects from progressive unrecognized growth of nodes did not occur, one cannot infer from these studies that therapeutic management of enlarged nodes is inferior to elective treatment. One further point not resolved is the possibility that clinical development of neck node metastases is paralleled by an increase in distant metastases. The incidence of such metastases appears to increase by about 10% in patients who develop neck nodes in a previously uninvolved region [45,46].

Nahum [47] reviewed the surgical literature relating to elective neck node dissection and concluded that the benefits of such surgery were not clearly definable on the available evidence. Most of his cited papers suggested that no more than 2 to 5% of patients would have benefited from elective neck dissection and that since the mortality of radical neck dissection was also of the order of 1 to 5%, such dissection was not justified. However, if surgical resection of the primary tumor is undertaken, additional dissection of the neck may not add significantly to perioperative mortality. Farr and Arthur's report [21] described a five-year survival rate of 33% for patients who had elective neck dissection and were found to have positive occult nodes. This was similar to the 32% survival of patients in whom late clinical node involvement developed. It has not been determined whether any advantage might result from postoperative irradiation of patients found to have subclinical node metastases at elective neck dissection, although combined radiation and surgery is more effective in preventing recurrence in patients with clinically involved nodes. Elective neck node irradiation and elective neck dissection have not been formally compared. Although the rates of failure in the neck are less in some series after irradiation than after surgery, most likely such series did not include patients identical in terms of primary tumor size and site and other important prognostic factors.

The efficacy of irradiation in preventing the late conversion of the clinically negative neck has been reported by several authors [39,48–52], yet the benefits in terms of survival are unclear. Without elective node irradiation about 35% patients with primary tumors of the oral tongue or floor of mouth develop homolateral nodes if they were initially node negative [48–50], and a similar number develop contralateral nodes if they present with ipsilateral involvement [48]. A dose of 3,000 to 4,000 cGy in three to four weeks resulted in late failure in the neck in 5 to 10% [48,51] and doses of 5,000 cGy in five weeks [50] or 6,000 cGy in six weeks [49] further reduced this number to nearly zero. Since two-thirds of patients would not have developed metastases if untreated, this may be restated as 70% control of subclinical disease at 3,000 to 4,000 cGy, and better than 95% control at 5,000 cGy or greater. Delivery of doses of the order of 5,000 cGy by external beam to the appropriate nodes may be difficult if a substantial part of treatment is to go to the primary tumor by interstitial therapy.

With well-lateralized primary tumors, appropriate treatment is of the homolateral neck only [38], but if the lesion lies near the midline, or if lymphatic pathways have been interrupted by surgery or tumor involvement, both sides of the neck should be treated [38,46,48]. Although discontinuous lymph node group involvement was noted in 6 of 21 neck dissection specimens [53], clinical observation suggests that the sequence of node involvement in the neck is usually orderly from superior to inferior. In most patients with oral cavity cancer, therefore, it is appropriate to treat the submandibular and upper deep cervical nodes to the level of the upper border of the thyroid cartilage. Even so, if full doses of radiation are used, further radiation probably cannot be given if the patient should develop a subsequent malignancy in the region.

Unfortunately, it is technically difficult to encompass the relevant lymph nodes and at the same time spare the sensitive salivary gland tissue, although xerostomia and other associated morbidity are reduced if unilateral radiation only is required. Some late atrophy of the sternocleidomastoid muscle has been seen after full neck irradiation to 6,600 cGy given dose in six weeks [49], and excessive soft tissue morbidity was noted when anterior-posterior opposed neck fields were used to deliver 5,500 to 6,000 cGy midplane at 1,100 cGy per week [52].

Despite the inconclusive nature of the evidence concerning improved survival following elective irradiation, the practice at the Princess Margaret Hospital is to extend radiation fields to cover at least those lymph nodes above the level of the thyroid cartilage if radiation is chosen as the treatment for the primary tumor. When surgery is used for the primary, then radiation may be given to the neck if elective treatment is considered advisable. However, the fields are usually similar to those used when radiation is the primary therapeutic modality, and while the dose to the oral cavity may possibly be lower, the sensitivity of the salivary glands is such that morbidity may be unchanged.

### 3.2. Therapeutic radiation

Therapeutic radiation may be used for patients with clinically involved nodes. Approximately one-half of all patients with carcinoma of the oral cavity have clinically positive cervical lymph nodes at the time of presentation [39], and a five-year survival rate of only 25% is common whether treatment is by surgery or irradiation [21,54,55]. These patients are more likely to develop later recurrence at the primary tumor site and in the neck and distant metastases [46,56]. Control of neck nodes is maintained more frequently when the primary tumor also remains controlled [55]. The rate of recurrence is high in the neck after radical neck dissection alone for clinically involved lymph nodes [57].

Where radiation has been used to treat neck nodes, some correlation has been established between the degree of control, the number and size of involved nodes, and the dose. Less than 10% of nodes were controlled by 4,000 cGy in three to four weeks [51], while for single nodes 3 cm or less in diameter 5,000 cGy in five weeks controlled approximately 50%, and 6,500 cGy in 6 1/2 to 7 weeks 90% [46,58]. However, where mobile nodes were greater than 3 cm diameter or multiple, failure occurred in 20% or more even when doses were greater than 6,500 cGy [58]. When fixed or bilateral nodes were present, either persistent or recurrent neck nodes were found in half of those patients in whom the primary was controlled. It has been demonstrated that even extensive node masses can be controlled by radiation therapy although larger nodes require greater doses of radiation for control. For example, only one of nine patients who received less than 7,000 cGy in seven weeks for node masses greater than 5 cm was controlled, while 11 of 15 were controlled at doses above 7,000 cGy [59]. The risks of morbidity following later surgery are increased by high radiation doses to the neck, however.

Cachin [60] demonstrated that capsular rupture was present in 70% of nodes greater than 3 cm in size and that local recurrence was significantly more common when such extension was present (27% versus 14%). Although large nodes may be reduced to impalpable levels after radiation, there is still a likelihood of finding tumor in about one-half of patients at subsequent neck dissection [46,61]. For these reasons many centres prefer to treat patients with neck node involvement more extensive than a single small node by combined surgery and radiation therapy [126]. In a randomized trial to evaluate preoperative irradiation, 2,000 cGy in five treatments in one week to the ipsilateral neck in patients with or without enlarged neck nodes reduced the rate of neck recurrence from 29% in those having surgery only, to 18% in the combined treatment group [57]. Higher preoperative doses to 5,000 cGy in five weeks in patients with enlarged nodes reduced the rate of recurrence in the neck from 26% to 8% [62]. Surgical morbidity was not increased at either of these dose levels. By treating both sides of the neck, the risk of later involvement of the clinically negative regions may be greatly reduced [48].

#### 4. THE PREDICTION OF RESPONSE TO TREATMENT

An indicator to predict the likelihood of satisfactory response to irradiation, either prior to treatment or as soon as possible after irradiation is completed, would greatly improve the selection of appropriate treatment modalities. Several attempts have been made to develop a suitable indicator.

Biochemical assays, including such tests as serum copper/zinc ratios [63], and carcinoembryonic antigen (CEA) levels [64], and skin tests of delayed hypersensitivity response to agents such as dinitrochlorobenzene (DNCB) [65] have failed to correlate sufficiently well to responses to specific treatment modalities to permit their use in selecting therapy.

Molinari [66] studied "potential proliferative activity" using tritiated thymidine techniques in biopsies obtained before and during radiation therapy. The results have been inconclusive.

The reports on the value of assessing the degree of tumor regression during and immediately following irradiation have been conflicting. Earlier reports suggested that neither the degree of regression of the primary tumor at the completion of irradiation, nor the degree of posttreatment induration, was a sensitive prognostic indicator [67,68]. However, others found that recurrence was more likely in those patients who had residual tumor present at the end of a course of fractionated radiation [69,70]. Sobel [71] suggested that the rate of tumor regression during the course of treatment was of less significance than complete tumor disappearance within three months of the end of treatment. Of 60 patients with oral cancer, only 16% had clearance of tumor before treatment was completed, while 43% had clearance at the end of treatment; this figure had risen to a plateau of 69% 90 days after treatment was completed. At intervals of 30 to 90 days after treatment, complete tumor clearance was predicted for local control in 78%. Persistent induration and surface irregularity at 30 to 90 days were almost 100% predictive of local failure, whereas induration at the completion of treatment was followed by local control in about 25%.

Review of these studies indicated that tumor doses and treatment volumes should be chosen on the basis of the pretreatment extent of the tumor, and not on the presence or absence of residual tumor at the completion of the planned course. However, unless combined radiotherapeutic-surgical management has been determined as the policy for a particular patient prior to any treatment, decisions concerning the need for attempted surgical "salvage" can probably be deferred until three months after irradiation.

## 5. INVESTIGATIONAL TECHNIQUES

The generally unsatisfactory results of primary radiation therapy and/or surgery for advanced oral cavity carcinoma have stimulated interest in the development of methods to improve tumor control and survival. These may be considered in three groupings: (1) chemotherapy and radiation therapy, (2) efforts to overcome the relative radioresistance of hypoxia in tumors, and (3) investigation of unconventional radiation fractionation.

### 5.1. Chemotherapy and radiation therapy (see also chapter 7)

Oral cavity tumors are among the more favorable in terms of response by site to present chemotherapy protocols. The most effective drugs appear to be methotrexate, cis-diamminedichloroplatinum (cis-platinum), adriamycin, and bleomycin, although reported rates of response vary widely for all drugs [72, 127]. The most effective sequencing of multimodality treatment programs remains to be determined, although the need for adequate vascular access for the chemotherapeutic agents would seem to favour the use of chemotherapy prior to irradiation or surgery when improved primary tumor or cervical node control is the major consideration. Increased toxicity has been seen in several combined chemotherapy-radiation therapy protocols [73,74,75]. Most results suggest that the responses obtained to each modality are additive although enhancement of radiation response by some drugs may be possible [76]. Where the results are additive, toxicity is usually less with sequential than with simultaneous multimodality treatment.

The general subject of combined modality treatment with radiotherapy and chemotherapy has recently been reviewed [77], and extensive reviews of the clinical results of combined radiation and chemotherapy have been published [72,78]. Although quantitative studies are limited, concurrent administration of radiation and methotrexate, bleomycin, 5-fluorouracil, actinomycin-D, or hydroxyurea increases the severity and shortens the time to onset of mucositis [79]. Skin reactions are enhanced to a lesser extent [79].

Several studies of methotrexate and radiation therapy have been reported. The RTOG noted toxicity-related failure to complete radiation therapy in 19%, and no differences in control rates or survival were found [73]. In common with most authors, Chassagne [80] found that control rates were better when radiation treatment following methotrexate was given to the volume involved by tumor prior to chemotherapy, and not to residual tumor only.

Bleomycin used in combination with radiation in oropharyngeal cancer caused delays in treatment and increased acute reactions without any improvement in tumor regression or in survival to 15 months when compared with radiation alone [81]. However, Shanta and Krishnamurthi [82] reported a randomized trial in advanced buccal squamous cancer comparing radiation alone (5,500–6,000 cGy in seven weeks cobalt-60) to concurrent radiation and bleomycin (10–15 mgm two or three times weekly to total 150 to 250 mgm). Total tumor clearance eight weeks after irradiation was 78% versus 19%, and recurrence-free five-year survival rates were 72% and 17% for the combined-treatment and radiation-only groups, respectively. Four of 64 patients who received bleomycin suffered fatal pneumonitis. A previous study in similar patients by these authors showed no benefit from combined methotrexate and irradiation.

Several studies of multiple-agent chemotherapy have reported response rates of 50 to 70%; although the toxicity of many combination chemotherapy programs has been high, and the duration of response of the order of only a few months and not greatly longer than that of single-agent chemotherapy, there has been continued interest in combining such programs with irradiation [72,83]. Where toxicity requires modification of dose for either chemotherapy or radiation therapy, comparison with single-modality treatment given without dose modification may be very difficult.

The treatment by chemotherapy of late recurrences after prior radiation therapy has been generally disappointing, and response rates to single or multiple agents are lower in these irradiated patients than in previously untreated patients. The low response rates, and the toxicity sometimes encountered, suggest that stricter criteria than simple reduction in tumor bulk for short periods may be appropriate in assessing the palliative benefits of such treatment.

In an attempt to determine effective combinations, most studies of combined radiation therapy and chemotherapy so far reported have concentrated on patients with advanced disease, and little is known yet about possible late toxicity. Studies of combined modalities require careful recording of the characteristics of the patients eligible for such treatments and the reasons for exclusion, since it is possible that only highly selected patients may enter complex protocols and many patients may withdraw during treatment.

### 5.2. Hypoxic cells as a cause of radiation failure

Many causes for the failure of radiation treatment to control tumors have been suggested. One such cause is believed to be the presence of hypoxic cells in human tumors. Gray [84] has demonstrated that the absence of oxygen requires an increase in radiation dose by a factor of 2.5 to 3.0 to produce the same radiation effect achieved in the presence of full oxygenation. Several of the techniques studied in an attempt to overcome the adverse effects of hypoxic cells on local control by irradiation are outlined here.

#### *5.2.1. Oxygen breathing and hyperbaric oxygen (HBO)*

A study comparing the treatment of patients who breathed either air or carbogen (95% oxygen, 5% carbon dioxide) at atmospheric pressure during irradiation showed no differences in tumor control, survival, or toxicity [85]. Several studies have also been conducted using hyperbaric oxygen chambers. Patients were placed in these chambers and irradiated under pressures of 3 atmospheres absolute in oxygen. To be eligible for such treatment, patients must be able to tolerate 30 to 60 minutes within the chamber, and some may require bilateral myringotomy to permit middle ear pressure equalization. Elderly and medically unfit patients may not be able to tolerate treatment in these chambers.

The series of randomized trials reported by the Medical Research Council (United Kingdom) have included two devoted to head and neck cancer patients. In the first trial [86] treatment was given either in air or in HBO in 10 fractions over 22 days on 3 days a week to a dose between 3,500 and 4,600 cGy according to field size. Patients were stratified by site, and for reporting purposes oral cavity patients were grouped with oropharynx, nasopharynx, and nasal sinus patients. In this "nasal and oral" subgroup, the recurrence-free rate at five years for those treated in HBO was 57% compared with 25% for those treated in air ($p < 0.01$), but survival was not improved [87]. Delayed complications were found more frequently in the HBO group, although this was significant only in the numbers developing laryngeal perichondritis.

In the second trial [87] the same fractionation scheme in HBO was compared with conventional fractionation in air (5,700 to 6,600 cGy in 30 treatments for most patients). At the time of reporting, both local control and survival showed a significant improvement for the HBO group. Those with oral cavity primary sites were not identified separately. No significant difference in toxicity was seen in this second trial, the dose to the larynx having been reduced by 10%.

Other randomized trials of HBO and radiation therapy for sites in the head and neck have included relatively few patients compared to the studies noted above. None have reported statistically significant results, although in general some benefit was noted for HBO both for local tumor control and survival. Long-term follow-up is not yet available from any of these studies.

The balance of available information is in favour of the use of HBO. The cumbersome and time-consuming techniques, however, prevent general application, but treatment in HBO will presumably be compared in appropriate trials with other measures designed to overcome the effects of hypoxic tumor cells. Dische [88] has suggested that an improvement in tumor control of the order of magnitude seen with HBO in the U.K. Medical Research Council trials could not be achieved by simple increase of the radiation dose in air with conventional fractionation without unacceptable increases in normal tissue morbidity.

*5.2.2. Heavy particle radiation beams*

A number of heavy particle radiation beams are undergoing radiobiological and clinical evaluation. These include fast neutrons, negative pi mesons, protons, and heavy ions. Interest in the use of such beams is related to the potential clinical application either of radiobiological factors, which increase the differential response of normal and tumor tissues, or of improved spatial distribution of radiation within the tumor and surrounding tissues [89]. None of these beams has yet been used extensively in clinical practice, and most information relates to fast neutron radiation.

In comparison to photons, fast neutron beams are less dependent on the presence of oxygen during radiation, in general have greater relative biological effectiveness, and have less repair of intracellular damage produced by such high linear energy transfer radiation. Two randomized trials in patients with advanced head and neck tumors compared neutron irradiation with photon irradiation [90,128]. Neutron irradiation did not improve survival in either trial, and although Hammersmith reported improved local control with neutrons, this result was not duplicated in Edinburgh and may have resulted from the difficulty in matching photon and neutron radiation doses. In some series there has been considerable late toxicity after neutron irradiation.

Several centres are studying combined photon and neutron radiation, and some have noted improved control of tumor masses in neck nodes and fewer complications than after neutron therapy alone [91,129].

The comparison of conventional radiation (where there is no standard time-dose scheme) with the many variables associated with new particle beams is complex, and at present all such radiation must be considered experimental.

### *5.2.3. Radiation sensitizers*

A number of chemical compounds are available that enhance the response to radiation of hypoxic cells [92]. Most interest has been in the nitroimidazole group of drugs, which belong to the electron-affinic class of sensitizers. The nitroimidazoles are examples of drugs that increase the response of hypoxic cells to radiation but not the response of normally oxygenated cells. In addition to being sensitizers, some of these drugs have a direct cytotoxic action on hypoxic cells. Since they are metabolized in a different way from oxygen, they can frequently reach the relevant hypoxic tumor regions. The major clinical toxicity of the nitroimidazoles is neurotoxicity. The maximum tolerable total dose for misonidazole, the agent currently undergoing major testing, is approximately 12 $gm/m^2$ body area. At present there is little agreement on how best to combine these drugs with radiation. In theory, a high pulse of the radiation sensitizing drug combined with a high single dose of irradiation would give the best result. However, intermittent high doses of radiation produce increased normal tissue toxicity, and experience gained over many years favours daily fractionated irradiation for most human tumors. Recent theoretical and laboratory studies suggest that useful sensitizer enhancement ratios could be achieved by combining small daily doses of a sensitizing drug with conventional external radiation [93], and a number of studies are presently in progress.

In a phase II study of misonidazole and radiotherapy in locally advanced carcinomas of the oral cavity, oropharynx, and hypopharynx, misonidazole was given once each week for five weeks, initially at 2.5 $gm/m^2$/week but later at 2.0 $gm/m^2$/week because of neurotoxicity [94]. The radiation fractionation used during the period the patient received misonidazole was unusual. Two doses four hours apart (250 cGy and 210 cGy) were given on the day of misonidazole, together with 180 cGy on each of three other days each week. This was designed to allow two treatments while serum misonidazole levels were relatively high, and the four-hour interval was intended to allow repair of sublethal damage in normally oxygenated tissues. Complete disappearance of tumor was noted in 67% of 36 patients who completed at least three doses of misonidazole and minimally acceptable radiation therapy, and this was considered better than would have been expected from conventional radiation alone. Randomized studies using this RTOG schedule have been commenced, in comparison with conventional daily fractionated radiation [130]. A randomized study is also continuing under the direction of the U.K. Medical Research Council using either intermittent or daily fractionated misonidazole. A schedule combining misonidazole with twice weekly radiation fractionation showed no improvement in local control rates [95].

There is a need for less toxic, and possibly more effective, hypoxic cell radiation sensitizers. Such drugs offer the possibility of improved tumor control and survival using conventional radiation sources, compared to the requirements of increased manpower, space, and cost for treatment in hyperbaric oxygen or with particle radiation beams. One concern with present drugs is the selection that must be made before patients can be treated with neurotoxic agents such as misonidazole. In a study from Princess Margaret Hospital, only about one-third of patients with oral cavity or oropharyngeal carcinomas were eligible to receive these drugs if strict criteria were applied—age less than 70 years, no prior history of neuropathy or central nervous system abnormality, no significant impairment of renal function, and no history of intractable alcoholism [131].

### *5.2.4. Smoking and hemoglobin oxygen-carrying capacity*

Anemia during radiation treatment has been demonstrated to be an important factor in decreasing local control [96]. Few patients with head and neck cancer are anemic on presentation, but other factors that reduce the oxygen-carrying capacity of the blood may affect tumor control by irradiation. Hb bound carbon monoxide (HbCO) reduces the capacity of blood to release oxygen to the tissues, and inhaled cigarette smoke is a major source of carbon monoxide. In an experimental system the control rate by irradiation of transplanted KHT sarcoma in mice was reduced when the animals were exposed to cigarette smoke to produce HbCO levels similar to those found in humans [97].

Although most physicians advise patients to discontinue smoking to reduce the risk of subsequent malignancy elsewhere in the aerodigestive tract and of other tobacco-related illness, there may also be other potential advantages to the patient who stops smoking.

### 5.3. Unconventional radiation dose schedules

Some investigators have attempted to improve control rates through a number of "unconventional" techniques. Various radiobiological justifications have been suggested, including alterations in oxygen enhancement ratios at low dose rates and different fraction sizes, differential repair of sublethal radiation damage in hypoxic and oxygenated cells, rapidly changing ratios of oxygenated and hypoxic cells after irradiation, and different growth patterns in normal tissues and in tumors favoring extended course treatment. Whether any of the attempts to exploit these principles will become applicable to clinical radiotherapy is as yet unclear.

In studies with continuous low dose rate, cobalt-60 irradiation patients were treated for six to eight hours per day at 90 to 130 cGy per hour, to total doses of 6,500 to 7,000 cGy [98]. Split course treatment gave more tolerable mucosal reactions, but the necrosis rate was high. Local control rates were sufficiently encouraging to support a randomized trial in comparison with conventional fractionation, which is still in progress.

Multiple daily fraction regimens using two [99], three [100,101], or eight [102] daily fractions have been reported. While some tolerable dose schedules have been established, serious necrosis has also occurred [101]. No convincing advantages over conventional fractionation have been established [132,133].

Split course treatment programs [103,104] have sometimes been reported to produce local tumor control rates similar to conventional treatments. The lower toxicity seen has been considered an advantage in palliative treatment [104,105]. However, others have described inferior tumor control levels following split course treatment [105,106], and planned interruptions in treatment have not found favour generally.

Few of these unconventional programs have been formally tested in randomized trials.

## 6. MINOR SALIVARY GLAND MALIGNANT TUMORS

Tumors of the minor salivary glands are uncommon but at least one-half are malignant. The commonest site for such tumors is the posterior half of the palate, reflecting the greater number of salivary glands in that site relative to other intraoral areas. In general, the primary treatment of these malignant tumors is surgical excision, although radiation therapy may be used either where surgical margins are inadequate or where excision is not practical. There are mixed opinions on the radiocurability of tumor types such as adenoid cystic carcinoma, although useful clinical responses have sometimes been seen. Combined surgery and postoperative radiation reduced the incidence of local failure compared to surgery alone in high-grade parotid gland tumors [16], and a similar result might be expected with minor salivary gland carcinomas. Wang [107] described control of disease for 3 years or longer in 6 of 22 patients with oral salivary gland tumors who were treated with radiation to doses of 6,500 cGy in 6 to 7 weeks.

## 7. MUCOSAL MELANOMAS

These rare melanomas are occasionally considered too extensive for surgical excision. Radiation produced local control to last follow up or death from other causes in four of nine patients treated at the Princess Margaret Hospital. The realization that melanomas are more likely to respond to large radiation fractions of the order of 400 cGy or more suggests that the traditional classification of melanomas as "radio resistant" is unjustified [108].

## 8. COMPLICATIONS OF RADIATION THERAPY

"Complications" and "side effects" following radiation therapy to the oral cavity are often difficult to distinguish and will be considered together. Detailed accounts of the histological and physiological changes associated with irradiation of the oral cavity have been published [109,110].

The most frequently found postradiation symptom is xerostomia secondary to decreased salivary gland function. When all major salivary glands have been irradiated to a dose equivalent to 6,000 cGy in six weeks, salivary output may decrease by more than 90%; although some symptomatic improvement may occur with time, the saliva never returns to normal quantity or composition. Many younger patients may tolerate doses of 4,500 to 5,000 cGy without developing permanent symptomatic xerostomia. Attempts to produce artificial salivary substitutes have had only mixed success [110]. The possible effects of adding xerostomia to a patient's other symptoms should be considered, especially where the chances of cure are very small or where "palliation" only is intended.

The development of drugs that reduce radiation damage to normal tissues preferentially to that in tumor would afford the possibility of improving the therapeutic ratio, and of reducing morbidity. A number of agents, especially sulfhydryl compounds such as WR2721 and related drugs, have produced alterations in dose response effects in both oral mucosa and salivary glands in animal systems. These agents appear to exert greater protective effects on normally oxygenated cells and to localize in greater concentration in normal tissues than in tumors [112]. At present, the available agents are too toxic to permit general use.

One of the major effects of changes in the volume and quality of saliva is an increase in dental caries; the consequent need for dental extractions in relation to radiation therapy has not been determined. Some authors have suggested that the interval between extractions and radiation therapy is not significant [113], whereas others recommend that at least two weeks should be allowed for local tissue healing [114]. Other factors, such as the volume of mandible irradiated, and the techniques of dental extraction are probably equally important [111]. Extractions performed following radiation have been said to produce a higher rate of bone infection and necrosis [114], but others [115] believe the risk is low when the procedure is performed carefully. Although most centres have adopted a conservative approach to dental management rather than indiscriminate total extractions prior to radiation, such a policy requires an awareness by the patient of the need for lifelong cooperation in the program since xerostomia and its effects are permanent.

Necrosis of bone or soft tissues is the major complication reported after irradiation of the oral cavity and adjacent tissues. Soft tissue necrosis occurs most commonly in the tongue, especially after interstitial implants [8,15], and will usually heal with conservative management. When soft tissue erosions appear over the gingiva, it may be unclear when bone necrosis begins: one definition of bone necrosis is exposure of bone in the irradiated field for at least two months in the absence of local neoplastic disease [111]. Necrosis is more common in the mandible than in the maxilla, probably because of differences in vascular supply and proximity to tumor. The causes, management, and prevention of radiation necrosis of the mandible have recently been discussed [116,117]. The overall incidence of bone necrosis described in the literature was found to be 4 to 35%. From this, and previous studies [14], apparently, the greatest risk was associated with the treatment of tumors of the retromolar trigone or floor of mouth which were adjacent to bone and teeth; the risk was also greater with more advanced tumors that were treated with higher doses to greater volumes. Necrosis was more likely as dose rose over 5,000 cGy in five weeks. The preventive and conservative dental programs introduced during the study period were identified as reducing the incidence of osteoradionecrosis. However, a relationship was also noted between the incidence of necrosis in the mandible and the presence of dental disease prior to irradiation [118], such that a policy of conserving severely decayed teeth may not be advisable.

The management of radionecrosis of the mandible is primarily conservative. Over a period of time, about 50 to 70% heal by such techniques [5,117]. Pain, trismus, and severe infection have been regarded as indications for surgery, with particular attention to resecting through unirradiated bone when possible. A recently introduced alternative for treating resistant soft tissue and bone necrosis is hyperbaric oxygen therapy administered at between 2.0 and 3.0 atmospheres absolute pressure, although optimum scheduling has not yet been determined [119].

Serious surgical morbidity associated with planned combined radiation and surgery is usually reported to be about 35% [25,120] and is less than that observed when primary radiation treatment is followed by salvage surgery where complication rates of up to 70% [25,120] have been recorded. These differences may be at least partly related to different definitions of morbidity, to the different radiation doses used, and to the intervals between radiation and surgery.

A major nonspecific effect of radical irradiation of the oral cavity is the exacerbation of alterations in nutrition. Although the immediate contributing causes may be dysphagia associated with radiation mucositis and alterations in salivary secretion and taste sensation, the nutritional and physiological changes seen during and after irradiation are complex [121], and their correction and management may be difficult [122]. Weight loss during irradiation may be considerable and may continue for at least three months after the completion of irradiation. There is no evidence as yet that maintaining the patient's weight during treatment by techniques such as intravenous hyperalimentation will increase survival, although the radiation may be better tolerated.

Conflicting evidence has been presented on the possible carcinogenic effects of radiation used to treat primary head and neck malignancies. Although the use of radiation treatment for the initial lesion was suggested to carry an increased risk of male patients' developing another primary 10 years or more later [123], others found similar rates of new cancers in the oral cavity or upper aerodigestive tract when comparing patients treated by surgery and by irradiation [124]. Combined treatment with radiation and chemotherapy, or other treatment methods described in the section on investigational techniques, may lead to an increase in tumor induction although adequate long-term follow-up is not yet available in most series.

## 9. SUMMARY

Radiation therapy is an effective means of treating squamous cell carcinomas of the oral cavity, although control rates decrease as the primary tumor enlarges and as lymph node involvement becomes more extensive. The appropriate indicators for combined surgery and radiation have not yet been established. Planned combined treatment and surgery deferred until the tumor recurs after radiation therapy fail to cure a substantial number of patients with advanced tumors.

Elective irradiation of the clinically uninvolved neck node regions is effective in preventing late node development but has not yet been proven to improve survival when compared to the treatment of only those patients who develop clinical node involvement.

The use of radiation therapy to treat more than one side of the oral cavity usually results in xerostomia. This physiological morbidity affects patients to different degrees and cannot be compared directly with the anatomical and cosmetic morbidity that accompanies surgical treatment of carcinomas in this region.

A number of investigational techniques are under study, but none has yet shown consistently improved results nor been accepted for general use. Carefully designed studies are needed to determine whether the good response rates described with some of these techniques in patients with advanced tumors will lead to improved survival rates. Finally, it will also be necessary to establish which patient groups can tolerate and benefit from potentially toxic multiple modality treatment programs.

## REFERENCES


1. Lederman M. Cancer of the oral cavity: Observations on classification and natural history. Int J Radiat Oncol Biol Phys (6): 1559–1565, 1980.
2. Gilbert H, Kagan AR. Recurrence patterns in squamous cell carcinoma of the oral cavity, pharynx, and larynx. J Surg Oncol (6): 357–380, 1974.
3. Frazell EL. A review of the treatment of cancer of the mobile portion of the tongue. Cancer (28): 1178–1181, 1971.
4. Fletcher GH. Place of irradiation in the management of head and neck cancers. Semin Oncol (4): 375–385, 1977.
5. Fitzpatrick PJ, Tepperman BS. Carcinoma of the floor of the mouth. J. Can Assoc Radiol (33): 148–153, 1982.
6. Hintz B, Charyulu K, Chandler JR, Sudarsanam A, Garciga C. Randomized study of local control and survival following radical surgery or radiation therapy in oral and laryngeal carcinomas. J Surg Oncol (12): 61–74, 1979.
7. Ange DW, Lindberg RD, Guillamondegui OM. Management of squamous cell carcinoma of the oral tongue and floor of mouth after excisional biopsy. Radiology (116): 143–146, 1975.
8. Fu KK, Chan EK, Phillips TL, Ray JW. Time, dose and volume factors in interstitial radium implants of carcinoma of the oral tongue. Radiology (119): 209–213, 1976.
9. Chu A, Fletcher GH. Incidence and causes of failures to control by irradiation the primary lesions in squamous cell carcinomas of the anterior two-thirds of the tongue and floor of mouth. AJR (117): 502–508, 1973.
10. Lees AW. The treatment of carcinoma of the anterior two-thirds of the tongue by radiotherapy. Int J Radiat Oncol Biol Phys (1): 849–858, 1976.
11. Mendenhall WM, Million RR, Cassisi NJ. Elective neck irradiation in squamous-cell carcinoma of the head and neck. Head Neck Surg (3): 15–20, 1980.
12. Gilbert EH, Goffinet DR, Bagshaw MA. Carcinoma of the oral tongue and floor of mouth: Fifteen years' experience with linear accelerator therapy. Cancer (35): 1517–1524, 1975.
13. Pierquin B, Chassagne D, Baillet F, Castro JR. The place of implantation in tongue and floor of mouth cancer. JAMA (215): 961–963, 1971.
14. Bedwinek JM, Shukovsky LJ, Fletcher GH, Daley TE. Osteonecrosis in patients treated with definitive radiotherapy for squamous cell carcinomas of the oral cavity and naso- and oropharynx. Radiology (119): 665–667, 1976.
15. Fayos JV. The role of radium implants in cancer of the oral cavity and oral pharynx. Int J Radiat Oncol Biol Phys (6): 423–429, 1980.
16. Fletcher GH. Textbook of Radiotherapy, 3rd ed. Philadelphia: Lea and Febiger, 1980.
17. Sahatchiev A, Moushmov M, Kirov S. Results of radical treatment of cancer of the anterior two-thirds of the tongue. Cancer (30): 703–707, 1972.
18. Richaud P, Tapley ND: Lateralized lesions of the oral cavity and oropharynx treated in part with the electron beam. Int J Radiat Oncol Biol Phys (5): 461–465, 1979.
19. Barker JL, Fletcher GH. Time, dose and tumor volume relationships in megavoltage irradiation of squamous cell carcinomas of the retromolar trigone and anterior tonsillar pillar. Int J Radiat Oncol Biol Phys (2): 407–414, 1977.
20. Chung CK, Rahman SM, Lim ML, Constable WC. Squamous cell carcinoma of the hard palate. Int J Radiat Oncol Biol Phys (5): 191–196, 1979.
21. Farr HW, Arthur K. Epidermoid carcinoma of the mouth and pharynx, 1960–1964. Elective radical neck dissection. Clin Bull (1): 130–135, 1971.
22. Cachin Y, Eschwege F. Combination of radiotherapy and surgery in the treatment of head and neck cancers. Cancer Treat Rev (2): 177–191, 1975.
23. Ketcham AS, Hoye RC, Chretien PB, Brace KC. Irradiation twenty-four hours preoperatively. Am J Surg (118): 691–697, 1969.
24. Lawrence WJr, Terz JJ, Rogers C, King RE, Wolf JS, King ER. Preoperative irradiation for head and neck cancer: A prospective study. Cancer (33): 318–323, 1974.
25. Kramer S. Comparison of preoperative and postoperative radiation therapy for patients with

carcinoma of the head and neck—The RTOG Study. Presented at Am Soc Ther Radiol, 1980.
26. Hamberger AD, Fletcher GH, Guillamondegui OM, Byers RM. Advanced squamous cell carcinoma of the oral cavity and oropharynx treated with irradiation and surgery. Radiology (119): 433–438, 1976.
27. Marcus RB, Million RR, Cassisi NJ. Postoperative irradiation for squamous cell carcinomas of the head and neck: Analysis of time-dose factors related to control above the clavicles. Int J Radiat Oncol Biol Phys (5): 1943–1949, 1979.
28. Vikram B. Importance of the time interval between surgery and postoperative radiation therapy in the combined management of head and neck cancer. Int J Radiat Oncol Biol Phys (5): 1837–1840, 1979.
29. Looser KG, Shah JP, Strong EW. The significance of "positive" margins in surgically resected epidermoid carcinomas. Head Neck Surg (1): 107–111, 1978.
30. Fletcher GH, Evers WT. Radiotherapeutic management of surgical recurrences and postoperative residuals in tumors of the head and neck. Radiology (95): 185–188, 1970.
31. Kraus FT, Perez-Mesa C. Verrucous carcinoma. Cancer (19): 26–38, 1966.
32. Memula N, Ridenhour G, Doss LL. Radiotherapeutic management of oral cavity verrucous carcinoma. Proc. 22nd Annual Meeting Amer Soc Ther Radiol, Int J Radiat Oncol Biol Phys (6): 1404, 1980.
33. Burns HP, Van Nostrand AWP, Palmer JA. Verrucous carcinoma of the oral cavity: Management by radiotherapy and surgery. Can J Surg (23): 19–25, 1980.
34. Fayos JV. Carcinoma of the mandible. Result of radiation therapy. Acta Radiol (Ther) (12): 378–386, 1973.
35. Porter EH. The local prognosis after radical radiotherapy for squamous carcinoma of the alveolus or the floor of the mouth. Clin Radiol (22): 139–143, 1971.
36. Henk JM. Radiosensitivity of lymph node metastases. Proc R Soc Med (68): 85–86, 1975.
37. del Regato JA, Spjut HJ. Ackerman and del Regato's Cancer Diagnosis, Treatment, and Prognosis, 5th Ed. St. Louis: C.V. Mosby, 1977.
38. Lindberg R. Distribution of cervical lymph node metastases from squamous cell carcinoma of the upper respiratory and digestive tracts. Cancer (29): 1446–1449, 1972.
39. Mendenhall WM, Million RR, Cassisi NJ. Elective neck irradiation in squamous cell carcinoma of the head and neck. Head Neck Surg (3): 15–20, 1980.
40. Beahrs OH, Barber KW Jr. The value of radical dissection of structures of the neck in the management of carcinoma of the lip, mouth, and larynx. Arch Surg (85): 49–56, 1962.
41. Lyall D, Shetlin CF. Cancer of the tongue. Ann Surg (135): 489–496, 1952.
42. Sako K, Pradier RN, Marchetta FC, Pickren JW. Fallibility of palpation in the diagnosis of metastases to cervical nodes. Surg Gynecol Obstet (118): 989–990, 1964.
43. Vandenbrouck C, Sancho-Garnier H, Chassagne D, Saravane D, Cachin Y, Micheau C. Elective versus therapeutic radical neck dissection in epidermoid carcinoma of the oral cavity. Cancer (46): 386–390, 1980.
44. Pointon, RC. Personal communication.
45. Jesse RH, Barkley HT Jr, Lindberg RD, Fletcher GH. Cancer of the oral cavity. Is elective neck dissection beneficial? Am J Surg (120): 505–508, 1970.
46. Northrop M, Fletcher GH, Jesse RH, Lindberg RD. Evolution of neck disease in patients with primary squamous cell carcinoma of the oral tongue, floor of mouth, and palatine arch, and clinically positive neck nodes neither fixed nor bilateral. Cancer (29): 23–30, 1972.
47. Nahum AM, Bone RC, Davidson TM. The case for elective prophylactic neck dissection. Trans Am Acad Ophtholmol Otolaryngol (82): 603–612, 1976.
48. Fletcher GH. Elective irradiation of subclinical disease in cancers of the head and neck. Cancer (29): 1450–1454, 1972.
49. Bagshaw MA, Thompson RW. Elective irradiation of the neck in patients with primary carcinoma of the head and neck. JAMA (217): 456–458, 1971.
50. Million RR. Elective neck irradiation for TxNo squamous carcinoma of the oral tongue and floor of mouth. Cancer (34): 149–155, 1974.
51. Horiuchi J, Adachi T. Some considerations on radiation therapy of tongue cancer. Cancer (28): 335–339, 1971.
52. Goffinet DR, Gilbert EH, Weller SA, Bagshaw MA. Irradiation of clinically uninvolved cervical lymph nodes. Can J Otolaryngol (4): 927–933, 1975.

53. Toker C. Some observations on the distribution of metastatic squamous carcinoma within cervical lymph nodes. Ann Surg (157): 419–426, 1963.
54. Wizenberg MJ, Bloedorn FG, Weiner S, Gracia J. Treatment of lymph node metastases in head and neck cancer. A radiotherapeutic approach. Cancer (29): 1455–1462, 1972.
55. Hanks GE, Bagshaw MA, Kaplan HS. The management of cervical lymph node metastasis by megavoltage radiotherapy. AJR (105): 74–82, 1969.
56. Merino OR, Lindberg RD, Fletcher GH. An analysis of distant metastases from squamous cell carcinoma of the upper respiratory and digestive tracts. Cancer (40): 145–151, 1977.
57. Strong EW. Preoperative radiation and radical neck dissection. Surg Clin North Am (49): 271–276, 1969.
58. Schneider JJ, Fletcher GH, Barkley HT Jr. Control by irradiation alone of nonfixed clinically positive lymph nodes from squamous cell carcinoma of the oral cavity, oropharynx, supraglottic larynx, and hypopharynx. AJR (123): 42–48, 1975.
59. Bataini JP, Brugere J, Ghossein NA, Bernier J, Jaulerry C, Brunin F. Radiotherapeutic control of subclinical and clinical neck disease in patients with cancers of supraglottic larynx and pharynx. Proc. International Head and Neck Oncology Research Conference, Rosslyn, Virginia, Sept. 8–10, 1980. Abstract 1.2.
60. Cachin Y, Sancho-Garnier H, Micheau C, Marandas P. Nodal metastasis from carcinomas of the oropharynx. Otolaryngol Clin North Am (12): 145–154, 1979.
61. Goodwin WJ Jr, Chandler JR. Indications for radical neck dissection following radiation therapy. Arch Otolaryngol (104): 367–370, 1978.
62. Barkley HT Jr, Fletcher GH, Jesse RH, Lindberg RD. Management of cervical lymph node metastases in squamous cell carcinoma of the tonsillar fossa, base of tongue, supraglottic larynx, and hypopharynx. Am J Surg (124): 462–467, 1972.
63. Garofalo JA, Erlandson E, Strong EW, Lesser M, Gerold F, Spiro R, Schwartz M, Good RA. Serum zinc, serum copper, and the Cu/Zn ratio in patients with epidermoid cancers of the head and neck. J Surg Oncol (15): 381–386, 1980.
64. Silverman NA, Alexander JC Jr, Chretien PB. CEA levels in head and neck cancer. Cancer (37): 2204–2211, 1976.
65. Osoba D, Kersey PA, Clark RM, Rosen IB. Prognostic value of skin testing with dinitrochlorobenzene in patients with head and neck cancer. Can J Surg (23): 43–44, 1980.
66. Molinari R. Study for a possible monitoring of radiosensitivity of oral and oropharyngeal carcinoma using evaluation of potential proliferative activity (L.I.). Proc. International Head and Neck Oncology Research Conference, Rosslyn, Virginia, Sept. 1980. Abstract 4.4.
67. Suit H, Lindberg R, Fletcher GH. Prognostic significance of extent of tumor regression at completion of radiation therapy. Radiology (84): 1100–1107, 1965.
68. Fazekas JT, Green JP, Vaeth JM, Schroeder AF. Postirradiation induration as a prognosticator. A retrospective analysis of squamous-cell carcinomas of the oral cavity and oropharynx. Radiology (102): 409–412, 1972.
69. Barkley HT Jr, Fletcher GH. The significance of residual disease after external irradiation of squamous-cell carcinoma of the oropharynx. Radiology (124): 493–495, 1977.
70. Mantyla M, Kortekangas AE, Valavaara RA, Nordman EM. Tumor regression during radiation treatment as a guide to prognosis. Br J Radiol (52): 972–977, 1979.
71. Sobel S, Rubin P, Keller B, Poulter C. Tumor persistence as a predictor of outcome after radiation therapy of head and neck cancers. Int J Radiat Oncol Biol Phys (1): 873–880, 1976.
72. Taylor SG. Head and neck cancer. In Cancer Chemotherapy 1979, Annual 3, Pinedo HM (ed). New York: Elsevier, 1981, pp. 263–278.
73. Fazekas JT, Sommer C, Kramer S. Adjuvant intravenous methotrexate or definitive radiotherapy alone for advanced squamous cancers of the oral cavity, oropharynx, supraglottic larynx or hypopharynx. Int J Radiat Oncol Biol Phys (6): 533–541, 1980.
74. Fu KK, Silverberg IJ, Phillips TL, Friedman MA. Combined radiotherapy and multidrug chemotherapy for advanced head and neck cancer: Results of a Radiation Therapy Oncology Group Pilot Study. Cancer Treat Rep (63): 351–357, 1979.
75. Lo TCM, Wiley AL Jr, Ansfield FJ, Brandenburg JH, Davis HL Jr, Gollin FF, Johnson RO, Ramirez G, Vermund H. Combined radiation therapy and 5-fluorouracil for advanced squamous cell carcinoma of the oral cavity and oropharynx: A randomized study. AJR (126): 229–235, 1976.

76. Elkind MM. Fundamental questions in the combined use of radiation and chemicals in the treatment of cancer. Int J Radiat Oncol Biol Phys (5): 1711–1720, 1979.
77. Combined Modalities. Chemotherapy/radiotherapy—Meeting summary. Int J Radiat Oncol Biol Phys (5): 1721–1723, 1979.
78. Goldsmith MA, Carter SK. The integration of chemotherapy into a combined modality approach to cancer therapy. V. Squamous cell cancer of the head and neck. Cancer Treat Rev (2): 137–158, 1975.
79. Fu KK. Normal tissue effects of combined radiotherapy and chemotherapy for head and neck cancer. Front Radiat Ther Oncol (13): 113–132, 1979.
80. Chassagne D, Richard JM, Le Floch O. Results of interstitial curietherapy in $T_3$ and $T_4$ floor of the mouth and tongue cancers after previous arterial infusion chemotherapy. Panminerva Med (18): 45–49, 1976.
81. Cachin Y, Jortay A, Sancho H, Eschwege F, Madelain M, Desaulty A, Gerard P. Preliminary results of a randomized EORTC study comparing radiotherapy and concomitant bleomycin to radiotherapy alone in epidermoid carcinomas of the oropharynx. Eur J Cancer (13): 1389–1395, 1977.
82. Shanta V, Krishnamurthi S. Combined bleomycin and radiotherapy in oral cancer. Clin Radiol (31): 617–620, 1980.
83. O'Connor AD, Clifford P, Dalley VM, Durden-Smith DJ, Edwards WG, Hollis BA. Advanced head and neck cancer treated by combined radiotherapy and VBM cytotoxic regimen—four-year results. Clin Otolaryngol (4): 329–337, 1979.
84. Gray LH, Conger AD, Ebert M, Hornsey S, Scott OCA. The concentration of oxygen dissolved in tissues at the time of irradiation as a factor in radiotherapy. Br J Radiol (26): 638–648, 1953.
85. Rubin P, Hanley J, Keys HM, Marcial V, Brady L. Carbogen breathing during radiation therapy. Int J Radiat Oncol Biol Phys (5): 1963–1970, 1979.
86. Henk JM, Kunkler PB, Smith CW. Radiotherapy and hyperbaric oxygen in head and neck cancer. Final report of first controlled clinical trial. Lancet (II): 101–103, 1977.
87. Medical Research Council Working Party. Radiotherapy and hyperbaric oxygen. Lancet (II): 881–884, 1978.
88. Dische S. Hyperbaric oxygen: The Medical Research Council trials and their clinical significance. Br J Radiol (51): 888–894, 1979.
89. Raju MR. Heavy Particle Radiotherapy. London: Academic Press, 1980.
90. Catterall M, Bewley DK. Fast Neutrons in The Treatment of Cancer. New York: Academic Press, 1979.
91. Griffin TW, Weisberger EC, Laramore GE, Tong D, Blasko JC. Complications of combined surgery and neutron radiation therapy in patients with advanced carcinoma of the head and neck. Radiology (132): 177–178, 1979.
92. L.W. Brady (ed). Radiation Sensitizers, Their Use in The Clinical Management of Cancer. Masson Publishing U.S.A., 1980.
93. Denekamp J, McNally NJ, Fowler JF, Joiner MC. Misonidazole in radiotherapy: Are many small fractions best? Br J Radiol (53): 981–990, 1980.
94. Fazekas JT, Goodman RL, McLean CJ. The value of adjuvant misonidazole in the definitive irradiation of advanced head and neck squamous cancer. An RTOG pilot study (78-02). Int J Radiat Oncol Biol Phys (7): 1703–1708, 1981.
95. Sealy R, Williams A, Levin W, Blair R, Flockhart I, Stratford M, Minchinton A, Cridland S. Progress in investigations in the use of misonidazole in head and neck cancer as a hypoxic cell radiation sensitizer and in combination with hyperbaric oxygen or hyperthermia. In Radiation Sensitizers: Their Use in the Clinical Management of Cancer, Brady LW (ed). Masson Publishing U.S.A., 1980, pp. 361–365.
96. Bush RS, Jenkin RDT, Allt WEC, Beale FA, Bean H, Dembo AJ, Pringle JF. Definitive evidence for hypoxic cells influencing cure in cancer therapy. Br J Cancer (37) (Suppl III): 302–306, 1978.
97. Siemann DW, Hill RP, Bush RS. Smoking: The influence of carboxyhemoglobin (HbCO) on tumor oxygenation and response to radiation. Int J Radiat Oncol Biol Phys (4): 657–662, 1978.
98. Pierquin BM, Mueller WK, Baillet F. Low dose rate irradiation of advanced head and neck cancers: Present status. Int J Radiat Oncol Biol Phys (4): 565–572, 1978.

99. Shukovsky LJ, Fletcher GH, Montague ED, Withers HR. Experience with twice-a-day fractionation in clinical radiotherapy. AJR (126): 155–162, 1976.
100. Backström A, Jakobsson PA, Littbrand B, Wersall J. Fractionation scheme with low individual doses in irradiation of carcinoma of the mouth. Acta Radiol (Ther) (12): 401–406, 1973.
101. Peracchia G, Salti C. Radiotherapy with thrice-a-day fractionation in a short overall time: Clinical experiences. Int J Radiat Oncol Biol Phys (7): 99–104, 1981.
102. Au SC, Archambeau JO. Continuous external irradiation. Int J Radiat Oncol Biol Phys (5): 253–255, 1979.
103. Holsti LR. Clinical experience with split-course radiotherapy. A randomized clinical trial. Radiology (92): 591–596, 1969.
104. Abramson N, Scruggs RP, Cavanaugh PJ. Short-course radiation therapy in the treatment of head and neck tumors. Radiology (118): 175–178, 1976.
105. Pilepich MV, Munzenrider JE, Rene JB. Unorthodox fractionation in the treatment of head and neck tumors. Int J Radiat Oncol Biol Phys (5): 249–252, 1979.
106. Million RR, Zimmermann RC. Evaluation of University of Florida split-course technique for various head and neck squamous cell carcinomas. Cancer (35): 1533–1536, 1975.
107. Wang CC. Radiation therapy in the management of oral malignant disease. Otolaryngol Clin North Am (12): 73–80, 1979.
108. Harwood AR, Cummings BJ. Radiotherapy for mucosal melanomas. Int J Radiat Oncol Biol Phys (8): 1121–1126, 1982.
109. Rubin P, Casarett GW. Clinical Radiation Pathology. Philadelphia: W.B. Saunders, 1968.
110. Beumer J III, Curtis T, Harrison RE. Radiation therapy of the oral cavity: Sequelae and management, Part 1. Head Neck Surg (1): 301–312, 1979.
111. Beumer J, Curtis T, Harrison RE. Radiation therapy of the oral cavity: Sequelae and management, Part 2. Head Neck Surg (1): 392–408, 1979.
112. Phillips TL. Rationale for initial clinical trials and future development of radioprotectors. Cancer Clin Trials (3): 165–173, 1980.
113. Starcke EN, Shannon IL. How critical is the interval between extractions and irradiation in patients with head and neck malignancy? Oral Surg (43): 333–337, 1977.
114. Daley TE, Drane JB. Management of Dental Problems in Irradiated Patients. Houston: University of Texas Press, 1972.
115. Carl W, Schaaf NG. Dental care for the cancer patient. J Surg Oncol (6): 293–310, 1974.
116. Murray CG, Herson J, Daly TE, Zimmerman S. Radiation necrosis of the mandible: A 10-year study. Part I. Factors influencing the onset of necrosis. Int J Radiat Oncol Biol Phys (6): 543–548, 1980.
117. Murray CG, Herson J, Daly TE, Zimmerman S. Radiation necrosis of the mandible: A 10-year study. Part II. Dental factors; onset, duration and management of necrosis. Int J Radiat Oncol Biol Phys (6): 549–553, 1980.
118. Murray CG, Daly TE, Zimmerman SO. The relationship between dental disease and radiation necrosis of the mandible. Oral Surg (49): 99–104, 1980.
119. Davis JC, Dunn JM, Gates GA, Heimbach RD. Hyperbaric oxygen: A new adjunct in the management of radiation necrosis. Arch Otolaryngol (105): 58–61, 1979.
120. Joseph DL, Shumrick DL. Risks of head and neck surgery in previously irradiated patients. Arch Otolaryngol (97): 381–384, 1973.
121. Donaldson SS. Nutritional consequences of radiotherapy. Cancer Res (37): 2407–2413, 1977.
122. Sobol SM, Conoyer JM, Zill R, Thawley SE, Ogura JH. Nutritional concepts in the management of the head and neck cancer patient. II. Management concepts. Laryngoscope (89): 962–979, 1979.
123. Wynder EL, Dodo H, Bloch DA, Gantt RC, Moore OS. Epidemiologic investigation of multiple primary cancer of the upper alimentary and respiratory tracts. I. A retrospective study. Cancer (24): 730–739, 1969.
124. Kogelnik HD, Fletcher GH, Jesse RH. Clinical course of patients with squamous cell carcinoma of the upper respiratory and digestive tracts with no evidence of disease 5 years after initial treatment. Radiology (115): 423–427, 1975.
125. Cummings BJ, Clark RM. Cancer of the oral cavity. J Otolaryngol (11): 359–364, 1982.
126. Decroix Y, Ghossein NA. Experience of the Curie Institute in treatment of cancer of the mobile tongue. II Management of the neck nodes. Cancer (47): 503–508, 1981.

127. Glick JH, Taylor SG. Integration of chemotherapy into a combined modality treatment plan for head and neck cancer: A review. Int J Radiat Oncol Biol Phys (7): 229–242, 1981.
128. Duncan W, Arnott SJ, Orr JA, Kerr GR. The Edinburgh experience of fast neutron therapy. Int J Radiat Oncol Biol Phys (8): 2155–2157, 1982.
129. Griffin TW, Lawrence GE, Hussey DH, Hendrickson FR, Rodriguez-Antunez A. Fast neutron beam radiation therapy in the United States. Int J Radiat Oncol Biol Phys (8): 2165–2168, 1982.
130. Phillips TL, Wasserman TH, Stetz J, Brady LW. Clinical trials of hypoxic cell sensitizers. Int J Radiat Oncol Biol Phys (8): 327–334, 1982.
131. Cummings BJ, Thomas GM, Rauth AM, Sorrenti V, Black B, Bush RS. Neurotoxic radiosensitizers and head and neck cancer patients - how many will benefit? Int J Radiat Oncol Biol Phys (8): 343–345, 1982.
132. Kotalik JF. Multiple daily fractions in radiotherapy. Cancer Treat Rev (8): 127–146, 1981.
133. Withers HR, Peters LJ, Thames HD, Fletcher GH. Hyperfractionation. Int J Radiat Oncol Biol Phys (8): 1807–1809, 1982.

# 7. CHEMOTHERAPY OF SQUAMOUS HEAD AND NECK CANCER

SUSAN W. PITMAN
JOSEPH R. BERTINO

## 1. INTRODUCTION

The role of chemotherapy in the management of cancers of the oral cavity continues to be defined through active ongoing clinical investigation. Since most series combine oral cavity with the other head and neck regions—namely, oropharynx, hypopharynx, larynx, nasopharynx, and paranasal sinuses—this chapter will review the use of chemotherapy in head and neck cancer and, where possible, cite oral cavity region-specific differences if such exist.

When chemotherapy is used in some advanced neoplastic diseases and complete responses are achieved a high probability of the time, chemotherapy results in significant prolongation of survival or cure. Such neoplasms include gestational trophoblastic tumors, Burkitt's tumor, testicular tumors, Wilm's tumor, acute lymphoblastic leukemia, non-Hodgkin's lymphoma, pediatric rhabdomyosarcoma, and advanced Hodgkin's disease. In other advanced neoplasms that respond to chemotherapy, palliation is associated with moderate prolongation of life, and these include prostate carcinoma, breast adenocarcinoma, acute myeloblastic leukemia, chronic lymphocytic leukemia, osteogenic sarcoma, and small-cell lung cancer. Yet in other cancers, such as chronic granulocytic leukemia, multiple myeloma, ovarian adenocarcinoma,

*I. van der Waal and G.B. Snow (eds), ORAL ONCOLOGY.* 

endometrial cancer, and neuroblastoma, chemotherapy achieves palliation with uncertain prolongation of life.

When chemotherapy is used in head and neck cancer that has metastasized or recurred either locally or regionally, palliation has not been associated with a significant prolongation of life beyond a few months. Complete remissions are seldom achieved and, when they are, tend to be short-lived. Drug combinations of active single agents are increasingly being evaluated, however, and hold promise to increase the percentage of patients responding to chemotherapy together with significantly improving their survival.

Patient debility may be an important factor limiting drug effectiveness. If there is either patient delay in reporting new symptoms or subsequent delay in referral for chemotherapy once biopsy confirms local or regional node recurrence, increasing dysphagia or odynophagia can lead to further weight loss and debility, further compromising patient performance status and drug effectiveness. Local infection, intermittent bleeding, and obstruction may further delay drug administration until these acute problems are resolved. Protein/calorie malnutrition may need to be reversed with nasogastric tube feeding, if a small diameter tube can be passed, by gastrostomy feeding, or by parenteral nutrition [1]. Dehydration must be reversed if nephrotoxic agents such as methotrexate or cis-platinum are to be safely administered without undue toxicity.

The past decade has witnessed a resurgence of interest in chemotherapy as an adjuvant to the surgical and radiation treatment of advanced stage III, IV disease. Its use in this setting will be reviewed.

## 2. GENERAL ASPECTS OF RESPONSE TO CHEMOTHERAPY

### 2.1. Definition of response to chemotherapy

Tumor responses are assessed by careful measurement of lesions prior to and during drug administration. Recording of these measurements on flow sheets helps ensure careful assessment at each visit. Accessible lesions are measured and recorded as the product of their two greatest perpendicular diameters. When medical, radiation, and surgical oncologists collaborate in multidisciplinary clinics, tumor measurements can be agreed upon and are subsequently subject to interobserver scrutiny when response to chemotherapy is assessed.

An indirect mirror examination together with manual palpation may be necessary to assess tumor dimensions. The physician giving chemotherapy should be proficient in this technique of physical examination. If fiberoptic nasopharyngo-laryngoscopy best assesses tumor dimensions, it may be necessary to use this technique as well. Nodal recurrence in a previously irradiated neck is particularly difficult to quantify, occurring as it does in indurated fibrotic tissue. CT scanning may be useful in these situations, particularly for lesions greater than 3 cm in size [2,3]. An additional benefit that CT scanning or ultrasound affords is the measurement of a third dimension to assess tumor size [4,5].

Response rates are intended to convey the relative efficacy of therapies in producing remissions of disease. By convention, there are four response grades: complete response (CR), partial response (PR), no change (NC), and progressive disease (PD). A complete response (or remission) (CR) is defined as disappearance of all measurable disease. Usually in the head and neck literature, CR refers to clinical disappearance of disease, rather than pathologic CR when microscopic verification of response as by a needle biopsy is attempted. A partial response (PR) is defined as 50% or greater regression of measurable disease without the development of new lesions. Response rate is expressed as a percentage and could be expressed for patients having CR or PR alone or together (CR + PR) for total response rate. Response with less than 50% regression of measurable disease is labeled no change or stable disease. Progressive disease (PD) is usually defined as >25% increase in measurable disease and/or appearance of new lesions during therapy. No change and progressive disease may be combined into a no-response (NR) category.

In addition to response rate other objective criteria for assessment of drug efficacy include patient survival and response duration. Of these, overall survival is the most objective and the least ambiguous.

### 2.2. Factors that affect response to chemotherapy

Both performance status and prior radiation therapy significantly affect response to chemotherapy in head and neck cancer. A recent review of 148 patients with advanced squamous cancer of the head and neck treated with a variety of chemotherapy protocols found that out of 74 patients with a Karnofsky performance status of 70% or greater, there were 24 CRs and PRs for an overall response rate of 32% and with a median survival of 28 weeks [6]. In contrast, of 38 patients with a Karnofsky performance status of 40% or less, there were 5 CRs and PRs (13% response rate) with a median survival of nine weeks ($P = 0.01$). Chemotherapy responders survived significantly longer than nonresponders. Cortes also found a higher percentage of responding patients (86%) when a combination of bleomycin, cytoxan, methotrexate, and 5-fluorouracil was given to active or ambulatory rather than to bedridden patients (45%) [7]. Others have observed a similar association [8,9].

Figure 7–1 shows the effect of performance status on survival in 35 patients treated with sequential methotrexate-leucovorin-5-fluorouracil at Yale, 23 of whom had had prior radiation therapy and 12 of whom were previously untreated. Using a Cox life table regression analysis, pretreatment performance status was found to be significantly ($P < 0.0001$) related to survival, with individuals either ambulatory or active (ECOG 0 or 1) surviving longer than individuals bedridden in part or completely (ECOG 2–4). Improving performance status of such patients, with intensive respiratory care, physiotherapy, or parenteral alimentation, may improve drug response rate, duration, and possibly prolong survival. Thus, performance status, although imprecise, must be assessed when comparisons are made between the results of

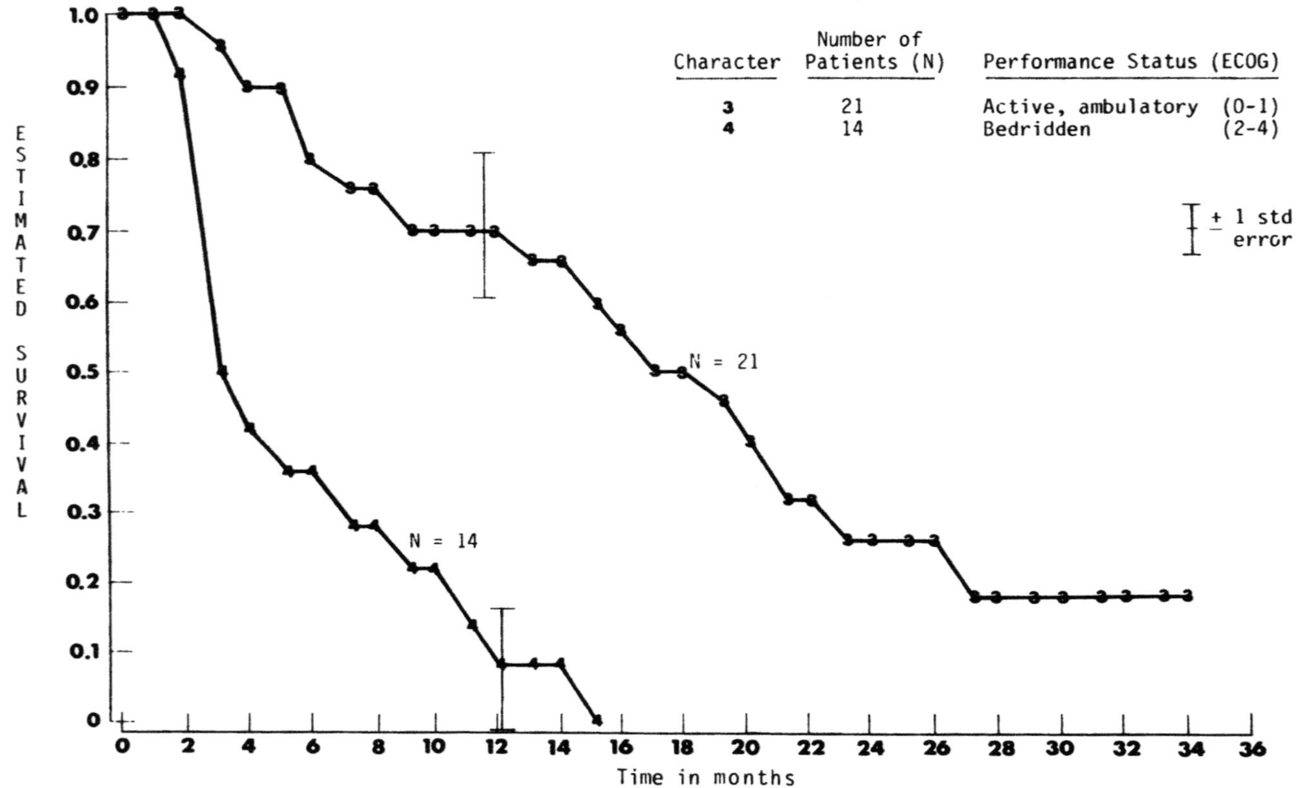


**Figure 7–1.** Effect of performance status on survival in 35 advanced squamous head and neck cancer patients given sequential methotrexate–5-fluorouracil with leucovorin rescue.

chemotherapy trials in head and neck cancer. Intertrial variation in the percentage of active or bedridden patients may well account for discrepancies in response rates and survival from institution to institution.

Prior radiation and/or surgical therapy may have significant impact on the effectiveness of a drug or drug combinations in head and neck cancer. Sealy and Helman [10] compared the efficacy of intra-arterial methotrexate in patients with and without prior radiotherapy. Sixty-four of 72 (84%) untreated patients responded with a median survival of 12 months compared to 16 of 36 (44%) with a one-month median survival.

Table 7–1 lists response rates as a function of prior treatment from series that analyzed for this variable [11–25]. In general, prior radiation and/or surgery seems to confer a relative therapeutic disadvantage, although there appears to be variability from series to series. Molinari [26], while not giving patient numbers, reported an equally large difference in responses (88% vs. 51%) among those without or with prior radiation or surgical treatment who received vincristine, bleomycin, and methotrexate in sequence. Prior chemotherapy also significantly affects response to subsequent chemotherapy [8,23].

Chemotherapeutic responsiveness may also depend on stage and extent of disease at the time of drug administration. Among 237 head and neck patients randomized between methotrexate, methotrexate-leucovorin, and methotrexate-leucovorin-araC, 40% of stage III patients achieved response, whereas only 17% of stage IV ($T_4$, $N_{2-3}$, $M_1$ disease) patients responded, and this was statistically significant ($P = 0.001$) [27]. Most patients had metastatic or recurrent disease in this series, as 92% had received prior radiation.

Among previously untreated head and neck cancer patients, stage may be less important. No response differences between stages III and IV disease have thus far been appreciated [16,28]. Some observers have noted more frequent responses among smaller $T_3$ lesions when compared to more extensive $T_4$ ones (84% vs. 56%). These investigators found no differences in response between $N_{-1}$ and $N_{2-3}$ nodal disease [16].

Although it is generally taught that locoregional disease responds more readily than disease at distant sites, some have seen similar response rates in distant and locoregional sites while others, surprisingly, have found that distant metastases are significantly more likely to respond than locoregional disease [29].

Table 7–2 presents pooled site-specific responses from recent series in the literature which analyzed for this variable [7,15–17,21,22,26,30–33]. Of 501 cases, 138 (28%) were given the single agent methotrexate or methotrexate with leucovorin rescue; the remainder received a variety of drug combinations. Within the oral cavity region, some series analyzed floor of mouth, buccal mucosa, and tongue (presumably anterior two-thirds) separately. Most, however, reported responses for oral cavity as a whole. Oral cavity and oropharynx, which comprise over one-half of reported cases, have similar response rates when either single agent methotrexate or drug combinations are

**Table 7–1.** Effect of prior radiation or surgical treatment on response rates in squamous head and neck cancer

| | | Prior therapy | | | No prior therapy | | |
|---|---|---|---|---|---|---|---|
| Investigator | Drugs | Evaluable cases | Responses CP + PR | % | Evaluable cases | Responses CR + PR | % |
| Wittes et al. [11,12] | Cis-platinum | 26 | 8 | ( 31%) | 22 | 9 | ( 41%) |
| Mills [13] | Methotrexate | 12 | 4 | ( 33%) | 11 | 7 | ( 64%) |
| Woods [9] | Methotrexate, methotrexate-leucovorin | 56 | 30 | ( 53%) | 16 | 5 | ( 30%) |
| Frei et al. [14] | Methotrexate-leucovorin | 28 | 14 | ( 50%) | 32 | 16 | ( 50%) |
| Randolph [15], Hong [16] | Cis-platinum, bleomycin | 12 | 4 | ( 33%) | 76 | 54 | ( 71%) |
| Brown et al. [17] | Velban, bleomycin, cis-platinum | 22 | 10 | ( 45%) | 23 | 17 | ( 74%) |
| Forastiere et al. [18] | Cis-platinum, cytoxan | 20 | 9 | ( 45%) | 7 | 5 | ( 71%) |
| Price [19], Hill [20] | Vincristine, bleomycin, methotrexate, hydrocortisone, 5-fluorouracil | 58 | 24 | ( 41%) | 76 | 57 | ( 75%) |
| Vogl et al. [21] | Mitomycin, methotrexate, bleomycin, cis-platinum | 21 | 9 | ( 43%) | 13 | 11 | ( 85%) |
| Vogl et al. [21] | Methotrexate, bleomycin, cis-platinum | 37 | 23 | ( 62%) | 9 | 6 | ( 67%) |
| Pitman | Methotrexate-leucovorin, 5-fluorouracil | 23 | 15 | ( 65%) | 12 | 10 | ( 83%) |
| Amer et al. [22] | Vincristine, bleomycin, cis-platinum | 22 | 11 | ( 50%) | 5 | 2 | ( 40%) |
| Decker [23], Kish [24] | Cis-platinum, 5-fluorouracil | 30 | 21 | ( 70%) | 34 | 30 | ( 88%) |
| Ervin et al. [25] | Methotrexate-leucovorin, cis-platinum, bleomycin | 11 | 11 | (100%) | 15 | 15 | (100%) |
| Totals | | 378 | 193 | ( 51%) | 355 | 244 | ( 69%) |

**Table 7–2.** Effect of site on response rates in squamous head and neck cancer

| | Chemotherapy | | | | | |
|---|---|---|---|---|---|---|
| | Methotrexate and methotrexate-leucovorin | | | Combinations | | |
| Site | Evaluable cases | Responses (CR + PR) | % | Evaluable cases | Responses (CR + PR) | % |
| Oral cavity (total) | 55 | 25 | (45%) | 136 | 79 | (58%) |
| Tongue | 18 | 9 | (50%) | 20 | 8 | (40%) |
| Floor of mouth | 23 | 10 | (43%) | 14 | 10 | (71%) |
| Buccal mucosa | 5 | 1 | (20%) | 4 | 1 | (25%) |
| Other oral cavity | 9 | 5 | (56%) | 98 | 60 | (61%) |
| Oropharynx | 35 | 17 | (50%) | 95 | 63 | (66%) |
| Hypopharynx | 17 | 3 | (18%) | 27 | 13 | (48%) |
| Nasopharynx | 8 | 2 | (25%) | 30 | 23 | (77%) |
| Larynx | 23 | 8 | (35%) | 57 | 28 | (49%) |
| Paranasal sinuses | — | — | — | 10 | 5 | (50%) |
| Other (including unknown site) | 6 | 2 | (33%) | 8 | 3 | (38%) |
| Totals | 144 | 57 | (41%) | 363 | 214 | (59%) |

Data extracted from the following series: Amer [22], Brown [17], Cortes [7], Creagan [32], Hong [16], Molinari [26], Presant [33], Randolph [15], Vogl [21].

given. Buccal mucosa appears to respond less well than other sites in the oral cavity. While Coker [28] found wide variation in response rates based on site (82% oral cavity, 61% oropharynx, and 54% larynx) in 51 previously untreated patients, the data presented in table 7–2 with larger number of patients fail to confirm a response advantage for oral cavity squamous cancers over other sites. When Amer [6] analyzed site-specific responses in a group of 158 cases treated primarily with single agents from 1967 to 1976, responses ranged from 16% in laryngeal primaries to 28% in tongue and 25% in oral cavity.

The impact on response of histologic differentiation has only recently been addressed. No relationship between histologic grading of head and neck tumors and regression after chemotherapy was found by Jorgensen [34] among 43 previously untreated tumors. Hong [16], likewise, found no difference in overall response rates among 29 well-differentiated and 26 poorly differentiated lesions. Complete responses were achieved more commonly in the well-differentiated group (34% vs. 8%) in these previously untreated tumors. Ohnuma [35], using bleomycin and dibromodulcitol, reported more frequent regression in well-differentiated tumors. Molinari [26] reported better responses in poorly differentiated lesions, Coker [28] more responses in well- or moderately well differentiated lesions. In view of these conflicting results, what role histologic differentiation plays, if any, in a tumor's response to chemotherapy remains to be defined.

## 3. SINGLE-AGENT CHEMOTHERAPY

Methotrexate, cis-platinum, bleomycin, and 5-fluorouracil are among the most commonly used chemotherapeutic agents in squamous head and neck cancer. Each will be reviewed, its mechanism of action, pharmacology, and toxicology discussed together with an assessment of their current usage in the management of these tumors.

### 3.1. Methotrexate

Methotrexate has been used in head and neck cancer for over a quarter of a century. Controversy still exists regarding its optimal use. Because of its unpredictable toxicity, it has been used extensively with leucovorin "rescue" in patients with this disease. The rationale behind the use of leucovorin was that it could reverse methotrexate action by (1) supplying reduced folate, thus bypassing methotrexate's imposed block on dihydrofolate reductase and (2) decreasing the uptake of methotrexate by cells.

#### *3.1.1. Current use*

Table 7–3 outlines clinical experience with "low-dose" methotrexate (without leucovorin rescue), at the dose and weekly schedule generally regarded as optimal [9,27,29,36–44]. With a total of 566 evaluable cases, the overall response rate is 29%. While the median duration of response is generally quoted at approximately two months, two more recent trials report five-month median response durations [29,41,45]. Thus, since 1975 when Goldsmith and

**Table 7–3.** Head and neck squamous cancer: Activity of methotrexate

| Investigator | Dose-Schedule | Evaluable cases | Responses (CR + PR) |
|---|---|---|---|
| Papac [36] | .8 mg/kg IV, IM biw | 15 | 8 |
| Lane [37] | 40-50 mg q 4 d | 27 | 14 |
| Leone [38] | 50 mg/m$^2$ IV q wk | 34 | 20 |
| DePalo [39] | 50-60 mg/m$^2$ IV q wk | 23 | 8 |
| Papac [40] | .8 mg/kg IV, IM biw | 35 | 7 |
| Vogler [41] | 15 mg/m$^2$ po q 6 h × 4 q wk | 44 | 12 |
| Vogler [41] | 60 mg/m$^2$ IV q wk | 61 | 19 |
| Woods [42] | 45 mg/m$^2$ IV q wk | 59 | 6 |
| DeConti [27] | 45 → 60 mg/m$^2$ IV q wk | 77 | 21 |
| Woods [9] | 50 mg/m$^2$ IV q wk | 23 | 6 |
| Williams [29] | 45 mg/m$^2$ IV q wk × 4 → 60 mg/m$^2$ IV q wk | 68 | 11 |
| Hong [43] | 40 → 60 mg/m$^2$ IV q wk | 17 | 4 |
| Vogl [44] | 40 → 60 mg/m$^2$ IV q wk | 83 | 29 |
| Totals | | 566 | 165 (29%) |

Carter [46] tabulated 100 cases and reported 50% responses, additional accrual, using the same dose and schedule, suggests a lower overall rate of response. Few responses are complete. The original 50% figure, however, has made low-dose unrescued methotrexate (40–60 mg/m$^2$ IV weekly) the gold standard to which other single agents or combinations are compared in this disease. For example, methotrexate on a monthly schedule had produced a response rate of 29% in 107 patients [47–53], but when this percentage was compared to the gold standard figure of 50%, it was judged inferior.

Early trials suggested that leucovorin could improve the therapeutic index to methotrexate through rescue [54]. Furthermore, it was empirically found that normal cells were rescued preferentially. Leucovorin "rescue" did not abrogate methotrexate's antitumor effect.

Further nonrandomized studies evaluating the efficacy of moderate-dose methotrexate with rescue (250–500 mg/m$^2$) on a weekly or twice weekly schedule [55] and high-dose methotrexate with rescue (≥1000 mg/m$^2$) on a weekly schedule produced responses in 50 to 60% of patients [14]. Additional toxicity, particularly nephrotoxicity with the higher doses, was described, however, including acute nonoliguric renal failure [56]. Nephrotoxicity had previously been reported only sporadically with lower doses [57]. During high-dose infusion, rapid drug excretion may lead to high methotrexate concentrations in the urine, which exceed the solubility of the drug below a urinary pH of 7.0 and which are believed to be responsible for intrarenal precipitation of the drug, leading to renal failure [56,58]. Thus, in high-dose regimens, hydration and alkalinization of the urine are recommended in order to avoid renal toxicity [59], and routine monitoring of drug level may be useful in predicting and preventing drug toxicity [60].

Four randomized trials (table 7–4) have been undertaken to confirm the superiority of methotrexate-leucovorin to low-dose unrescued methotrexate in head and neck cancer [9,27,41,61]. The earliest study suggested an improved therapeutic index following methotrexate-leucovorin, a finding not subsequently confirmed [61]. In the ECOG study, similar response rates were seen in the two arms and toxicity was likewise similar [27]. The study concluded that there was no advantage to methotrexate with leucovorin rescue. Unfortunately, while the low-dose methotrexate was given on an optimal weekly schedule, the methotrexate-leucovorin arm was administered on a suboptimal every other week basis. Cytofluorometry has documented marrow recovery within one week of methotrexate leucovorin [62], and clinical results have confirmed that a weekly schedule is well tolerated [63].

The Ludwig Cancer Institute study randomized patients to receive methotrexate at either 50 mg/m$^2$, 500 mg/m$^2$, or 5,000 mg/m$^2$ doses, all on a weekly schedule [9]. Leucovorin rescue was administered identically. Whether unnecessary leucovorin administration to those receiving the lowest methotrexate dose might have affected its antitumor activity in these patients remains conjectural. A higher response rate of 45% was observed following the 5,000 mg/m$^2$ methotrexate arm, but was associated with more drug-related deaths. All patients on this study were not carefully monitored for toxicity with 24-hour serum creatinine levels or serum methotrexate levels, possibly accounting for the higher mortality rate following the high-dose therapy. Responses lasted a median of 12 weeks with 5,000 mg/m$^2$ methotrexate and 6 weeks following 500 mg/m$^2$ and 50 mg/m$^2$.

Vogler and the Southeastern Cancer Study Group also concluded that methotrexate-leucovorin offered no therapeutic advantage [41]. One hundred fifty-four evaluable head and neck cancer patients were randomized to receive methotrexate with or without leucovorin (table 7–4). While similar response rates (27%, 27%, and 34%) and similar median response durations (6.3, 5.8, and 5.4 months) were observed, the oral route of methotrexate administration may have resulted in variability of absorption at the doses employed in this study. Furthermore, serum concentrations of methotrexate were not measured. In summary, while flaws in study design or execution are present in the three largest randomized trials, none shows a significant enough therapeutic advantage for methotrexate-leucovorin to justify the extra cost, risk of extra toxicity, or patient monitoring which methotrexate-leucovorin requires.

Use of low-dose unrescued methotrexate on a weekly schedule at a dose of 40 to 60 mg/m$^2$ is reasonable palliative chemotherapy for patients with locally recurrent or widely metastatic disease. Since a 5% mortality figure is quoted with its use [27], its use must be tempered with cautious monitoring of hematologic and renal function in these patients. Many are found to be prerenally azotemic on the basis of poor oral intake secondary to either anorexia or tumor-induced dysphagia or odynophagia. A pretreatment creatinine clearance should be routinely obtained since methotrexate is primarily excreted via

**Table 7–4.** Randomized trials of methotrexate vs. methotrexate-leucovorin rescue in squamous head and neck cancer

| Investigator | Dose-Schedule | Evaluable cases | Responses (CR+PR) | % | Drug-related deaths |
|---|---|---|---|---|---|
| Levitt [61] | MTX 80 $mg/m^2$ IV 30 hr infusion q 2 wk | 16 | 7 | 44% | 4 |
| | MTX-LCV 240-360 $mg/m^2$ IV 36–42 hr → 1080 $mg/m^2$ | 25 | 15 | 60% | 2 |
| Vogler [41] | MTX-LCV 125 $mg/m^2$ po q 6 h × 4 q wk | 49 | 11 | 22% | 1 |
| | MTX 15 $mg/m^2$ po q 6 h × 4 q wk | 44 | 12 | 27% | 1 |
| | MTX 60 $mg/m^2$ IV q wk | 61 | 20 | 33% | 1 |
| DeConi [27] | MTX 40 $mg/m^2$ IV q wk | 77 | 21 | 27% | 2 |
| | MTX-LCV 240 $mg/m^2$ IV q 2 wk | 74 | 19 | 25% | 5 |
| Woods [9] | MTX-LCV 50 $mg/m^2$ IV q wk | 23 | 6 | 26% | 1 |
| | MTX-LCV 500 $mg/m^2$ IV q wk | 27 | 7 | 26% | 0 |
| | MTX-LCV 5000 $mg/m^2$ IV q wk | 22 | 10 | 45% | 3 |

the kidneys (see the following discussion on mechanism of action and pharmacology). If methotrexate-leucovorin is administered, monitoring of renal function with a serum creatinine 24 hours after treatment together with a serum methotrexate concentration should be routine. If drug-induced nephrotoxicity, nausea, or vomiting-induced dehydration is present, appropriate hydration and/or extension of leucovorin rescue can be considered early enough to prevent untoward toxicity. For patients who have failed low-dose methotrexate, occasional responses with higher methotrexate-leucovorin doses have been reported [9].

### *3.1.2. Mechanism of action*

Methotrexate is a tight binding inhibitor of the enzyme dihydrofolate reductase (folate reductase) [64]. As a consequence of this inhibition, the formation of tetrahydrofolate—the active coenzyme form of folic acid—is prevented, thus resulting in a decrease in synthetic reactions requiring a one-carbon transfer (the synthesis of thymidylate and purine synthesis). Thus, DNA synthesis is impaired and, to a lesser extent, RNA as well.

Methotrexate also competes for uptake into cells with reduced folate, in particular, 5-methyl tetrahydrofolate and 5-formyl tetrahydrofolate (leucovorin, citrovorum factor, folinic acid) [65–67]. Therefore, in addition to preventing tetrahydrofolate coenzyme synthesis, the drug decreases reduced folate uptake into cells, preventing possible bypass of the methotrexate-induced block by endogenous or exogenously administered reduced folates. Recent studies indicate that the persistence of methotrexate in certain body tissues (liver, kidney, for example) may be explained not only by its tight binding to dihydrofolate reductase, but also by its conversion to polyglutamate forms (additional glutamates added in $\gamma$-carboxyl linkages to the molecule, for example) [68]. These polyglutamate forms are also tight binding inhibitors of dihydrofolate reductase [69]. The role of polyglutamate formation of methotrexate in regard to selectivity of action as well as toxicity—both acute and chronic—is being explored.

Inasmuch as methotrexate is a potent inhibitor of DNA synthesis, the drug is most effective when cells are in the DNA synthetic or S-phase [70]. Thus, cells in plateau or resting phase, characteristic of large bulky tumors, or tumors with many cells not in cycle ($G_0$ cells), are less susceptible to pulses of methotrexate. Other variables determine natural sensitivity of a cell to methotrexate; these include the level of reduced folates in the cell, the level of DHFR and its rate of synthesis, the transport of methotrexate, and the amount of drug retained as polyglutamates.

### *3.1.3. Pharmacokinetics*

Absorption of methotrexate from the gastrointestinal tract is almost complete when doses up to 30 $mg/m^2$ are ingested. Doses of methotrexate higher than

30 mg/m$^2$ are proportionally less well absorbed, and the drug should be administered parenterally if predictable blood levels are desired at high doses [71]. The drug is well tolerated by intravenous administration, and may also be administered by the SG, IM, or IP route. After oral administration to a fasting subject, peak blood levels are reached in one to two hours, and absorption is complete by three to four hours [71–73].

After an intravenous bolus of methotrexate is administered, the drug disappears from the blood in three distinct phases [74]. The initial phase of drug disappearance in plasma has a half-life of approximately 30 to 40 minutes and is thought to reflect the distribution of the drug, initially in the extracellular space and then in the total body water. The $t_{1/2}$ of the second phase is approximately 2.5 hours and reflects renal clearance of the drug. A third phase can also be measured, especially when high doses of drug are administered, with a half-life of approximately 10 hours. This third phase is most likely due to enterohepatic circulation of the drug (excretion in bile and reabsorption in the small bowel) [75]. If levels of methotrexate are greater than $10^{-7}$M, this prolonged third phase can lead to toxicity since it has been shown that marrow and gastrointestinal tract DNA synthesis continues to be inhibited until levels fall below this serum concentration [76]. Additional evidence of this phase's importance derives from experiments in mice in which this terminal phase is eliminated by administration of carboxypeptidase G, a drug that rapidly hydrolyzes and inactivates methotrexate, thus decreasing methotrexate [77]. Approximately 16% of the drug is estimated to be lost by biliary excretion; this percentage may increase with larger doses [78].

Distribution of methotrexate into tissues reflects the presence or absence of transport systems, the level of the major binding proteins for methotrexate dihydrofolate reductase, and the intracellular conversion to polyglutamate forms of methotrexate. Recent information indicates that virtually every tissue examined has the ability to convert methotrexate as well as folates to polyglutamate forms. The predominant forms for methotrexate are the methotrexate ($Glu_2$) and methotrexate ($Glu_3$) while naturally occurring folates are converted to the pentaglutamate. The importance of the conversion is that it presumably leads to prolonged retention of the drug since it is effluxed from the cell less readily than unbound methotrexate [79]. Liver and kidney contain the highest amount of methotrexate and retain it for the longest period of time. Erythrocytes also contain large amounts of methotrexate as polyglutamates as a result of incorporation of the drug into developing forms in the marrow and conversion of polyglutamates [80]. The role of these large depots of methotrexate that are retained for long periods of time after methotrexate (months) in chronic toxicity observed (for example, liver) is not clear [80].

Polyglutamates of methotrexate are not found in plasma or urine since plasma contains a potent conjugase that rapidly hydrolyzes these compounds to the monoglutamate of methotrexate. In plasma approximately 50% of the methotrexate is weakly bound by proteins, mainly albumin. Since this binding can be decreased by drugs such as sulfonamides and aspirin, this binding more likely is related to the p-aminobenzoylglutamate part of methotrexate.

Methotrexate also is distributed slowly into body cavities such as the CSF, pleural, and peritoneum. Distribution into pleural or peritoneal effusions and retention with slow subsequent release may result in prolonged plasma methotrexate concentrations and an increase in systemic toxicity [81].

For many years it was believed that little or no metabolism of methotrexate occurred. With small doses most of the drug was found to be excreted unchanged in the urine, with a small amount of breakdown product noted, apparently a pteroate derivative. This compound, identified as 2,4-diamino-$N_{10}$methylpteroic acid (DAMPA) in plasma and urine during the third phase of drug disappearance, presumably arises due to metabolism of the drug by bowel bacteria [82]. With higher doses of drug in addition to DAMPA, a second metabolite may be formed in relatively high concentrations, namely, 7-hydroxymethotrexate [83]. Both of these products are much less potent than methotrexate in binding to dihydrofolate reductase and are therefore less active metabolites of the drug. Jacobs et al. [83] have proposed that since the 70H metabolite is less soluble than methotrexate and since after high doses as much as 30% of the drug excreted during the second 12 hours of administration may be in this form, it could contribute to the nephrotoxicity that may occur with high-dose treatment.

Conversion to polyglutamate forms intracellularly, as mentioned above, occurs rapidly and to a large extent in many tissues. However, rather than leading to inactivation of the drug, these polyglutamate forms bind to the target enzyme dihydrofolate reductase as tightly as does methotrexate [83]. Polyglutamates may be responsible for inhibition of other enzymes (for example, thymidylate synthetase), thus explaining the possible broadened spectrum of methotrexate action in high doses.

Methotrexate is excreted primarily by the kidney [84], but a small amount is also excreted into the bile, with some reabsorption as noted above. After oral absorption fecal elimination is proportional to dose; at doses of greater than 30 $mg/m^2$, proportionally greater amounts of the drug are found in the feces [71]. Except for low plasma concentrations, methotrexate clearance by the kidney is greater than inulin clearance; thus the drug appears to be actively secreted by the tubules as well as filtered. Urinary excretion of 7-OH methotrexate increases with time, and greater amounts are found after the first 6 to 12 hours in urine.

### 3.2. Cis-platinum

Cis-platinum (cis[II]platinumdiamminedichloride) was first discovered in a serendipitous manner by Rosenberg and his colleagues in 1965 [85]. They astutely followed up an observation that bacteria were killed when electric current was applied; the cause was found to be the generation of cis-platinum by platinum from the electrodes combining with substances in the media.

**Table 7–5.** Cis-platinum: activity in squamous head and neck cancer

| Investigator | Dosage-Schedule (IV) | Evaluable cases | Responses CR + PR |
|---|---|---|---|
| Hill [87] | .2-2.5 mg/kg q 5-10 d | 31 | 7 (23%) |
| Wittes [11] | 120 mg/m$^2$ q 3-4 wk | 26 | 8 (31%) |
| Randolph [15] | 40 mg/m$^2$ q 1 wk | 13 | 4 (31%) |
| Jacobs [88] | 80 mg/m$^2$ q 3 wk (infusion) | 18 | 7 (39%) |
| Sako [89] | 120 mg/m$^2$ q 3 wk | 15 | 5 (33%) |
| | 20 mg/m$^2$ d 1-5 q 3 wk | 15 | 4 (27%) |
| Hayat [90] | 100 mg/m$^2$ q 3 wk | 14 | 2 (14%) |
| Aribas [91] | 20 mg/m$^2$ d 1-5 q 4 wk | 52 | 18 (34%) |
| Davis [92] | 120 mg/m$^2$ q 4 wk | 30 | 4 (13%) |
| Pannettiere [93] | 50 mg/m$^2$ d 1, 8 q 4 wk | 65 | 16 (25%) |
| Hong [43] | 50 mg/m$^2$ d 1, 8 q wk | 21 | 6 (29%) |
| Totals | | 300 | 81 (27%) |

Initially discarded after phase I trials indicated that the drug caused nephrotoxicity, cis-platinum is now used safely with forced diuresis.

### 3.2.1. *Current use*

Table 7–5 lists the single-agent activity of cis-platinum when administered at the dosage and schedule of 80–120 mg/m$^2$ q for three to four weeks in 300 evaluable cases reported thus far [11,15,43,87–93]. Median duration of response in most series is approximately four months. It is one of the most widely used agents in combined drug regimens in this disease.

### 3.2.2. *Mechanism of action*

Overwhelming evidence favors the target of cis-platinum to be DNA. The active form of cis-platinum may act as an alkylating agent, and it has been shown to react with several nucleophilic sites on DNA. Like most alkylating agents, cis-platinum has no cell cycle specificity [94].

### 3.2.3. *Pharmacokinetics*

After administration, there is a rapid clearance of this drug ($t_{1/2} \simeq 35$ minutes) followed by a very slow second phase ($t_{1/2} \simeq 34$ days). Less than 30% of the drug is excreted within the first 24 hours, and even after 5 days less than 50% of the drug is found in the urine. The long half-life is probably explained by the extensive binding of the drug to plasma protein(s). Whether the drug is active once bound to plasma protein is not clear [95].

### 3.2.4. *Toxicity*

The dose-limiting toxicity of cis-platinum, despite forced diuresis, is nephrotoxicity. The use of infusions (24 hours or longer) using large amounts of fluid (urine output > 300 cc/hour) lessens renal toxicity; alternatively, the drug is used with prehydration (four to six hours) with concomitant administration of mannitol or furosemide [96–98]. Recently, even doses of 200 mg/m$^2$, twice the average dose, have been used safely in patients with high-risk embryonal cell carcinoma, using hypertonic saline infusions [99].

With higher doses of the drug, hematologic toxicity may also be seen. Other side effects are nausea and vomiting, which are difficult to control with anti-emetics, and hearing loss.

### 3.3. Bleomycin

Bleomycin refers to a family of polypeptide antibiotics isolated from a Streptomyces by Umezawa and coworkers [100]. Because of the relative lack of myelosuppression caused by this agent, it has been utilized mainly in combination with other active agents in this disease.

#### *3.3.1. Current use*

Several dosage schedules of bleomycin have been utilized; either pulse dose (once or twice weekly or five-day courses repeated every two to four weeks) or continuous intravenous doses (usually five days or longer). Even daily small doses have been used SC for extended periods of time. The effect of schedule on tumor response has not been completely resolved, but continuous infusions of the drug may produce the best response [101,102].

#### *3.3.2. Mechanism of action*

The bleomycins have been shown recently to be capable of degrading DNA. Certain organs such as bone marrow are presumably protected from this action because of the presence of an inactivating enzyme [100]. Bleomycin is most active against cells in the $G^2$ phase of the cell cycle [103], and some attempts have been made to synchronize or hold up cells in $G^2$ with other agents (for example, vincristine) and then to treat with bleomycin.

#### *3.3.3. Pharmacokinetics*

The development of a radioimmunoassay has led recently to studies of the pharmacokinetics of this drug. These studies are complicated by the fact that bleomycin is a mixture of several polypeptides; the radioimmunoassay measures $A^2$ and $B^2$ fractions, which are the predominant forms. The drug disappears with an initial rapid phase ($t_{1/2}$ = 1.4), and a second slower phase ($t_{1/2} \simeq$ 9 hours [104]. Approximately 60% of the drug is excreted unchanged [105]. In patients with renal function impairment, prolonged excretion with increased host toxicity was observed. Apparently, therefore, bleomycin should be used with caution in patients with compromised renal function.

#### *3.3.4. Toxicity*

Skin toxicity may occur with schedules that utilize high-dose intensive regimens. Skin toxicity usually consists of erythema, mainly on the fingers. These changes may progress to desquamation and ulceration if the drug is continued. The major toxicity noted with this drug is pulmonary fibrosis, and usually is not seen, unless the cumulative dose of the drug exceeds 400 mg. Patients over 70 years of age or those who have underlying pulmonary disease appear to be at higher risk to develop this complication [106].

### 3.4. 5-Fluorouracil

5-Fluorouracil in head and neck cancer has marginal activity when used intravenously [107]. In fact, the 15% response rate reported is not too different from the response rate for gastrointestinal cancer [108]. Higher response rates have been reported with intra-arterial administration [109].

#### *3.4.1. Mechanism of action*

5-Fluorouracil must be converted to nucleotides in order to be active. The important nucleotide forms of this analog are 5-fluorodeoxyuridylate (FdUMP), a potent inhibitor of thymidylate synthetase, and 5-fluorouridine triphosphate (FUTP), which may be incorporated into RNA. The inhibition of DNA synthesis that results from FdUMP binding to thymidylate synthetase is well understood and is thought to be more important in terms of the antitumor effects of this compound [110]. The consequences of 5-fluorouracil incorporation into RNA is less well understood, but may be important in toxic effects due to this drug. Recently, it has also been shown that inhibition of thymidylate biosynthesis by this drug as well as methotrexate leads to incorporation of dUTP into DNA [111].

The synergistic effect of methotrexate followed by 5-fluorouracil, first demonstrated in the S180 tumor by Bertino et al. [112], may be due to enhanced inhibition of thymidylate synthetase that could result from the increase in dihydrofolate polyglutamates that pile up as a consequence of methotrexate inhibition of dihydrofolate reductase [113]. This coenzyme has been shown to markedly enhance FdUMP binding to thymidylate synthetase. In addition, as a result of methotrexate inhibition of purine biosynthesis, phosphoribosyl pyrophosphate levels increase; and when 5-fluorouracil is subsequently administered, more of this drug is taken up because of the increased levels of fluorouridine monophosphate that are formed [114]. Not only is more FdUMP subsequently formed, but more 5-fluorouracil is incorporated into RNA as a consequence of increased levels of FUTP that result. Not yet clear is whether the biochemical basis of the synergy that results is predominantly an RNA or a DNA effect of whether cells differ in this regard.

*3.4.2. Pharmacokinetics*

Inactivation of 5-fluorouracil occurs primarily in the liver [115]. The products formed—fluoro-α-alanine, urea, ammonia, and carbon dioxide—are primarily excreted in the urine.

Following a single rapid IV dose, peak plasma levels occur immediately, and the drug is rapidly cleared with a half-life of 15 minutes. When a standard dose is administered (15 mg/kg), peak levels produced are $10^{-3}$ to $10^{-4}$ M [116]. The drug diffuses rapidly into all body compartments and is distributed in a volume equivalent to the total body water [117]. Approximately 20% of the drug is excreted unchanged in the urine in the first few hours, and the remainder is metabolized by the liver and excreted within the first 24 hours after administration [118]. As most of the drug is normally inactivated in the liver, dose modification would seem prudent if patients have liver function abnormalities.

*3.4.3. Toxicity*

The major toxicities associated with this drug usage are mucositis, diarrhea, and bone marrow impairment. Oral ulceration and mild diarrhea are the first signs of early toxicity, and the drug should be withheld if these occur. Pancytopenia, especially leukopenia, may occur more commonly with five-day courses of this drug; the nadir of the platelet and white blood cell count depression occurs approximately 10 days after the last dose is administered. Cerebellar toxicity may occur in a small number of patients, especially with larger doses of the drug, presumably as a consequence of metabolism of 5-fluorouracil to fluorocitrate, an inhibitor of the Krebs cycle [119]. Occasionally, skin rash may also be produced by this drug.

### 3.5. Remaining active single agents

The remaining active single agents in head and neck cancer are listed in table 7–6 and are derived from the several major classifications of neoplastic compounds, including antimetabolites, antibiotics, bifunctional alkylating agents, and plant alkaloids [120].

## 4. COMBINATION CHEMOTHERAPY IN ADVANCED DISEASE

Early studies combined methotrexate and bleomycin given weekly or twice weekly. Neither response rates nor response duration appeared to be superior to the single-agent activity of methotrexate in nonrandomized trials and mucositis was usually dose limiting [121–125]. One promising combination, which adds hydroxyurea to weekly low-dose methotrexate and bleomycin, reports a 70% response rate in 32 patients, with complete remissions in 30% [126]. Among previously untreated patients, 55% (6 out of 11) achieved complete response compared to 24% among those previously irradiated or who had had prior surgery.

**Table 7–6.** Cumulative single-agent activity in squamous head and neck cancer*

| Drug | Evaluable cases | Responses (CR+PR) | % |
|---|---|---|---|
| Bleomycin | 346 | 73 | 21% |
| 5-fluorouracil | 118 | 18 | 15% |
| Cyclophosphamide | 77 | 28 | 36% |
| Vinblastine | 35 | 10 | 29% |
| Adriamycin | 34 | 8 | 23% |
| Chlorambucil | 34 | 5 | 15% |
| Procarbazine | 31 | 3 | 10% |
| Hydroxyurea | 18 | 7 | 39% |

*Excluding cis-platinum and methotrexate.
Table from Wolf GT and Chretien PB, "The chemotherapy and immunotherapy of head and neck cancer," *Cancer of the Head and Neck,* JR Suen and EN Myers, ed. (NY: Churchill-Livingstone, 1981.)

The advent of cis-platinum as an active agent has witnessed a rapid proliferation of combination drug regimens, some of which combine cis-platinum and methotrexate, others combining cis-platinum and bleomycin with other active agents. When cis-platinum and methotrexate have been combined, most regimens have resulted in greater toxicity than when either drug is administered alone, despite attempts at minimizing additional nephrotoxicity [127,128]. One well-tolerated regimen combining small individual doses of these agents is that of Tejada [129].

When cis-platinum and bleomycin have been combined, both drugs can be given at full single-agent doses with acceptable toxicity. Addition of methotrexate to cis-platinum and bleomycin has usually resulted in a significant increase in toxicity [130,131]. Two regimens with significant activity that appear well tolerated are those of Vogl [132] and Ervin [133], the former easily administered on an outpatient schedule and the latter, which uses methotrexate-leucovorin, requiring hospitalization and close monitoring.

While many combinations induce tumor regression in more than 50% of patients, particularly in those previously untreated (see table 7–1), no combination has significantly increased the number of complete responses in patients with metastatic or recurrent disease. Some promising drug combinations, active in recurrent or metastatic disease, are listed in table 7–7 [18,24,134,135]. Of these, the cis-platinum–5-fluorouracil combination has achieved a large number of complete remissions (30%) [24]. The cytoxan–adriamycin–cis-platinum combination in patients with excellent performance status has resulted in a median survival of eight months, superior to any other published reports [134]. Using the same agents as Holoye but on a different schedule, Cortes [7] reported a similarly high response rate, Plasse [136] a substantially lower one. Holoye's study, however, found an 11% incidence of drug-related deaths.

**Table 7–7.** Promising drug combinations in metastatic or recurrent advanced squamous head and neck cancer

| Investigator | Drugs | Dose ($mg/m^2$)-schedule | No. of patients | Responses CR + PR | % |
|---|---|---|---|---|---|
| Creagan[134] | Cyclophosphamide<br>Adriamycin<br>Cis-platinum | 400 d 1<br>40 d 1 } q 4 wk<br>40 d 1 | 25 | 16 | (64%) |
| Kish[24] | Cis-platinum<br>5-fluorouracil | 100 d 1 with hydration, mannitol<br>1000 d 1 → 5 infusion with allopurinol | 30 | 21 | (70%) |
| Forastiere[18] | Cis-platinum<br>Cyclophosphamide | 60 d 1 } q 3 wk<br>600 d 1 } | 23 | 14 | (60%) |
| Holoye[135] | Bleomycin<br>Cytoxan<br>Methotrexate<br>5-fluorouracil | 30 mq (total) d 1 → 4 infusion<br>200 IV d 1 → 5<br>30 IV d 1, d 5<br>400 IV d 1 → 5 | 22 | 13 | (59%) |

In general, most three- and four-drug combinations result in more toxicity than that reported with individual single agents. The median duration of most responses with combination chemotherapy is four to seven months [21,29,126]. Overall median survival for patients receiving combination chemotherapy in the best of series is six to eight months [134]. Thus, although dramatic increases in regression rates may be achieved using more toxic combination programs, such treatment may not yet confer a meaningful survival advantage.

Furthermore, two prospective randomized trials have compared drug combinations to the best single-agent treatment in head and neck cancer. Both fail to show a statistically significant advantage for the combination regimens [29,45]. The ECOG compared methotrexate 40–60 $mg/m^2$ IV weekly to methotrexate–bleomycin–cis-platinum (MBP), consisting of methotrexate 40 $mg/m^2$ days 1 and 15; bleomycin 10 iu IM days 1, 8, and 15; and cis-platinum 50 $mg/m^2$ day 4 on a 21-day cycle. There were 15 of 83 (35%) responders in the MTX arm vs. 22 of 88 (48%) responders in the MBP arm, with 16% complete responses to MBP and 8% to methotrexate. Duration of response was similar (5.8 months for MBP and 5 months for methotrexate). These differences are of borderline statistical significance [45].

Another prospective randomized study compared low-dose methotrexate (45 $mg/m^2$ IV weekly with escalation to 60 $mg/m^2$ at week five in the absence of toxicity) to PVB (cis-platinum–velban–bleomycin: cis-platinum 60 $mg/m^2$ day 1, vinblastine 0.1 mg/kg days 1 and 15, and bleomycin 15 iu IV weekly on a 28-day cycle) [29]. No difference in the groups was seen, with 11 of 68 patients (16.2%) responding to methotrexate vs. 13 of 66 (20%) to PVB. Of interest was a higher response rate to the drug combination in patients with distant metastases (43.5%) vs. 2 of 21 (9.5%) for methotrexate ($P < .05$). Response duration and survival were poor in both arms, toxicity was comparable, and no significant advantage was seen for the combination over single-agent methotrexate. Neurologic and mucous membrane toxicity were more severe with the combination of cis-platinum–velban–bleomycin while renal toxicity was equally frequent. Other randomized studies have compared combinations to single agent cis-platinum [92]. No differences were found in either response rate or durability of responses.

The comparability of drug combinations and single-agent therapy in randomized studies thus far is not unexpected, given the failure of these combinations to meaningfully increase complete responses in earlier phase II trials. Furthermore, when active agents are incorporated into combination regimens, accompanying dose reduction of individual agents may compromise the regimen. For example, with cis-platinum and bleomycin reduction in dose of both drugs reduces toxicity but appears to compromise response rates as well [137,138].

While most polychemotherapy regimens are designed to include agents with differing mechanisms of actions and with differing dose-limiting toxicities, another promising approach in head and neck cancer is the exploitation of biochemical or pharmacologic changes induced by sequencing agents. Table 7–8 lists three such promising drug combinations [19,26,139,140].

The observation that the cytotoxic effects of methotrexate and 5-fluorouracil were schedule dependent in vivo followed by the observation that methotrexate pretreatment increased levels of 5-fluorouracil intracellularly in vitro has led to our use of this combination in squamous head and neck cancer. A 71% response rate in patients with advanced disease has been confirmed in 36 patients (65%) at the Karolinska Institute [140]. While the response duration is 3.6 months, the median survival for all 23 previously irradiated patients with metastatic or recurrent disease is 11.5 months. While pretreatment performance status may be a factor in their improved survival, patients were equally divided between excellent (ECOG 0–1) and poor (ECOG 2–4) performance status groups. Toxicity was appreciable, with diarrhea and limiting toxicity. Failure of this sequence to achieve significant numbers of complete remissions suggests that further progress must be made in our understanding of time-sequence drug-induced perturbations in malignant cells.

Molinari [26] sequenced vincristine to arrest cells in $G^2$, bleomycin to induce progression into the S-phase of the cell cycle prior to administering the S-phase-active antimetabolite methotrexate. This vincristine-bleomycin-methotrexate sequence resulted in little toxicity, with median durations of response of 6.9 months in complete responders and 3.9 months in partial responders.

Price and Hill [141] have long used a kinetic-based sequential regimen (table 7–8), with 5-fluorouracil added to the vincristine-bleomycin-methotrexate-leucovorin sequence. Hydrocortisone was added to delay bleomycin-induced pulmonary fibrosis and to prevent immediate reactions to bleomycin. Particularly active in untreated disease, as is true in most combinations (see table 7–1), the sequence produces responses in fewer than half of patients with recurrent or metastatic disease. Using a schedule similar to that proposed by Price and Hill [141], Tannock reported only 11% responses among such recurrent or metastatic patients [142].

Further evidence that there may, indeed, be marked sequence and schedule dependency of squamous head and neck cancer comes from a clinical trial of cytoxan, adriamycin, and cis-platinum [134]. When all three drugs were given on day one (CAP 1), Creagan reported 64% responses; when adriamycin was given on day one, cytoxan on day three, and cis-platinum days one, two, and three (CAP 3), markedly inferior results were achieved. It was postulated that these divergent results may have been due to schedule dependency, as has been suggested from animal models in which the most effective combination was cytoxan followed by adriamycin [143].

In summary, new active agents in this disease are needed. Unfortunately, recent phase II trials have failed to suggest promising activity in head and neck

**Table 7–8.** Promising drug combinations used in sequence

| Investigator | Schema | Drug dosages | No. of patients | Response rate |
|---|---|---|---|---|
| Pitman et al. [139]<br>Ringborg et al. [140] | 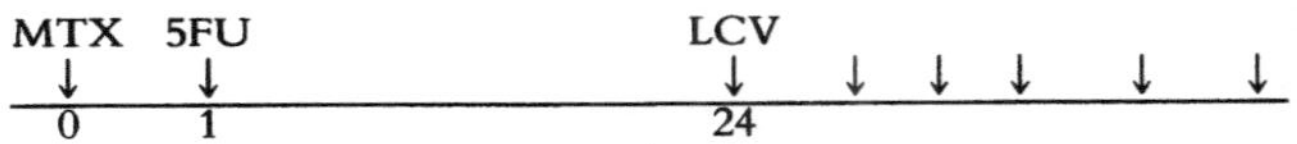 | Methotrexate 125–250 mg/m$^2$ IV<br>5-fluorouracil 500 mg/m$^2$ IV<br>Leucovorin 10 mg/m$^2$ IV then po q 6 h × 5<br>Repeat weekly | 35<br>36 | 71%<br>65% |
| Price et al. [19] | 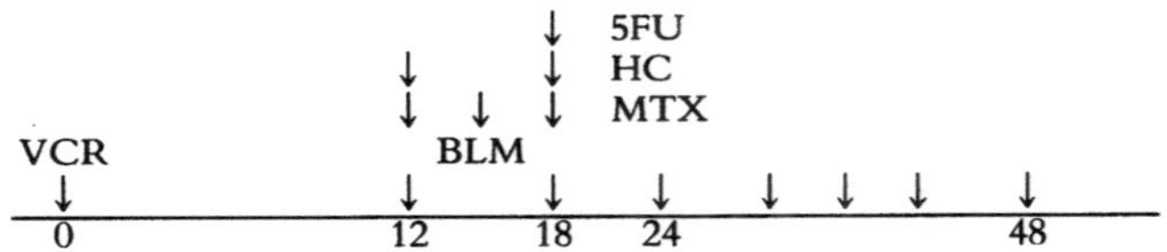 | Vincristine 2 mg IV<br>Bleomycin 60 mg infusion<br>Methotrexate 100 mg IV voles × 3<br>Hydrocortisone 500 mg IV × 2<br>5-fluorouracil 500 mg IV<br>Leucovorin 15 mg IM q 6 h × 4<br>Repeat q 3 weekly | 138 | 59% |
| Molinari et al. [26] | 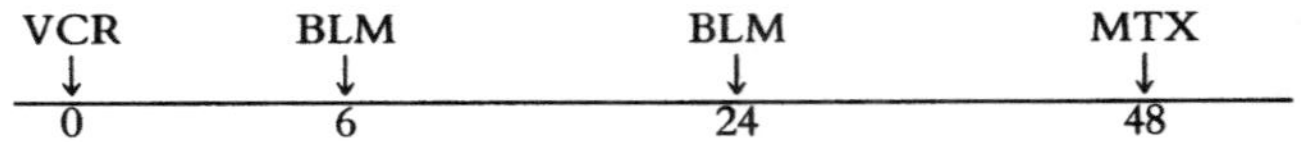 | Vincristine 1 mg IV<br>Bleomycin 15 mg IM<br>Methotrexate 20 mg/m po<br>Repeat weekly | 60 | 62% |

squamous cell cancer [144–146]. One exception may be infusion vindesine [147].

## 5. ADJUVANT CHEMOTHERAPY

Despite aggressive surgery and irradiation given preoperatively or postoperatively, large numbers of stage III and stage IV squamous head and neck cancer patients relapse, either with locoregional recurrence or with distant metastasis [148]. Reasoning that the addition of a third modality might decrease the incidence of local recurrence or incidence of distant metastases in these poor prognosis patients, investigators have long examined chemotherapy in this setting. In many randomized trials drugs and irradiation were given concurrently in an effort to potentiate radiation's cytocidal effects [149–156]. Additive toxicity to normal tissues usually resulted [151,152]. Only one study with concurrent 5-fluorouracil demonstrated improved five-year survival, with superior survival limited to oral cavity and tonsil sites [150].

In other randomized trials, the drug was given prior to irradiation [157,158]. Usually, no more than one or two weeks of chemotherapy were administered before irradiation was begun, insufficient time to achieve much tumor regression. Indeed, few early studies document the degree of tumor regression achieved prior to irradiation; in view of the low order of activity of the single agents used in these randomized trials (5-fluorouracil, methotrexate, bleomycin), it is unsurprising that no significant impact on survival has been demonstrated.

With the advent of cis-platinum as an active agent, together with achievement of clinical responses in 50 to 75% of patients following cis-platinum- or methotrexate-containing combinations (table 7–1), significant reduction of tumor bulk prior to radiation or surgery was reported by many clinical investigators and the feasibility of administering drug without hampering subsequent surgery or radiation was proven [15,16,19,159–161].

Initial enthusiasm with this neoadjuvant chemotherapy has been tempered by the poor survival of many of these patients, despite aggressive drug combinations [8,162,163]. Didolkar [8] reported a 15% overall two-year survival despite aggressive preoperative cis-platinum and bleomycin or cis-platinum, bleomycin, and methotrexate.

What is evident from many such preliminary trials is that chemotherapy may improve survival in the subset of patients who respond to it [19,164–166].

Rygaard and Hansen [164] administered bleomycin (.7 mg/kg) for two weeks prior to and during the first week of irradiation [164]. With a minimum follow-up of three years in 101 $T^3$ tumors, responders had a 47-month median survival compared to a 16-month median in nonresponders. Ervin [165] reported that partial or complete response to induction chemotherapy with methotrexate-leucovorin 3 $g/m^2$ weekly for four weeks allowed more aggressive definitive local treatment in responding patients when compared to nonresponders. Thus, median survival of responding patients was significantly better than of nonresponders (>38 months vs 15 months). In oral cavity tumors, infusion of intra-arterial methotrexate or bleomycin preoperatively improved survival in those patients who responded to it [166].

The observation that chemotherapy might affect survival in responding patients coupled with the high response rates following cis-platinum–bleomycin in previously untreated patients, using cis-platinum 100 mg/m$^2$ day 1 with hydration and mannitol diuresis and bleomycin 15 mg/m$^2$ bolus day 3 followed by 15 mg/m$^2$ infusion days [12,16], has led to the preoperative use of this regimen in a randomized half of stage III and IV patients participating in a large, multiinstitution trial in the United States. Preliminary results are that the 53% response rate of the first 68 patients receiving the induction regimen is lower than previously reported, while toxicity was minimal with no delays in surgery or significant changes in performance status or weight seen post-chemotherapy [138]. There was no significant difference in postoperative complications noted. It is, as yet, too early to assess impact on survival in this study. However, with only 50% of patients responding to chemotherapy, it will not be surprising if the cis-platinum–bleomycin combination fails to alter overall survival.

Perhaps increasing the number of cycles of effective regimens administered preoperatively or preradiation, as some have already done [23], will result in a further increase in the percentage of responding patients, which will be necessary before survival can be improved.

## 6. INTRA-ARTERIAL CHEMOTHERAPY

Intra-arterial cytotoxic therapy has been used for palliation of local or regionally recurrent squamous cell head and neck cancer for a quarter of a century. The rationale for prolonged arterial infusion is based on several theoretical advantages: (1) considering the volume of distribution, the concentration of antineoplastic agent, achieved in the region of the tumor, should be higher when administered intra-arterially than when the same drug was given orally or intravenously; (2) despite equivalent or higher tumor concentrations, systemic toxicity may be less pronounced when a drug is delivered intra-arterially than when it is delivered systemically. Schouwenburg et al. [167] could demonstrate in a rat model that prolonged intra-arterial infusion of bleomycin and 5-fluorouracil is superior to their systemic administration.

In Goldsmith and Carter's review [46] of 12 clinical trials in head and neck cancer using intra-arterial infusion, an overall response rate of 53% among 340 patients was reported. This degree of activity is higher than now reported with either single agent methotrexate and cis-platinum and is comparable to results with drug combinations. Its use is associated with significantly more local morbidity and toxicity. Most of the complications—including skin infection, leakage of drug, and kinking of the catheter—are related to the use of an indwelling catheter. Other difficulties are related to the vessel itself, such as thrombosis of the artery, together with hemorrhages or aneurysms. Despite these drawbacks, if sufficient technical expertise can be achieved, adjuvant chemotherapy via the intra-arterial route is worthy of further investigation in localized, advanced squamous head and neck cancer. When intra-arterial methotrexate was administered prior to radiation in 82 advanced oral cavity tumors, all of which had been followed a minimum of four years, a significant survival advantage was demonstrated for those methotrexate-responsive tumors that could be implanted with interstitial radium following external beam irradiation [168].

The vast majority of intra-arterial infusion treatments use methotrexate, 5-fluorouracil, or bleomycin. Use of intra-arterial cis-platinum [169], together with use of portable total transplantable infusion pumps [170], holds future promise. If reduced nephrotoxicity with intra-arterial cis-platinum can be achieved without deterioration of tumor response, the complications may well be worth the price.

## 7. SUMMARY

In summary, the chemotherapy of squamous oral cavity tumors has evolved rapidly over the past decade. It holds promise to achieve better and more long-lasting palliation in disease that has already recurred or metastasized. It holds promise, as well, to prevent recurrence or metastases in locally advanced stage III and stage IV disease, ultimately improving survival. To achieve these goals, inclusion of appropriate patients in well-designed clinical trials should be a priority for all physicians who treat this disease.

## REFERENCES

1. Sako K, Lore JM, Kaufman S, et al. Parenteral hyperalimentation in surgical patients with head and neck cancer: A randomized study. J Surg Onc (16): 391–402, 1981.
2. Miller EM, Norman D. The role of computed tomography in the evaluation of neck masses. Radiology (133): 145–149, 1979.
3. Son YH. Evaluation of neck mass: Computed tomography. Conn Med (45): 75–78, 1981.
4. Baker SR, Krause CJ. Ultrasonic analysis of head and neck neoplasms. Ann Otol (90): 126–131, 1981.
5. Gooding GAW. Gray-scale ultrasonography of the neck. JAMA (243): 1562–1564, 1980.
6. Amer MF, Al-Sarraf M, Vaitkevicius VK. Factors that affect response to chemotherapy and survival of patients with advanced head and neck cancer. Cancer (43): 2202–2206, 1979.
7. Cortes EP, Kalra J, Amin VC, Attie J, Eisenbad L, Khafif R, Wolk D, Aral I, Scrubba J, Akbijik N, Heller K. Chemotherapy for head and neck cancer relapsing after radiotherapy. Cancer (47): 1966–1981.
8. Didolkar MS, Coleman JJ, Elias EG, Gray WC, Cosentino E. Chemotherapy for advanced carcinoma of head and neck: An effective outpatient schedule of cytoxan, oncovin, methotrexate and bleomycin. Head & Neck Surg (4): 92–97, 1981.
9. Woods RL, Fox RM, Tattersall MHN. Advanced squamous cell carcinomas of the head and neck—A randomised study of three methotrexate doses. Brit Med J (282): 600–602, 1981.
10. Sealy R, Helman P. Treatment of head and neck cancer with intra-arterial cytotoxic drugs and radiotherapy. Cancer (30): 187, 1972.
11. Wittes RE, Cvitkovic E, Shah J, et al. Cis-dichlorodiammine-platinum (II) in the treatment of epidermoid carcinoma of the head and neck. Cancer Treat Rep (61): 359–366, 1977.
12. Wittes RE, Heller K, Randolph V, et al. Cis-dichlorodiammine-platinum (II)-based chemotherapy as initial treatment in advanced head and neck cancer. Cancer Treat Rep (63): 1533–1538, 1979.

13. Mills EED. Intermittent intravenous methotrexate in the treatment of advanced epidermoid carcinoma. S Afr Med J (46): 398–401, 1972.
14. Frei E, Blum R, Pitman SW, Kirkwood J, Henderson IC, Skarin AT, Mayer RJ, Bast R, Garnick M, Parker I, Canellos G. High-dose methotrexate with leucovorin rescue rationale and spectrum of antitumor activity. Amer J of Med (68): 270–276, 1980.
15. Randolph VL, Vallejo A, Spiro RH, et al. Combination therapy of advanced head and neck cancer: Induction of remissions with diamminedichloroplatinum (II), bleomycin and radiation therapy. Cancer (41): 460–467, 1978.
16. Hong WK, Shapshay SM. Treatment of previously untreated stage III and IV squamous cell carcinoma of the head and neck. Otolaryng Clin N Am (13): 521–528, 1980.
17. Brown AW, Blom J, Butler W, Guerrero GG, Richardson M, Henderson RL. Combination chemotherapy with vinblastine, bleomycin, and cis-diamminedichloroplatinum (II) in squamous cell carcinoma of the head and neck. Cancer (45): 2830–2835, 1980.
18. Forastiere AA, Crain SM, Coker DD, Elias EG, Amornmarn R, Wiernick PH. Cisplatin and cyclophosphamide combination chemotherapy in advanced head and neck squamous cell cancer. Proc Amer Soc Clin Onc (1): 196, 1982.
19. Price LA, Hill BT. Safe and effective 24-hour combination chemotherapy without cisplatin as initial treatment in head and neck cancer. Proc Amer Soc Clin Onc 1: 202, 1982.
20. Hill BT, Dalley VM, Shaw JH. 24-hour combination chemotherapy without cisplatin in recurrent or metastatic head and neck cancer. Proc Amer Soc Clin Onc (1): 202, 1982.
21. Vogl SE, Lerner H, Kaplan BH, Camacho F, Anberg J, Schoenfeld D. Mitomycin-C, methotrexate, bleomycin and cis-diamminedichloroplatinum II in the chemotherapy of advanced squamous cancer of the head and neck. Cancer (50): 6–9, 1982.
22. Amer MH, Izbicki R, Vaitkevicius VK, Al-Sarraf M. Cis-diamminedichloroplatinum, oncovin and bleomycin (COB) in advanced head and neck cancer, phase II. Cancer (45): 217–223, 1980.
23. Decker DA, Drelichman A, Jacobs J, Hoschner J, Kinzie J, Loh JJK, Weaver A, Al-Sarraf M. Adjuvant chemotherapy with high dose bolus cis-diammindichloroplatinum II and 120 hour infusion 5-fluorouracil in stage III and IV squamous cell carcinoma of the head and neck. Proc Amer Soc Clin Onc (1): 195, 1982.
24. Kish J, Drelichman A, Weaver A, Jacobs J, Bergsman K, Al-Sarraf M. Cis-platinum and 5-fluorouracil infusion in patients with recurrent and disseminated epidermoid cancer of the head and neck. Proc Amer Soc Clin Onc (1): 193, 1982.
25. Ervin RJ, Weichselbaum R, Miller D, et al. Treatment of advanced squamous cell carcinoma of the head and neck with cis-platin, bleomycin, and methotrexate (PBM). Cancer Treat Rep (65): 787–791, 1981.
26. Molinari R, Mattavelli F, Cantu G, Chiesa F, Costa L, Tancini G. Results of a low-dose combination chemotherapy with vincristine, bleomycin and methotrexate (V-B-M) based on cell kinetics in the palliative treatment of head and neck squamous cell carcinoma. Eur J Cancer (16): 469–472, 1980.
27. DeConti RC, Schoenfeld D. A randomized prospective comparison of intermittent methotrexate, methotrexate with leucovorin and a methotrexate combination in head and neck cancer. Cancer (48): 1061–1072, 1981.
28. Coker DD, Elias EG, Chretien PB, Gray WC, Coleman JJ, Zentai TA, Didolkar MS, Morris DM, Viravathana T, Hebel JR. Combination chemotherapy for advanced squamous cell carcinoma of the head and neck. Head & Neck Surg (4): 111–117, 1981.
29. Williams SD, Einhorn LH, Velez-Garcia E, Essessee I, Ratkin G, Birch R, Garrard J. Chemotherapy of head and neck cancer: Comparison of cisplatin and vinblastine and bleomycin (PVB) versus methotrexate (MTX). Proc Amer Soc Clin Onc (1): 202, 1982.
30. Woods RL, Fox RM, Tattersall MHN. Methotrexate treatment of advanced head and neck cancers: A dose response evaluation. Cancer Treat Rep (65) (Suppl): 155–159, 1981.
31. Bertino JR, Boston B, Capizzi RL. The role of chemotherapy in the management of cancer of the head and neck: A review. Cancer (36): 752–758, 1975.
32. Creagan ET, Fleming TR, Edmonson JH, Ingle J, Woods JE. Cyclophosphamide, adriamycin and cis-dichlorodiammineplatinum II in the treatment of patients with advanced head and neck cancer. Cancer (47): 240–244, 1981.
33. Presant CA, Ratkin G, Klahr C et al. Adriamycin, BCNU plus cyclophosphamide (ABC) in advanced carcinoma of the head and neck. Cancer (44): 1571–1575, 1979.

34. Jorgensen K, Schlichting J. Relationship between histologic grading of head and neck tumours and regression after chemotherapy. Acta Radiologica Oncology (19): 357–359, 1980.
35. Ohnuma, A. Effects of combination therapy with bleomycin (NSC-125066) and dibromodulcitol (NSC-104800) on squamous cell carcinoma in man. Cancer Chem. rep. (56): 625–633, 1972.
36. Papac RJ, Lefkowitz E, Bertino JR. Methotrexate (NSC-740) in squamous cell carcinoma of the head and neck. II. Intermittent intravenous therapy. Cancer Chemother Rep (51): 69–72, 1967.
37. Lane M, Moore JE, Levin H et al. Methotrexate therapy for squamous cell carcinoma of the head and neck. JAMA (204): 561–564, 1968.
38. Leone LA, Albala MM, Rege VB. Treatment of carcinoma of the head and neck with intravenous methotrexate. Cancer (21): 828–837, 1968.
39. DePalo GM, DeLana M, Molinari R, et al. Clinical evaluation of high weekly intravenous doses of methotrexate in advanced oropharyngeal carcinoma. Tumori (56): 259–268, 1970.
40. Papac R, Minor DR, Rudnick S, et al. Controlled trial of methotrexate and Bacillus Calmette-Guarin therapy for advanced head and neck cancer. Cancer Res (38): 3150–3153, 1978.
41. Vogler WR, Jacobs J, Moffitt S, Velez-Garcia E, Goldsmith A, Johnson L, Mackay S. Methotrexatee therapy with or without citrovorum factor in carcinoma of the head and neck, breast, and colon. Cancer Clin Trials (2): 227–236, 1979.
42. Woods. Personal communication.
43. Hong WK, Schaefer S, Issell B, Cummings C, Luedka D, Bromer R, Lavin L. A prospective randomized trial of methotrexate versus cisplatin in the treatment of recurrent squamous cell carcinomas of the head and neck. Proc Amer Soc Clin Onc (1): 202, 1982.
44. Vogl. Personal communication.
45. Vogl. Personal communication.
46. Goldsmith MA, Carter S. The integration of chemotherapy into a combined modality approach to cancer therapy. V. Squamous cell cancer of the head and neck. Cancer Treat Rev (2): 137–158, 1975.
47. Huseby RA, Downing V. The use of methotrexate orally in treatment of squamous cancers of the head and neck. Cancer Chemother Rep (16): 511–514, 1962.
48. Papac RJ, Jacobs EM, Foye LV Jr, et al. Systemic therapy with amethopterin in squamous carcinoma of the head and neck. Cancer Chemother Rep (32): 47–54, 1963.
49. Hellman S, Iannotti At, Bertino JR. Determination of the levels of serum folate in patients with carcinoma of the head and neck treated with methotrexate. Cancer Res (24): 105–113, 1964.
50. Vogler WR, Huseby CM Jr, Kerr W. Toxicity and antitumor effect of divided doses of methotrexate. Arch Intern Med (115): 285–293, 1965.
51. Kligerman MM, Hellman S, VonEssen DE, et al. Sequential chemotherapy and radiotherapy. Radiology (87): 247–250, 1966.
52. Andrews NC, Wilson WL. Phase II study of methotrexate (NSC-740) in solid tumors. Cancer Chemother Rep (51): 471–474, 1967.
53. Sullivan RD, Miller E, Sires MP. Antimetabolite-metabolite combination cancer chemotherapy—effects of intra-arterial methotrexate intramuscular citrovorum factor therapy in human cancer. Cancer (12): 1248–1262, 1959.
54. Capizzi RL, DeConti RC, Marsh JC, Bertino JR. Methotrexate therapy of head and neck cancer: Improvement in therapeutic index by the use of leucovorin "rescue." Cancer Res (30): 1782–1788, 1970.
55. Kirkwood JM, Canellos GP, Ervin TJ, Pitman SW, Weichelsbaum R, Miller D. Increased therapeutic index using moderate dose methotrexate and leucovorin twice weekly vs weekly high-dose methotrexate-leucovorin in patients with advanced squamous carcinoma of the head and neck: A safe new effective regimen. Cancer (47): 2414–2421, 1981.
56. Pitman SW, Parker LM, Tattersall MHN, Jaffe N, Frei E. Clinical trial of high-dose methotrexate (NSC-740) with citrovorum factor (NSC-3590)—Toxiologic and therapeutic observations. Cancer Chemo Rep (6): 43–49, 1975.
57. Condit PT, Chang RE, Joel W. Renal toxicity of methotrexate. Cancer (23): 126–131, 1969.
58. Stoller RG, Jacobs SA, Drake JC, et al. Pharmacokinetics of high-dose methotrexate. Cancer Chemother Rep (6): 19–24, 1975.

59. Pitman SW, Frei E III. Weekly methotrexate-calcium leucovorin rescue. I. Effects of alkalinization on nephrotoxicity. Cancer Treat Rep (61): 695–701, 1977.
60. Stoller RG, Hander KR, Jacobs SA, et al. Use of plasma pharmacokinetics to predict and prevent methotrexate toxicity. N Engl J Med (297): 630–634, 1977.
61. Levitt M, Mosher MB, DeConti RC, Farber LR, Skeel RT, Marsh JC, Mitchell MS, Papac RJ, Thomas ED, Bertino JR. Improved therapeutic index of methotrexate with "leucovorin rescue." Cancer Res (33): 1729–1734, 1973.
62. Krishan A, Pitman S, Tattersall MHN, et al. Flow micro-fluorometric patterns of human bone marrow and tumor cells in response to cancer chemotherapy. Cancer Res (36): 3813–3820, 1976.
63. Jaffe N, Frei E III, Traggis D, et al. Weekly high-dose methotrexate citrovorum factor in osteogenic sarcoma: Pre-surgical treatment of primary tumor and of overt pulmonary metastases. Cancer (39): 145–150, 1977.
64. Bertino JR. The mechanism of action of the folate antagonists in man. Cancer Res (23): 1286–1306, 1963.
65. Goldman ID, Lichenstein NS, Oliverio VT. Carrier mediated transport of the folic acid analogue, methotrexate, in the L1210 leukemia cell. J Biol Chem (243): 5007–5017, 1968.
66. Nahas A, Nixon PE, Bertino JR. Uptake and metabolism of $N^5$formyltetrahydrofolate by L1210 leukemia cells. Cancer Res (32): 1416–1421, 1972.
67. Huennekens FM, Vitols KS, Henderson GB. Transport of folate compounds in bacterial and mammalian cells. Adv in Enzymology: 313–344, 1978.
68. Baugh CM, Krumdieck CL, Nair MG. Polygammaglutamyl metabolites of methotrexate. Biochem Biophys Res Commun (52): 27–34, 1973.
69. Jacobs SA, Adamson RH, Chabner BA, Derr CJ, Johns DG. Stoichiometric inhibition of mammalian dihydrofolate reductase by the -glutamyl metabolite of methotrexate, 4-amino-4-deoxy-$N^{10}$-methyl-pteroylglutamyl-glutamate. Biochem Biophys Res Comm (63): 692–798, 1975.
70. Hryniuk WM, Fischer GA, Bertino JR. S-phase cells of rapidly growing and resting populations. Differences in response to methotrexate. Biol Pharmacol (5): 57–64, 1969.
71. Henderson ES, Adamson RH, Oliverio VT. The metabolic fate of tritiated methotrexate. II. Absorption and excretion in man. Cancer Res (25): 1018–1024, 1965.
72. Chungi VS, Bourne DWA, Dittert LW. Drug absorption VIII: Kinetics of GI absorption of methotrexate. J Pharmaceutic Sci (67): 560–561, 1978.
73. Pinkerton CR, Welshman SG, Dempsey SI, Bridges JM, Glasgow JFT. Absorption of methotrexate under standardized conditions in children with acute lymphoblastic leukeaemia. Br J Cancer (42): 613–615, 1980.
74. Huffman D, Wan SH, Azarnoff DL, Hoogstraten B. Pharmacokinetics of methotrexate. Clin Pharmacol Ther (14): 572–579, 1973.
75. Bischoff KG, Dedrick RL, Zaharko DS, Longstreth JA. Methotrexate pharmacokinetics. J Pharmaceutic Sci (60): 1128–1133, 1971.
76. Chabner BA, Young RC. Threshold methotrexate concentration for in vivo inhibition of DNA synthesis in normal and tumorous target tissues. Clin Invest (52): 1804–1811, 1973.
77. Chabner BA, Johns DG, Bertino JR. Enzymatic cleavage of methotrexate provides a method for prevention of drug toxicity. Nature 239: 395–397, 1972.
78. Creaven PJ, Hansen HH, Alford DA, Allen LM. Methotrexate in liver and bile after intravenous dosage in man. Br J Cancer (28): 589–591, 1973.
79. Gewirtz DA, White JC, Randolph JK, Goldman ID. Transport, binding and polyglutamylation of methotrexate in freshly isolate rat hepatocytes. Cancer Res (40): 573–578, 1980.
80. Kamen BA, Nylen PA, Camitta BM, Bertino JR. Methotrexate accumulation in cells as possible mechanism of chronic toxicity to the drug. Br J Hematol, in press.
81. Wan SH, Huffman DH, Azarnoff D, Stephens R, Hoogstraten B. Effect of route of administration and effusion on methotrexate pharmacokinetics. Cancer Res (34): 3487–3491, 1974.
82. Valerino DM, Johns DG, Zaharko DS, Oliverio VT. Studies of the metabolism of methotrexate by intestinal flora. I. Identification and study of biological properties of the metabolite 4-amino-4-deoxy-$N^{10}$-methylpteroid acid. Biochem Pharmacol (21): 821–831, 1972.
83. Jacobs SA, Stoller RG, Chabner BA, Johns DG. 7-hydroxymethotrexate as a urinary metabolite in human subjects and Rhesus monkeys receiving high-dose methotrexate. J Clin Invest (57): 534–538, 1976.

84. Huang KC, Enczak BA, Liu YK. Renal tubular transport of methotrexate in the Rhesus monkey and dog. Cancer Res (39): 4838–4848, 1979.
85. Rosenberg B, Van Camp L, Krigos T. Inhibition of cell division in Escherichia coli by electrolysis products from a platinum electrode. Nature (205): 698–699, 1965.
86. Rosenzweig M, Von Hoff DD, Slavik M et al. Cis-diamminedichloroplatinum II. Annals Int Med (86): 803–812, 1977.
87. Hill JM, Loeb E, MacLellan A, Hill NO, Khan A, King JI. Clinical studies of platinum coordination compounds in the treatment of various malignant diseases. Cancer (59): 647–659, 1975.
88. Jacobs C, Bertino JR, Goffinet DR, FU WW, Goode RL. 24-hour infusion of cis-platinum in head and neck cancers. Cancer (42): 2135–2140, 1978.
89. Sako K, Rizack MS, Kalmens I. Chemotherapy for advanced and recurrent squamous cell carcinoma of the head and neck with high and low dose cis-diamminedichloroplatinum. Am J Surg (136): 529–533, 1978.
90. Hayat M, Bayssas M, Brule G, et al. Cis-platinum-diamminodichloro (CDDP) in chemotherapy of cancers. Biochemic (60): 935–940, 1978.
91. Aribas E. Personal communication.
92. Davis S, Kessler W. Randomized comparison of cis-diamminedichloroplatinum vs cis-diamminedichloroplatinum, methotrexate and bleomycin in recurrent squamous cell carcinoma of the head and neck. Cancer Chemo Pharmacol (3): 57–59, 1979.
93. Pannettiere FJ, Lehane D, Fletcher WS, et al. Cis-platinum therapy of previously treated head and neck cancer: The Southwest Oncology Group's two-dose-per-month outpatient regimen. Med Pediatr Oncol (8): 221–225, 1980.
94. Drewinko B, Brown BW, Gottlieb JA. The effect of cis-diamminedichloroplatinum (II) on cultured human lymphoma cells and its therapeutic implications. Cancer Res (33): 3091–3095, 1973.
95. Deconti RC, Toftness BR, Lange RC, et al. Clinical and pharmacological studies with cis-diamminedichloroplatinum II. Cancer Res (33): 1310–1315, 1973.
96. Ward JM, Arabin ME, Berlin E, et al. Prevention of renal failure in rats receiving cis-diamminedichloroplatinum (II) by administration of furosemide. Cancer Res (37): 1238–1240, 1977.
97. Hayes DM, Critkovic E, Golbey RB, et al. High-dose cis-platinumdiamminedichloride. Cancer (39): 1372–1381, 1977.
98. Chary KK, Higby DJ, Henderson ES, et al. Phase I Study of high dose cis-dichlorodiammine platinum (II) with forced diuresis. Cancer Treat Rep (61): 367–370, 1977.
99. Ozols RF, Javadpour N, Messerschmidt EL, Young RC. Poor prognosis non-seminomatous testicular cancer: An effective "high-dose" cis-platinum regimen without increased renal toxicity. Proc Amer Soc Clin Oncol (1): 113, 1982.
100. Umezawa H. Chemistry and mechanism of action of bleomycin. Fed Proc (33): 2296–2307, 1976.
101. Sikic BI et al. Improved therapeutic index of bleomycin when administered by continuous infusion in mice. Cancer Treat Rep 62: 2011–2017, 1978.
102. Krakoff IH, Critkovic E, Currie E, Yeh S, Lamonte C. Clinical, pharmacologic and therapeutic studies of bleomycin given by continuous infusion. Cancer (40): 2027–2037, 1977.
103. Byfield JE, Lee YC, Tu L, et al. Molecular interactions of the combined effects of bleomycin and x-ray on mammalian cell survival. Cancer Res (36): 1138–1143, 1976.
104. Holoye PT, Broughton A, Strong JE, et al. Bleomycin: Pharmacokinetics of continuous intravenous infusion. Proc Amer Assoc for Canc Res (17): 70, 1977.
105. Broughton A, Strong JE. Radioimmunoassay of bleomycin. Cancer Res (36): 1418–1421, 1976.
106. Blum RH, Carter SK, Agre K. A clinical review of bleomycin: A new antineoplastic agent. Cancer (31): 903–913, 1973.
107. Bertino JR, Mosher MD, DeConti RC. Chemotherapy of cancer of the head and neck. Cancer (31): 1141–1149, 1973.
108. Moertel CG. Clinical management of advanced gastrointestinal cancer. Cancer (36): 675–682, 1975.
109. Johnson RD, Kisken WA, Curreri A. Squamous cell carcinoma of the oral cavity. Arch Surg (90): 760–763, 1965.

110. Heidelberger C. Fluorinated pyrimidines and their nucleosides. In Handbook of Experimental Pharmacology, Sartorelli and Johns (ed), New York: Springer-Verlug, pp. 193–231, 1974.
111. Goulean M, Bleile B, Tseng BY. Methotrexate-induced misincorporation of uracil into DNA. Proc Natl Acad Sci (77): 1956–1960, 1980.
112. Bertino JR, Sawicki WL, Lindquist CA, Gupta VS. Schedule dependent effects of methotrexate and 5-fluorouracil. Cancer Res (37): 327–328, 1977.
113. Fernandez DJ, Bertino JR. 5-fluorouracil-methotrexate synergy: Enhancement of 5-fluorodeoxyuridylate binding to thymidylate synthase by dihydropteroylpolyglutamates. Proc Nat'l Acad Sci (USA) (77): 5663–5667, 1980.
114. Cadman E, Heimer R, Davis L. Enhanced 5-fluorouracil nucleotide formation after methotrexate administration: Explanation for drug synergism. (205): 1135–1137, 1979.
115. Cooper GM, Dunning WF, et al. Role of catabolism in pyrimidine utilization for nucleic acid synthesis in vivo. Cancer Res (32): 390–397, 1972.
116. Finn C, Sadee W. Determination of 5-fluorouracil (NSC-19893) plasma levels in rats and man by isotope dilution-mass fragmentography. Cancer Chem Rep (59): 279–286, 1975.
117. Chaudhuri NK, Montag BJ, Heidelberger C. Studies on fluorinated pyrimidines. III. The metabolism of 5-fluorouracil-2-$^{14}$C and 5-fluorourotic acid-2-$^{14}$C in vivo. Cancer Res (18): 318–328, 1958.
118. Clarkson B, O'Connor A, Winston, et al. The physiologic disposition of 5-fluorouracil and t-fluoro-$^{21}$deoxyuridine in man. Clin Pharmacol Ther (5): 581–610, 1965.
119. Koenig H, Patel A. Biochemical basis for fluorouracil neurotoxicity. The role of Krebs cycle inhibition by fluoroacetate. Arch Neurology (32): 155–160, 1970.
120. Wolf GT, Chretien PB. The chemotherapy and immunotherapy of head and neck cancer. In Cancer of the Head and Neck, JR Suen and EN Myers (eds). New York: Churchill-Livingstone, 1981.
121. Medenica R, Alberto P, Lehman W. Traitement des carcinomes epidermoides oro-pharyngo-larynges dissemines par combinaison de methotrexate et de bleomycine a petites doses. Schwerz Med Wochesnchr (106): 799–802, 1976.
122. Yagoda A, Lippman AJ, Winn RF, et al. Combination chemotherapy with bleomycin (BLM) and methotrexate (MTX) in patients with advanced epidermoid carcinomas. Proc Am Assoc Cancer Res (16): 247, 1975.
123. Lekich JJ, Frei E III. Phase II study of concurrent methotrexate and bleomycin chemotherapy. Cancer Res (34): 2240–2242, 1974.
124. Mosher MB, DeConti RC, Bertino JR. Bleomycin therapy in advanced Hodgkin's disease and epidermoid cancers. Cancer (30): 56–60, 1972.
125. Broquet MA, Jacot-des-Combes E, Montandon A, et al. Traitement des carcinomes epidermoides oro-pharyngo-larynges par combinaison de methotrexate et de bleomycine. Schwerz Med Wocheschr (104): 18–22, 1974.
126. Medenica R, Albert P, Lehmann W. Combined chemotherapy of head and neck squamous cell carcinomas with methotrexate, bleomycin and hydroxyurea. Cancer Chemother Pharmacol (5): 145–149, 1981.
127. Jacobs C. High-dose methotrexate and cis-platinum in the treatment of recurrent head and neck cancer. Rec Res Can Res (76): 290–295, 1981.
128. Pitman SW, Minor DR, Papac R, et al. Sequential methotrexate leucovorin (MTX-LCV) and cis-platinum (CDDP) in head and neck cancer. Proc Am Assoc Cancer Res (20): 419, 1979.
129. Chandler JR, Tejada FJ. Triple therapy for advanced cancer of the head and neck. Arch Otolaryngol (107): 27–29, 1981.
130. Elias EG, Chretien PB, Monnard E, et al. Chemotherapy prior to local therapy in advanced squamous cell carcinoma of the head and neck. Preliminary assessment of an intensive drug regimen. Cancer (43): 1025–1031, 1979.
131. Caradonna R, Paladine W, Ruckdeschel JC, et al. Methotrexate, bleomycin and high-dose cis-dichlorociammineplatinum (II) in the treatment of advanced epidermoid carcinomas of the head and neck. Cancer Treat Rep (63): 489–491, 1979.
132. Vogl SH, Kaplan BH. Chemotherapy of advanced head and neck cancer with methotrexate, bleomycin, and cis-diamminedichloroplatinum II in an effective outpatient schedule. Cancer (44): 26–31, 1979.

133. Ervin TJ, Weichselbaum R, Miller D, et al. Treatment of advanced squamous cell carcinoma of the head and neck with cisplatin, bleomycin, and MTX (PBM). Cancer Treat Rep (65): 787–791, 1981.
134. Creagan E, Fleming T, Edmonson J, Ingle J, Woods J. Chemotherapy for advanced head and neck cancer with the combination adriamycin, cyclophosphamide and cis-diamminedichloroplatinum (II): Preliminary assessment of a one-day vs. three day drug regimen. Cancer (47): 2549–2551, 1981.
135. Holoye PY, Byers RM, Gard DA, Goepfert H, Guillamondegui OM, Jesse RH. Combination chemotherapy of head and neck cancer. Cancer (42): 1661–1669, 1978.
136. Plasse T, Ohnuma T, Goldsmith MA, Brooks S, Holland JF, Biller H. Bleomycin infusion followed by cyclophosphamide, methotrexate and fluorouracil in patients with head and neck cancer. Proc Amer Soc Clin Onc (1): 194, 1982.
137. Glick JH, Marcial V, Richter M, Velez-Garcia E. The adjuvant treatment of inoperable stage III and IV epidermoid carcinoma of the head and neck with platinum and bleomycin infusions prior to definitive radiotherapy: An RTOG pilot study. Cancer (46): 1919–1924, 1980.
138. Wolf GT, Makuch RW. Pre-operative cis-platinum (CDDP) and bleomycin (BLM) in patients with head and neck squamous carcinoma (HNSCC). Proc Am Soc Clin Onc (20): 400, 1980.
139. Pitman SW, Kowal CD, Papac RJ, et al. Sequential methotrexate–5-fluorouracil: A highly active drug combination in advanced squamous cell carcinoma of the head and neck. Proc Amer Soc Clin Onc (20): 473, 1980.
140. Ringborg U, Ewert J, Kinneman J, Lundquist PG, Strander H. Sequential methotrexate–5-fluorouracil treatment of advanced carcinoma of the head and neck. UICC Conf on Clin Onc (14): 1981.
141. Price LA, Hill BT, Calvert AG, et al. Kinetically based multiple drug treatment for advanced head and neck cancer. Br J Med (3): 10–11, 1975.
142. Tannock I, Sutherland D, Osoba D. Failure of short-course multiple drug chemotherapy to benefit patients with recurrent or metastatic head and neck cancer. Cancer (49): 1358–1361, 1982.
143. Corbett TH, Griswold DP, Mayo JG, et al. Cyclophosphamide-adriamycin combination chemotherapy of transplantable murine tumors. Cancer Res (35): 1568–1573, 1975.
144. Forastiere AA, Young CW, Wittes RE. A phase II trial of m-AMSA in head and neck cancer. Cancer Chemo Pharmacol (6): 145–146, 1981.
145. Cheng E, Currie V, Wittes RE. Phase II trial of pyrazofurin in advanced head and neck cancer. Cancer Treat Rep (63): 2047–2048, 1979.
146. Edmonson JH, Frytak S, Letendre L, Kvols LK, Egan RT. Phase II evaluation of dianhydrogalactitol in advanced head and neck carcinomas. Cancer Treat Rep (63): 2081–2083, 1979.
147. Byrne R, Popkin J, Licciardello J, Bromer R, Weinger R, Hong W. Continuous 48-hour infusion of vindesine (DVA) in head and neck squamous cell carcinoma. Proc Amer Soc Clin Onc (1): 194, 1982.
148. Snow JB, Gelber RD, Kramer S, et al. Comparison of preoperative and postoperative radiation therapy for patients with carcinoma of the head and neck. Interim Report. Acta Otolaryngol (91): 611–626, 1981.
149. Abe M, Shigematsu Y, Kimura S. Combined use of bleomycin with radiation in the treatment of cancer. Recent Res Cancer Res (63): 2, 169–178, 1978.
150. Lo T, Wiley AL, Ansfield FJ, Brandenburg JH, Davis HL, Gollin FF, Johnson RO, Famirez G, Vermund H. Combined radiation therapy and 5-fluorouracil for advanced squamous cell carcinoma of the oral cavity and oropharynx: A randomized study. Cancer (126): 229–235, 1976.
151. Bagshaw MA, Doggett RLS. A clinical study of chemical radiosensitization. In Frontiers of Radiation Therapy and Oncology, Korger S, Vaeth JM (eds). Baltimore: University Park Press, 1969, pp. 164–173.
152. Cachin Y, Jortay A, Sancho H, et al. Preliminary results of a randomized EORTC study comparing radiotherapy and concomitant bleomycin to radiotherapy alone in epidermoid carcinomas of the oropharynx. Eur J Cancer (13): 1389–1395, 1977.
153. Condit PT. Treatment of carcinoma with radiation therapy and methotrexate. Missouri Med (65): 832–835, 1968.

154. Kapstad B, Bang G. Rennaes S, et al. Combined preoperative treatment with cobalt and bleomycin in patients with head and neck carcinoma: A controlled clinical study. Int J Radiat Oncol Biol Phy 4: 85–89, 1978.
155. Richards GJ Jr, Chambers RG. Hydroxyurea: A radiosensitizer in the treatment of neoplasms of the head and neck. AJR (105): 555–565, 1969.
156. Stefani S, EElls RW, Abbate J. Hydroxyurea and radiotherapy in head and neck cancer: Results of prospective controlled study in 126 patients. Radiology (101): 391–396, 1971.
157. Knowlton AH, Percarpio B, Bobrow S, et al. Methotrexate and radiation therapy in the treatment of advanced head and neck tumors. Radiology (116): 709–712, 1975.
158. Kramer S. Methotrexate and radiation therapy in the treatment of advanced squamous cell carcinoma of the oral cavity, oropharynx, supraglottic larynx and hypopharynx (Preliminary report of a controlled clinical trial of the Radiation Therapy Oncology Group). Can J Otolaryngol (4): 213–218, 1975.
159. Arlen M. High-dose methotrexate in preoperative management. MY State J Med, 1384–1389, 1979.
160. Marcial VA, Velez-Garcia E, Figueroa-Valles NR, Cintron J, Vallecillo LA. Multidrug chemotherapy (vincristine-bleomycin-methotrexate) followed by radiotherapy in inoperable carcinomas of the head and neck: Preliminary report of a pilot study of the Radiation Therapy Oncology Group. Int J Radiation Oncology Biol Phys (6): 717–721, 1980.
161. Spaulding MB, Klotch D, Grillo J. Adjuvant chemotherapy in the treatment of advanced tumors of the head and neck. Amer J Surg (140): 538–542, 1980.
162. Vogl SE, Lerner H, Kaplan BH, et al. Failure of effective initial chemotherapy to modify the course of stage IV (MO) squamous cancer of the head and neck. Cancer (50): 840–844, 1982.
163. Tannock I, Cummings B, Sorrenti V, et al. Combination chemotherapy used prior to radiation therapy for locally advanced squamous cell carcinoma of the head and neck. Cancer Treat Rep (66): 1421–1424, 1982.
164. Rygaard J, Hansen HS. Bleomycin as adjuvant in radiation therapy of advanced squamous carcinoma in head and neck. Acta Otolaryngol Suppl (36): 161–166, 1979.
165. Ervin T, Kirkwood J, Weichselbaum R, Miller D, Pitman SW, Frei E. Improved survival for patients with advanced carcinoma of the head and neck treated with methotrexate-leucovorin prior to definitive radiotherapy or surgery. Laryngoscope (41): 1181–1190, 1981.
166. Richard JM, Snow GB. Present role of chemotherapy in head and neck cancer. Amsterdam Excerpta Medica, 14–21, 1975.
167. Schouwenburg, PF, van Putten LM, Snow GB. External carotid artery infusion with single and multiple drug regimens in the rat. cancer (45): 2258–2264, 1980.
168. Nervi C, Arcangeli G, Badaracco G. The relevance of tumor size and cell kinetics as predictors of radiation response in head and neck cancer. Cancer (41): 900–906, 1978.
169. Horn Y, Adam Y, Walack N, et al. Long-term remission of an advanced head and neck tumor following intra-arterial infusion with cis-dichlorodiammineplatinum. J Surg Onc (18): 189–192, 1981.
170. Baker SR, Wheeler RH, Ensminger ND. Intra-arterial infusion chemotherapy for head and neck cancer using a totally implantable infusion pump. Head and Neck Surg (5): 118–124, 1981.

# 8. RECONSTRUCTIVE SURGERY OF THE ORAL CAVITY

R.M. TIWARI

## 1. INTRODUCTION

The oral cavity has, anatomically speaking, two separate compartments, namely, the vestibule and the oral cavity proper. This division is provided by the dental arches of the upper and lower jaws. The vestibule is the space that lies between the dental arcade, on the one hand, and the lips, on the other, and communicates with the oral cavity proper in the presence of full dentition through the retromolar fossa [1]. The oral cavity proper consists of the floor of the mouth and the mobile anterior two-thirds of the tongue below and the hard and soft palate above. The palatoglossal arches behind form the boundary between the oral cavity and the oropharynx. It functions as a receptor organ for food and plays a vital role in mastication and articulation. Through the tongue and the palate it subserves the function of taste. Movements of the lips and the cheeks also participate in facial expression. In complete nasal obstruction and in case of air hunger, the oral cavity serves also as a pathway for respiration.

Each component of the oral cavity has a special structure to suit its function, and in attempting to reconstruct one or more areas of this anatomy, one must endeavour to provide not only the structure and appearance but also a return to function as far as possible. Eventually, this will depend upon the degree of surgical trauma and the proportionate defect before reconstruction is begun.

Although this chapter attempts to bring forward a general outline with regard to reconstruction of the different components of the oral cavity as separate groups, the clinician charged with reconstruction may have to undertake restoration of a defect involving more than one part simultaneously, using techniques most suitable to a particular case. The close relationship of the tongue and the floor of the mouth to the hyoid influences the function of swallowing. Following ablative surgery of these areas, steps at reconstruction must take this factor into account to avoid the problem of aspiration.

The planning for reconstruction should be discussed and preparations made before ablative surgery is begun [2]. Immediate reconstruction is the generally accepted policy today [3]. Histopathological control of the margins by frozen section examination is a sound policy in all doubtful cases.

Reconstruction in previously irradiated or operated tissues poses special problems [4]. These tissues have poor vascularity, and the process of healing in these subjects is slow [5].

Many notable advances have been made in the field of reconstructive surgery in the last decade, and the reconstructive surgeon today has a wide variety of methods available in his armamentarium [6,7,8]. On the other hand, the older established techniques are still available. In the final choice of method and technique, the clinician must take into account the age, general condition, and sociopsychological make-up of the patient as well as the site and extent of the primary lesion and the resulting defect. Every case has to be judged on its own merits. In this chapter an attempt has been made to include the salient features of each technique. The reader is referred to the appropriate literature for details of individual techniques.

## 2. PREOPERATIVE PREPARATION

The essential preoperative steps that bear on the final results in any surgical procedure in the oral cavity should be borne in mind. These are as follows:

1. Attention to oral hygiene.
2. Nutritional state of the patient.
3. Attention to any systemic conditions, such as diabetes, cardiac and/or pulmonary state.
4. Consultation with the prosthodontist.

## 3. THE LIPS

### 3.1. Surgical anatomy

Not only do the lips form the entrance to the oral cavity but they serve the extremely important function of keeping the oral cavity closed, thus allowing mastication and swallowing and preventing drooling. This function is due to the sphincter around the mouth formed by the orbicularis oris muscle. Its deep layer is formed by the fibers of the buccinator, reinforced by bundles of the incisive muscles, which give it an attachment to the nasal septum and maxilla

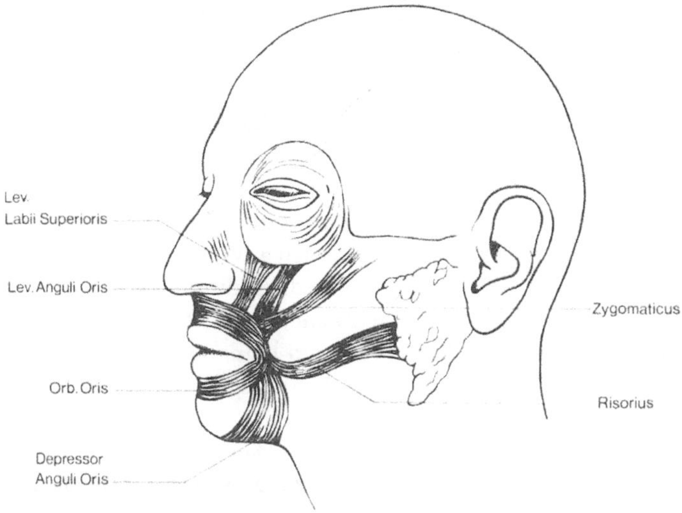


**Figure 8–1.** Muscular connections of the orbicularis oris.

[1]. The superficial bulk of the orbicularis oris is formed by the insertion of seven small muscles that act as elevators or depressors (figure 8–1). In addition, short oblique fibres travel from the skin to the mucus membrane. The orbicularis oris is supplied by the superior and inferior labial arteries and branches of the facial nerve. Most significantly, the orbicularis oris can be separated from its surrounding muscles without loss of its sphincteric competence as long as the vessels and nerves remain intact [9]. The vessels run just underneath the mucocutaneous junction. The recognition of the existence of certain conspicuous landmarks and junctional points between the lips and the surrounding areas is of considerable significance [10]. These areas and the lines of tension between them become more apparent with age, and the clinician must take these into consideration. As long as these aesthetic watersheds are not transgressed by lines of incision, healing occurs with a minimum of scarring. The lower lip is slightly fuller than the upper and appears to be tucked behind the upper lip at the commissure. The upper lip rolls gently upward at the commissure, but with advancing age this tends to drop. The lower lip exhibits a slight anterior protrusion along its entire length, and there is a subtle depression beneath its midpoint. The vermilion-cutaneous junction is the most noticeable area of the lips. It is also the area where most lesions begin. Its restitution after surgery is important if good cosmetic result is to be expected.

### 3.2. Surgical considerations

Reconstruction of the lips could be best considered under the following circumstances:

1. After excision of benign lesions of moderate dimensions.
2. After removal of small malignant lesions or fairly large benign lesions requiring sacrifice of up to 40% of the lip tissue.
3. After sacrifice of more than half of the lip.
4. After excision of lesions about the commissure.
5. When total lip reconstruction is apparent.

Small defects are closed primarily. One should attempt to obtain the scar, be it on the mucosal or the skin surface, in such a way that no puckering occurs. Much depends on how the incision is placed. Additionally, the incision should not be placed across the vermilion-cutaneous junction, as this will almost certainly lead to notching. Should this step be necessary, then the vermilion border should be carefully approximated. An angle of 30° is ideal for fusiform incisions [10].

Defects of the lip after excision of up to 40% of the tissue are corrected by direct approximation. The method of wedge excision has long been employed for excision of such lesions. Defects are closed in three layers. This ensures an acceptable reinnervation and virtually no disruptions of muscle function. The technique, however, has certain drawbacks. A wedge excision tends to transgress the anatomical junctional areas mentioned earlier, leading to a linear contraction of the scar [11]. This may eventually produce inversion of the vermilion border [12]. Certain modifications in the technique have been brought forward. The W plasty is the result of the application of the modified V-Y principle [13]. For small wedge excisions the arms of the W plasty are nearly vertical, but as the size of the wedge excision increases, the arms of the W should flare laterally to avoid crossing the lip-chin junction. Defects of this magnitude—that is, up to 40% loss of tissue—can also be reconstituted by the methods of Estlander [14], Abbé [15], and Stein [16] which were described in the last century. These methods had to be necessarily staged. They produce additional scarring and rounding of the commissure, which needs to be corrected later. The step technique overcomes these problems, and defects of up to two-thirds of the lower lip can be reconstituted with satisfactory cosmetic and functional results as regards the sensibility, mobility, symmetry, and the width of the oral orifice [17]. In this technique the lesion is excised in a rectangular fashion with generous margins. Downward bilateral step-shaped incisions of full thickness skin approximately 1 cm long are then taken in order to develop flaps. Two to four flaps are usually created. The total length of the first two flaps should equal the length of the defect. The incisions must not cross the labiomental line. When the defect is not central, the number of step flaps are fewer and the length of the first lateral flap is usually less than 1 cm (figure 8–2).

For larger defects Converse [18] described a technique of full thickness repair of an upper lip defect with preservation of the vermilion. Until the

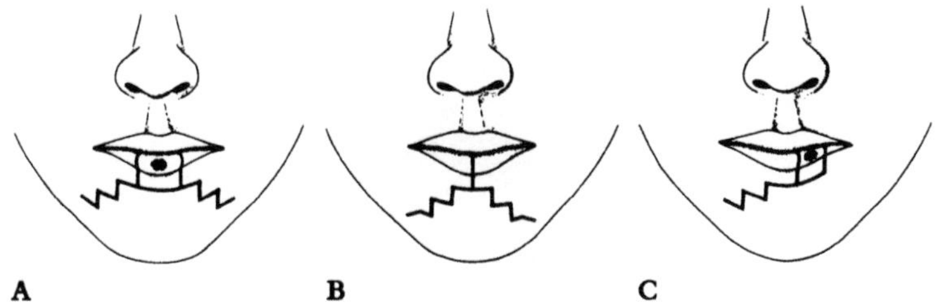


**Figure 8–2.** The step technique of lower lip reconstruction after excision for cancer after Johanson et al. [12].

description in 1974 by Karapandzic [19] of a method using lip tissue as myocutaneous flap with intact nerve supply, the advancement flap technique described by Bernard [20] in 1853 and its modifications [21–27] were used extensively. The procedure of Karapandzic takes advantage of the fact that the orbicularis oris can be released from its attachment to the surrounding muscles and moved along with the mucosa and skin as well as the attached vessels and nerves. It thus exclusively makes use of the local tissues for reconstruction; the only disadvantage seems to be a relative microstoma. Good results with this technique have also been reported by others [28]. As pointed out by Karapandzic, selection of patients is important.

Total replacment of the lower lip by full thickness advancement flaps was described by Dieffenbach [29,30] in 1843. This procedure, as well as some of the procedures for repair of subtotal defects, often lacks a mucosal lining, which can be obtained from the adjoining buccal mucosa or by the use of tongue flaps [31–33]. The use of nasolabial flaps as myocutaneous flaps for lower lip reconstruction offers all the three layers of the required tissues and avoids the need for a separate mucosal flap. The basic nasolabial flap was first described by Sushruta in 600 B.C [34,35]. Pierce and O'Connor [36] introduced this method to us in 1934. The procedure has recently been revived and modified by Meyer and Failat [37]. The technique permits an immediate repair, preserves more of the orbicularis oris muscle on the labial commissure, and provides adequate mucosal coverage. The resulting lip function is good.

Gillies fan flap has been used for lesions involving the commissure [38]. It results in a blunting of the angle of the mouth which needs correction. Brusati [39] recently described a technique that overcomes this problem.

Finally, situations arise when not enough local tissue is available for reconstruction or the tissue available is qualitatively not optimal to be utilised for the purpose of reconstruction. Distant flaps then offer the only alternatives, and while many other methods have been used in the past [40], the forehead flap [41], the deltopectoral flap [42], and the sternomastoid myocutaneous flap [43, 44] offer better alternatives and much more satisfactory results (figure 8–3).

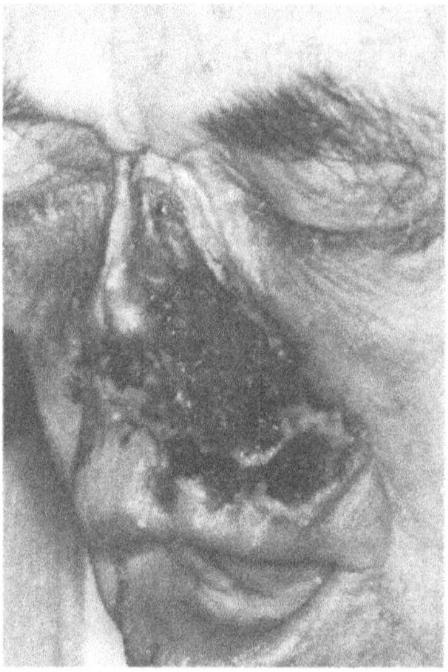

A

**Figure 8–3.** Preoperative photograph of a patient with recurrent ulcerative lesions of the externa nose involving the upper lip.

## 4. BUCCAL MUCOSA AND CHEEK

### 4.1. Surgical anatomy

In the surgical anatomy of this area, the points to be taken into account are the existence of the vestibule both above and below, the opening of the parotid duct, and the presence of a thick layer of soft tissues composed of the buccinator muscle, fibrofatty tissue, vessels, and nerves between the mucosa and the skin of the cheek. For this reason mucosal lesions do not easily involve the skin of the cheek.

### 4.2. Reconstruction

Primary closure of a defect in the buccal mucosa is to be considered after removal of benign mucosal or submucosal tumours. The mucosa should then be approximated in a horizontal plane. This gives the least noticeable scar without any puckering. Defects after removal of $T_1$ and $T_2$ lesions are reconstituted by skin grafts. Meticulous haemostasis is the first essential step. A skin graft 0.6 to 0.72 mm in thickness and free from perforation is taken from the medial surface of the thigh. The graft is carefully sutured to the edges, and a bolus dressing of antibiotic impregnated gauze is applied [45]. The graft should be generous, should loosely fit the defect, and should not be stretched. This is important if crimping is to be avoided [46]. The dressing is kept in

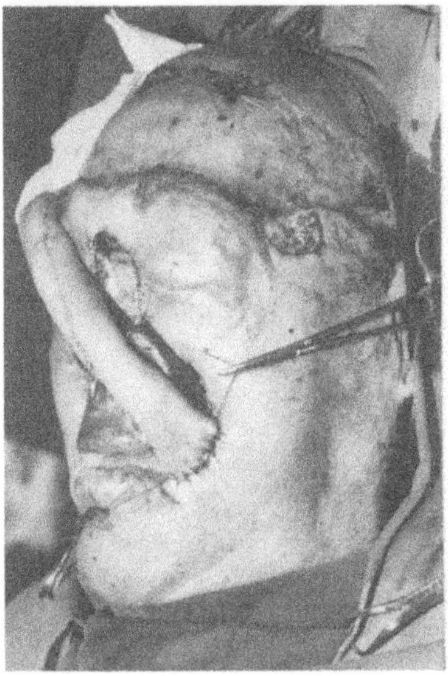

B

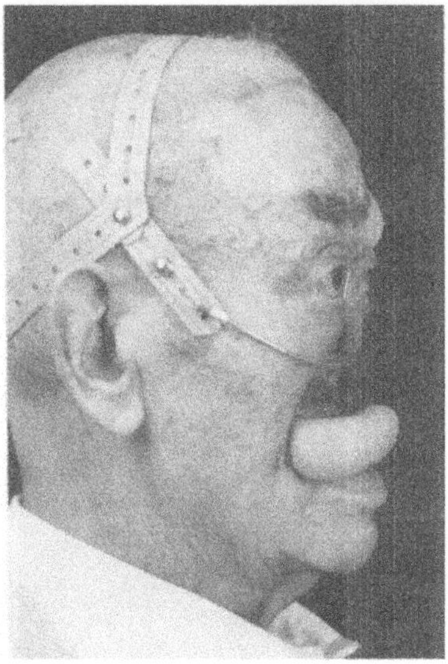

C

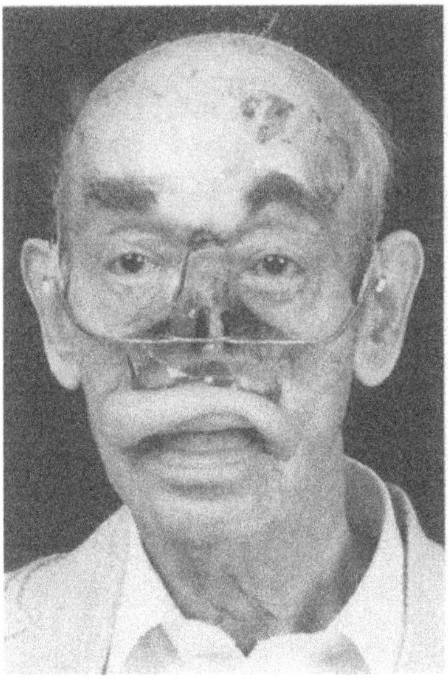

D

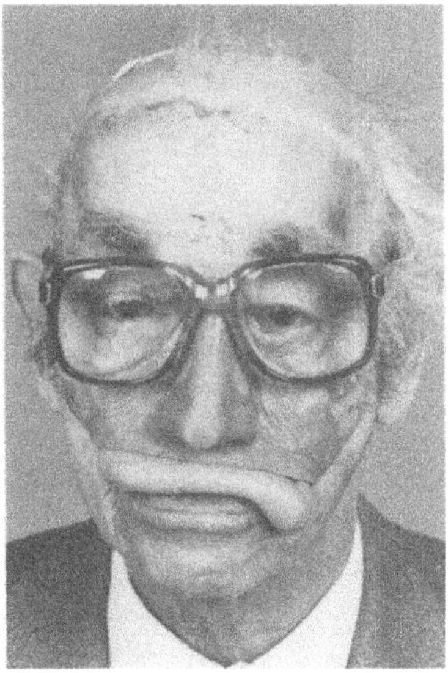

E

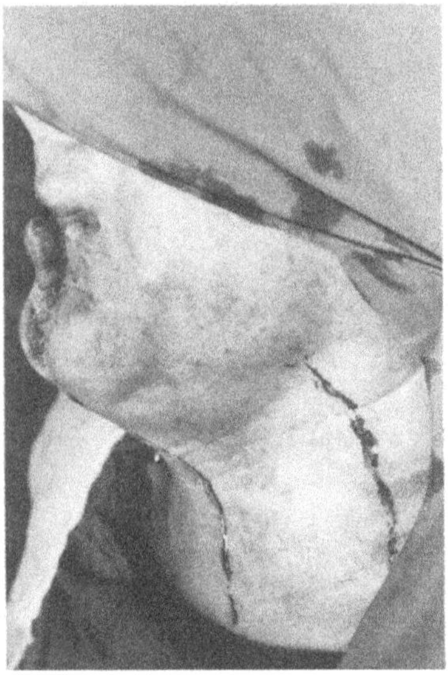

A

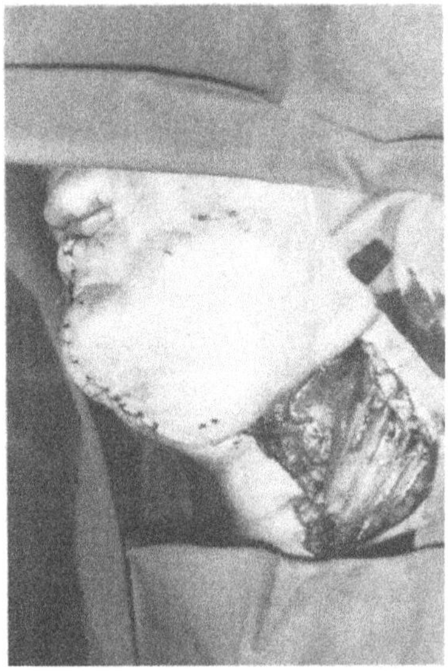

B

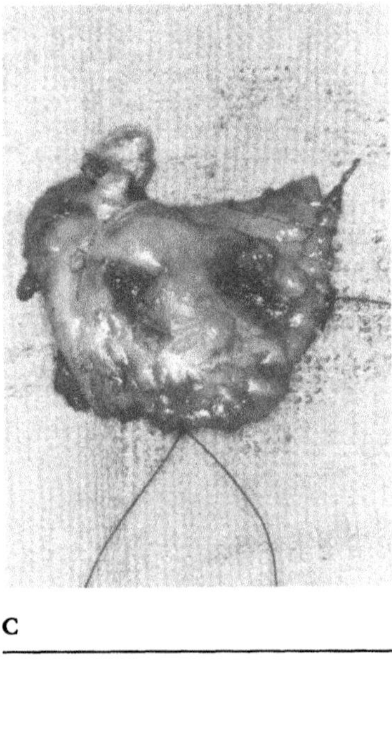

C

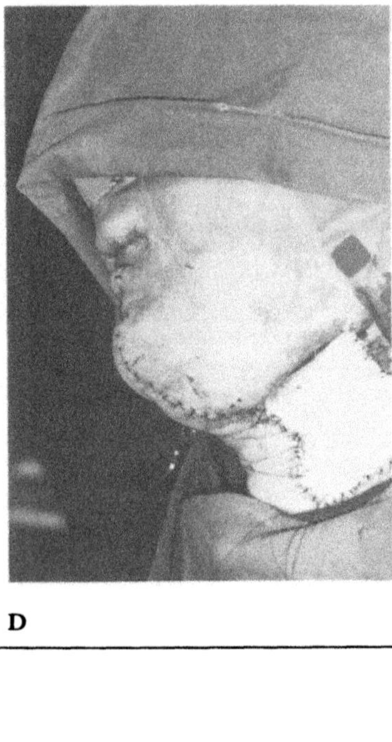

D

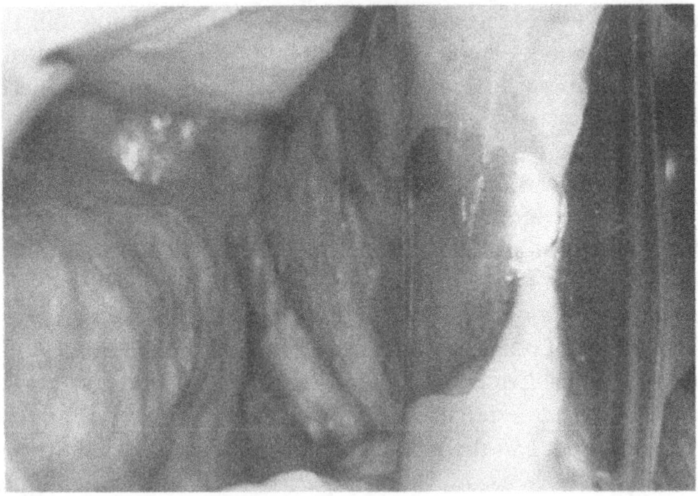

E

**Figure 8–4. A, B, C** show use of cervical skin flap for replacement of buccal lining.
**D.** Specimen of buccal mucosa with double primary cancers.
**E.** Postoperative intraoral appearance.

place for about eight days. A good contact between the graft and the tissues of the cheek provides a stable fibrin layer essential for the take of the graft [47]. Every effort should be made to keep a good oral hygiene, and antibiotics should be administered. A preoperative check of oral flora is essential since certain micro-organisms—notably, staphylococcus aureus, pseudomonas, and proteus—are known to produce more proteolytic enzymes that destroy the fibrin layer [48,49].

Larger mucosal defects and defects involving the soft tissues, but not the external skin are best closed by pedicle flaps. These flaps may be mucosal or pedicle skin flaps. The tongue flap described by Conley [50] and Gosserez [51] has been used extensively [52,53]. Although it is a reliable flap it should only be used when other substitutes are not available since it compromises with the function of an essential organ and results in the impairment of speech and swallowing. Two skin flaps have been most commonly used for restoring the buccal surface, namely, the temporal flap [54] and the cervical flap [55]. The forehead flap can be brought into the oral cavity through a tunnel into the cheek below the zygmatic arch, as introduced by McGregor, or deep to the zygoma [56]. The use of the cervical flap requires a split skin graft on the neck. Both procedures are necessarily staged (figure 8–4).

Full thickness defects of the cheek require a combination of flaps. The use of the forehead and the deltopectoral flap simultaneously was reported by McGregor and Reid [57]. These flaps are reliable because of their axial arterial supply and do not infringe upon the integrity of the cervical area. Shah [58] reported on the use of the forehead flap for both the lining and the outer coverage in total cheek defects. The compound neck pedicle described in 1955 by Owens made use of local cervical tissues for repair of cheek defects and is useful in selected cases where the use of larger flaps mentioned above may be considered mutilating or may be contraindicated because of the condition of the patient [59]. A scalp flap based on the posterior branch of the superficial temporal artery provides both lining and mass to the cheek. This can be used in combination with a bilobed skin flap from the pre- and postauricular area in the reconstruction of a total cheek defect (figure 8–5). It does have the disadvantage that the donor area is hair bearing but the forehead is spared. Other available methods of repair include the sternomastoid island flap [60] and the subcutaneous pedicle flap [61] for the lining, the cervicopectoral rotation flap [62] for coverage, the arterialised omental flap with free skin grafts for full thickness repair [63], and the unlined repairs [64]. The pectoralis major myocutaneous flap has been used for this purpose in the last few years (figure 8–6). The use of latissimus dorsi island myocutaneous flap has also been reported [65].

The wide variety of methods available today enables choice of the appropriate technique applicable to individual problems and thus the achievement of better results.

### 5. RECONSTRUCTION OF THE TONGUE

The structure of the tongue renders itself most amicably to reconstruction. Thus after partial glossectomy the tongue can be reconstituted by a careful three-layer closure without any noticeable functional disability. After hemiglossectomy of the mobile part of the tongue, the other half can be folded so as to bring the tip toward the base of the tongue and sutured in three layers. It results in a slightly small but a functionally adequate organ. After excision of moderately large lesions from the lateral margin, the defect is not suitable for closure by swinging the tip around. Closure by direct approximation of the edges produces a rather ugly longer tongue. These defects are best treated by skin grafting with the quilting technique of Mc Gregor [66].

Although reconstruction of the tongue by using the remaining organ is possible after sacrifice of three-fourths of the tongue, it is better to treat such defects surgically as total defects from the point of view of reconstruction and to bring outside tissue to provide mass and lining. Such defects of the tongue are often associated with loss of the adjoining floor of mouth. Sacrifice of three-fourths or more of the tongue is a crippling deformity. In the past pedicle skin tubes were attempted to provide the necessary replacement [67]. A pterygoid muscle sling was used by Washio [68] to restore deglutition. Matulic [69] reported a technique of reconstruction of the tongue in 1978 by a combination of sternomastoid muscle and a forehead flap. In the small series reported, a segment of the horizontal ramus of the mandible was removed in every case. Three months later activity of the muscle transplant during speech and deglutition could be verified by electromyography. Conley [70] has recently reported similar results with the use of a pectoralis major myocutaneous flap. He postulated that either the muscle adapts itself to the functions of its new surroundings, as in the case of Matulic's sternomastoid flap; or neurotization of the denervated muscle flap by axons from the intact segment of the remaining tongue occurs, and, lastly, that the possibility of fabrication of a "new tongue" by the transfer of hypoglossal nerves into the denervated segment of the peripheral aspect of the myocutaneous flap. The author has several patients who after subtotal loss of mobile tongue are adequately rehabilitated with neurotization of the myocutaneous flap. Achievement of good approximation of the muscle layers is important; 3-0 vicryl sutures are preferred.

### 6. THE FLOOR OF THE MOUTH

From the standpoint of reconstruction, the following points are of interest and worthy of attention:

1. The frequent bilateral involvement of cancers in the anterior part of the floor of the mouth.
2. The frequent extension of these cancers to the undersurface of the tongue.
3. The proximity of the mandible.
4. The mylohyoid muscle attached along the mylohyoid line forming a complete diaphragm, which forms a barrier except posteriorly in a small area where the floor of mouth lies just deep to the subcutaneous tissues.
5. The geniohyoid and the genioglossus muscles extending from the undersurface of the tongue to the hyoid and the genial tubercles on the mandible.
6. The possibility of a second primary in the area.
7. The openings of Wharton's ducts in the anterior compartment.

The division of the floor of the mouth into anteriormedial, anteriorlateral, and posterior compartments by Feind and Cole [71] is a practical one (figure 8–7).

Defects arising from excision of a small and early lesion may be closed primarily. Practically, most early lesions, however, require coverage after excision. This is provided by free split skin grafts. The technique is very similar to the one described earlier for the repair of defects of the buccal mucosa. Druck and Lurton [72] have described a technique for repair of the anterior floor of mouth defects with an island pedicle tongue flap. They recommend the procedure as an alternative to skin grafting in large $T_1$ and early $T_2$ lesions.

Although the oral cavity is the most easily visible part of the body, at least 50% of the patients are in an already advanced stage of the disease at the time of first examination [73–76].

Larger lesions need replacement of the soft tissues and lining which is largely

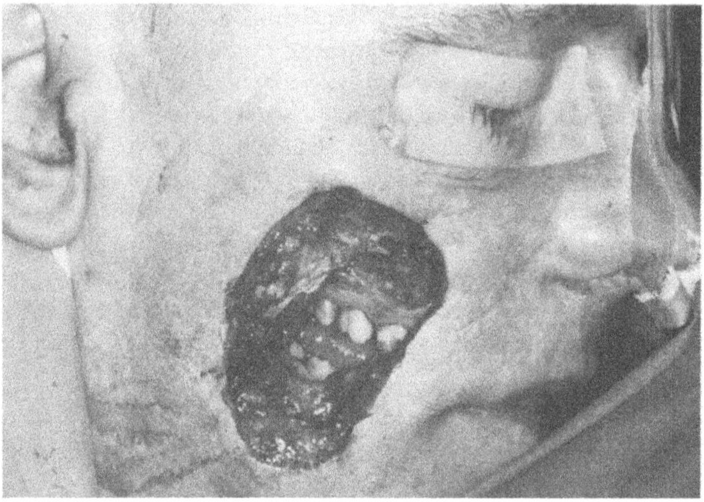

A

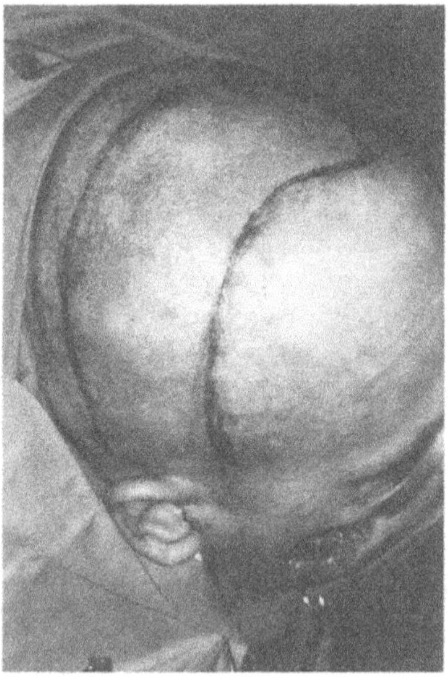

B

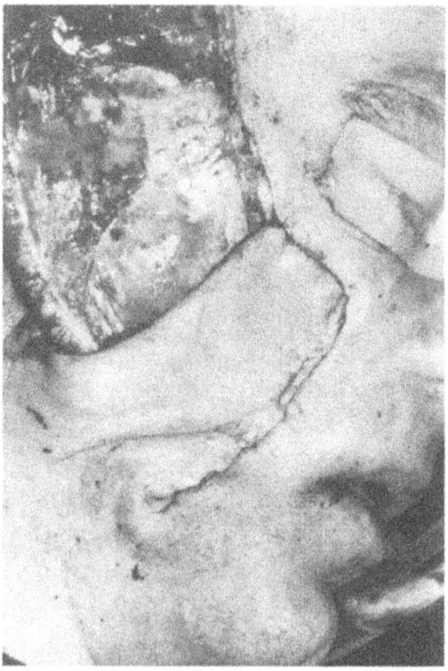

C

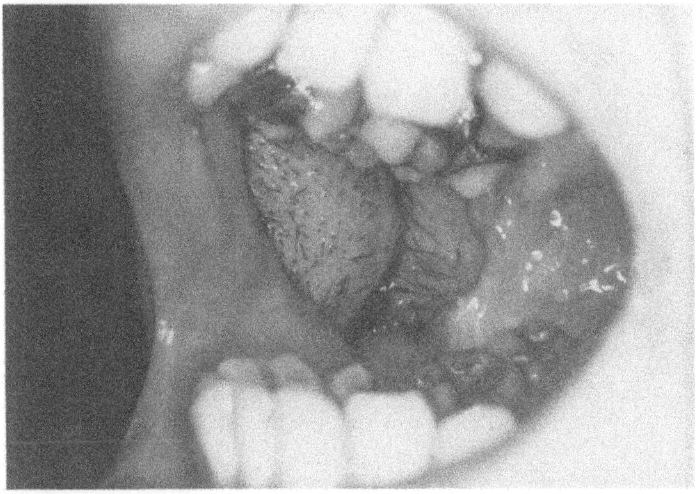

D

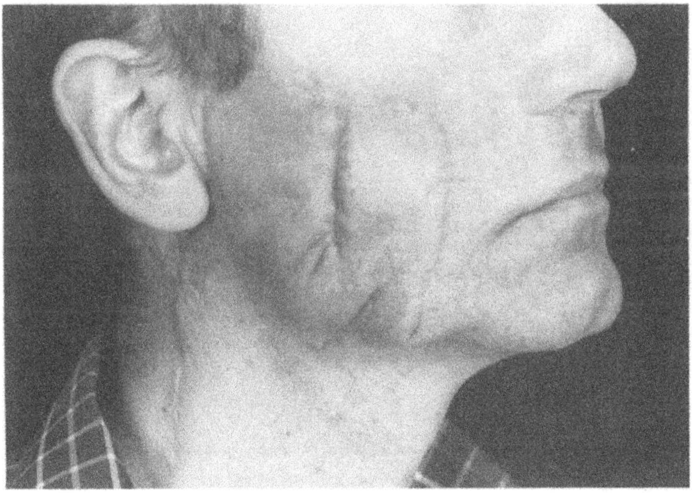

E

**Figure 8–5. A.** Total cheek defect after excision for recurrent cancer.
**B.** Planned scalp flap based on the posterior branch of the superficial temporal artery.
**C.** Stage in reconstruction.
**D.** Postoperative intraoral appearance.
**E.** Postoperative external appearance.

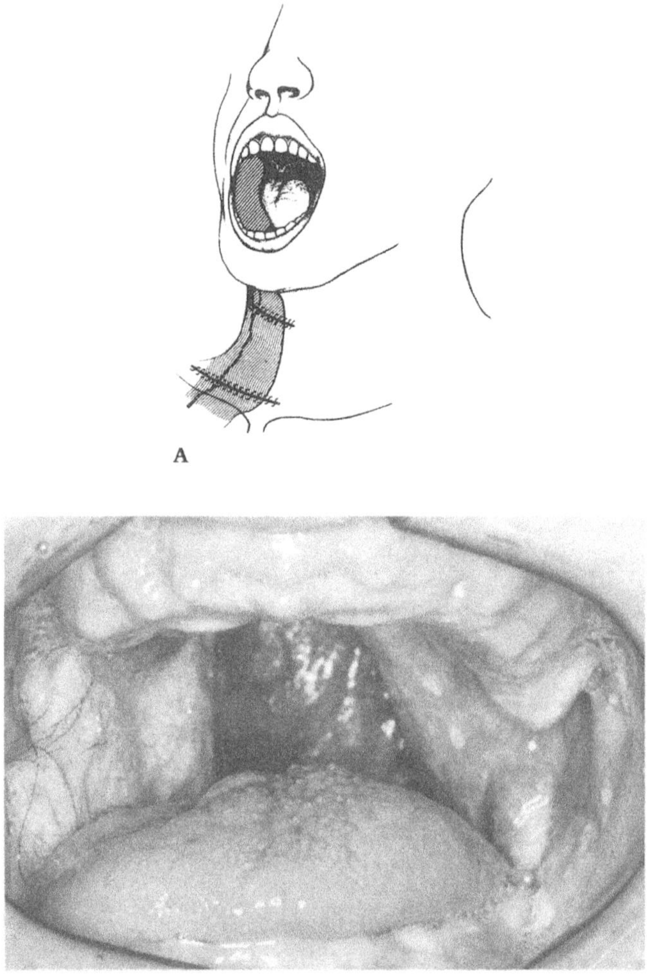

A

B

**Figure 8–6. A.** Use of the pectoralis major myocutaneous flap for replacement of soft tissues and mucosal lining; diagramatic.
**B.** Postoperative intraoral appearance.

composed of muscle. Up until a few years ago when the studies of McCraw and his colleagues [77] brought better understanding of myocutaneous flaps, the forehead flap and the deltopectoral flap were the mainstay in the repair of these defects [78,79]. These skin flaps are quite reliable, but their use in the oral cavity is not without problems. The disadvantage of the forehead flap is the occasional necrosis in irradiated patients and the objectionable scar on the forehead. The deltopectoral flap needs a large area of skin grafting, and its use

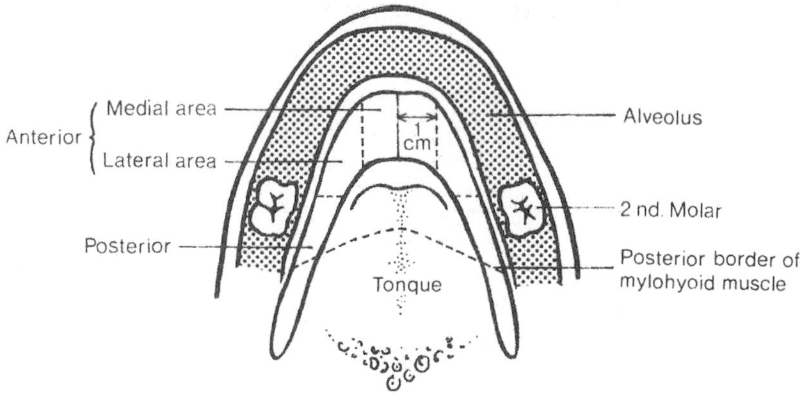


**Figure 8–7.** Divisions of the floor of mouth after Feind and Cole [71].

in the anterior floor of mouth is likely to be met with failure in about 10% of cases [80–82]. Nasolabial flaps can be easily deployed and are reliable [83–85]. Their use in the repair of the floor of mouth is, however, limited to relatively small lesions only. They are not suitable for use in the lateral part of the floor of mouth and in the presence of a normal dentition since patients tend to bite on them. The sternomastoid myocutaneous flap first mentioned in the literature by Owens and lately reintroduced by McCraw [86], Ariyan [87], and Sasaki [88] can be used for small lesions but it has a slightly higher incidence of complications [89]. The trapezius myocutaneous flap described by Demargasso [90] can be used for larger defects. Its vascular supply too is not entirely reliable, and a complication rate of up to 25% has been reported [91,92,93].

The pectoralis major myocutaneous flap described by Ariyan [94] and Baek [95] is the most reliable flap for this purpose. It has a dependable vascular pedicle, and a large amount of muscle and skin is available for use. Larger excisions are thus possible (figure 8–8). In the event of a cancer of the floor of the mouth infiltrating through the mylohyoid muscle and involving the subcutaneous tissue or skin of the neck, this flap can provide adequate skin coverage and if need be can be designed to provide both the lining of the oral cavity and the coverage for the skin defect in the neck. While using the myocutaneous flap, it is important to take the retraction of the skin into account. The maximum retraction takes place in a plane at right angles to the arrangement of the collagen fibres [96]. Thus on the thorax this occurs maximally in the transverse diameter of the flap. A margin of 25% should be added for this purpose. It is important to take at least two centimeters more of the muscle layer if at all possible beyond the skin edges since retraction of the muscle can lead to insufficient tissue available for the important second layer. Torsion of the pedicle should be avoided, as this almost certainly will lead to necrosis of the flap. Inclusion of a layer of the muscle around the vascular pedicle overcomes

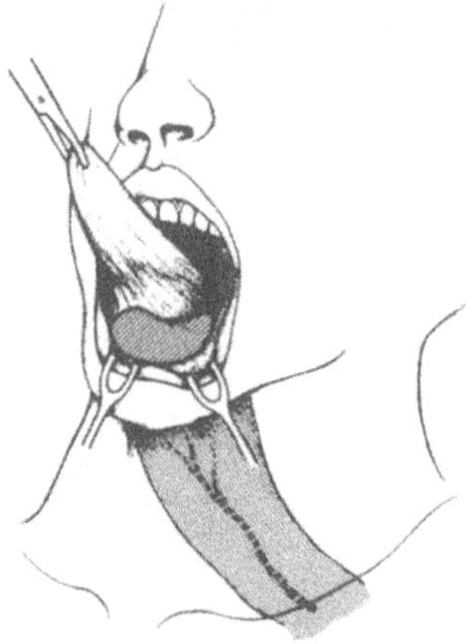

A

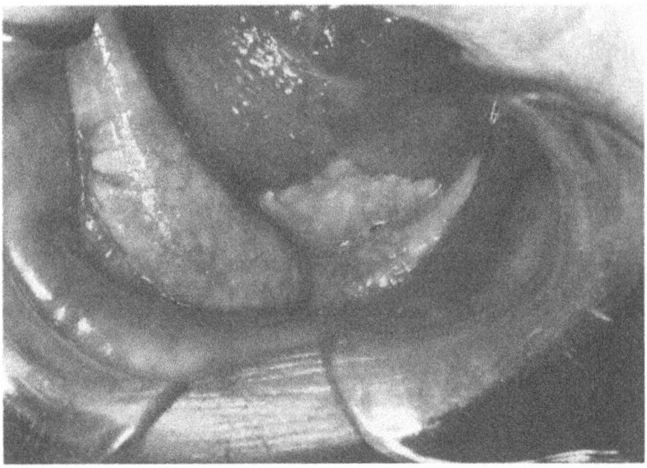

B

**Figure 8–8. A.** Total replacement of floor of the mouth with pectoralis major myocutaneous flap: diagramatic.
**B.** Postoperative clinical photograph with total reconstruction of floor of the mouth with pectoralis major myocutaneous flap.

this problem to some extent. These flaps may occasionally be too thick for the purpose of intraoral reconstruction [97,98]. Although complications such as orocutaneous fistulae may still occur, especially in irradiated patients, most of them heal spontaneously [99]. Futrell [100] described the platysma myocutaneous flap for intraoral reconstruction and used it for $T_2$ and $T_3$ lesions with good results. Its use has recently been reported by Cannon et al. [101]. It certainly has the advantages of a single-stage reconstruction with local tissues thereby reducing further scars, no new dissection fields are opened, and the time required for reconstruction is further reduced. However, like the sternomastoid flap it lies in the field of irradiation. The muscle is not always well developed, and the vascularity of the thin skin flap can be precarious. Moreover, its main blood supply comes from the submental branch of the facial artery and the transverse cervical artery. Both vessels are ligated in neck dissection.

The introduction of microvascular flaps has brought renewed interest and possibilities in this field of reconstruction. Free vascularised flaps based on the dorsalis pedis and superficial circumflex iliac arteries and free musculocutaneous flaps have been described [102–104]. A forearm flap with the radial artery has been described recently [105]. These flaps provide a single-stage repair. These procedures are at present limited to special centres since special teams are needed and the procedures are comparatively more time consuming. However, with increasing expertise and a two-team approach, the time factor has been largely overcome.

## 7. MANDIBLE

### 7.1. Surgical anatomy

Certain anatomical features need to be appreciated in the understanding of the spread of oral cancers to the bone and its therapeutic implications:

1. The thinness of the alveolar mucosa and its closeness to the bone.
2. The presence of the mandibular canal and the proximity of the mandibular foramen to tumours in the posterior part of the oral cavity.
3. The presence of the mental foramen and its proximity to the vestibule of the mouth.
4. The narrowing of the horizontal ramus of the mandible with age. Most of this takes place at the expense of the alveolar ridge with the result that the mandibular canal comes to lie closer to the alveolus while its distance from the lower border of the horizontal ramus remains unaltered. This also brings the mental foramen closer to and sometimes on the alveolar ridge itself.

Sacrifice of a part of the mandible in relation to cancers of the oral cavity may be indicated under the following circumstances:

1. When a tumour within the oral cavity arises from or extends to the mucosa over the mandible.
2. When a cancer is fixed to the bone with or without evidence of bony erosion
3. When a tumour invades the mental foramen, as for instance in lesions of the vestibule or recurrent advanced cancers of the lower lip.

4. In the presence of invasion of the mandibular canal.
5. When metastatic lymph nodes are adherent to the mandible.

A properly planned surgical approach includes the removal of a necessary amount of mandibular bone but should not necessarily be destructive [106].

**7.2. Surgical considerations**

When a part of the mandible has to be sacrificed, marginal resection of the bone below the level of the mylohyoid is possible in most cases and obviates the need for replacement of bone [107,108]. Sacrifice of a segment of the lateral part of the mandible leaves a defect that is cosmetically not significant. Replacement of soft tissues in most cases is enough. The decision to replace the bony loss immediately, later, or not at all depends upon the age, general condition, and nature of work and outlook of the patient, as well as state of the disease. Reconstruction of an anterior arch defect involving the symphysis and a varying length of one or both horizontal rami, on the other hand, is mandatory by virtue of the resulting functional and cosmetic deformity. An immediate repair offers the advantage of restoration of bony continuity and function, but carries an increased risk of failure because such a repair is undertaken in a contaminated field of operation [109,110]. This is certainly true for the free grafts. A planned secondary reconstruction does require the patient's cooperation and adds to the cost of hospitalisation. Moreover, in the presence of fibrosis the tissues in which such a repair is undertaken have diminished vascularity. However, since the approach is through a surgically clean field, the risks of failure are minimized. The two prime objectives of mandibular reconstruction are as follows:

1. To provide stable support eventually capable of supporting a denture.
2. To restore the appearance to as near normal as possible.

Autografts are the preferred source for the purpose of mandibular replacement. The superiority of the cancellous bone for this purpose has long been recognised [111,112]. The ileum and the ribs are the sources most commonly used. The former, however, provides an abundance of cancellous bone, is much more stable and yet malleable, and is most suitable for this purpose. Up to half of the mandible or more can be replaced by grafts from the iliac bone. Cancellous bone from ileum has been extensively used in combination with prosthesis made of titanium, vitallium, ticonium, and stainless steel. These prostheses serve as containers for the cancellous bone during the period of organization, calcification, and bony union [113–115]. Metallic implants have been used extensively in the past. Their use has not been without problems, however [116,117]. In an attempt to minimize the possibility of rejection, they have been used with silastic and teflon [118]. The last decade has witnessed an increasing interest in the use of autografts as free grafts, as pedicled osteomyocutaneous grafts, and as free vascularised osteocutaneous and osteomyocutaneous grafts. This field is rapidly advancing, and there is an increasing trend toward immediate reconstruction. Prosthetics may still play a role in situations where more than half of the mandible needs replacing.

In 1976 Snow et al. [119] published a series of 58 cases of free autogenous iliac crest grafts as a delayed procedure with 82% successful results and with complete rehabilitation including a dental prosthesis. Immediately after the ablative surgery has been carried out, the remaining mandible is immobilised by the application of maxillary and mandibular splints and intermaxillary fixation. Immobilisation of the mandibular segments is imperative. Three months later a graft from the ileum, in the form of a through and through piece of the crest and slightly longer than the defect to be bridged, is taken and preserved in a gauze soaked in the patient's own blood to ensure maximum viability. The stumps of the mandible are freed from surrounding scar tissue and the bone drilled away until vascular cancellous bone is exposed. The graft and the mandibular ends are prepared in a form to fit each other closely and are kept in this position by stainless steel wire suture. Intermaxillary fixation is again applied for another eight weeks. A vestibuloplasty is necessary at a later stage before the prosthesis can be fitted. The free skin graft is immobilised by an acrylic base built up with a gutta-percha and kept in place by circumferential wiring around the mandible.

Recently, after analysing the results of primary and delayed mandibular reconstruction in 54 patients, Lawson et al. [120] concluded that primary reconstruction succeeded in 46% of the cases as opposed to 90% when the repair was delayed and carried out as an elective secondary procedure. The methods used for reconstruction did not include free vascularised grafts. Recently, Piggot and Logan [121] have reported 70% successful results with primary free autogenous grafts using rib and iliac crest.

Several osteomyocutaneous pedicle flaps have been introduced in the last few years [122–125]. The possibilities for such flaps had already been put forward by Snyder [126] and Conley [127] a decade ago, and the development of the myocutaneous flaps was a logical stimulus to their development. The pioneer research of Medgyeshi [128], Brookes [129], Gothman [130], Rhinelander [131], and Cohen and Harris [132] has provided better understanding of circulation through bone in general and the relationship of periosteal and endosteal circulation in particular. This research has formed the physiological basis for the osteomyocutaneous pedicle flaps. The pectoralis major osteomyocutaneous flap with rib is especially useful for defects of the floor of mouth and anterior arch of the mandible. In using this flap it is advisable to take a little longer length of the rib than the defect. All fibrous tissue should be removed from the ends. The periosteum with the muscular attachment should be carefully preserved, and the cancellous bone should be properly approximated. Use of compression plates is not mandatory. The author has obtained good functional and cosmetic results with this flap (figure 8–9).

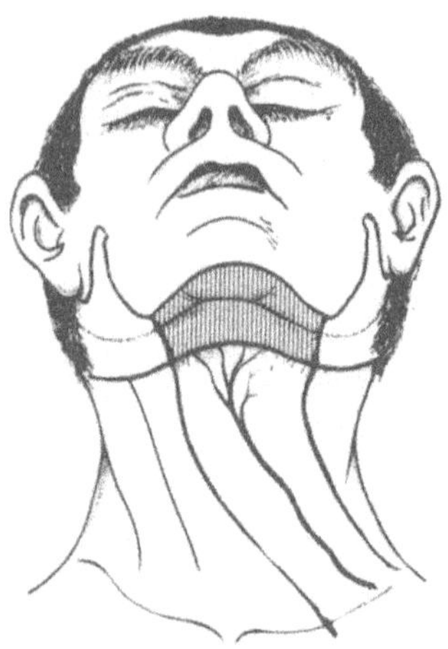

A

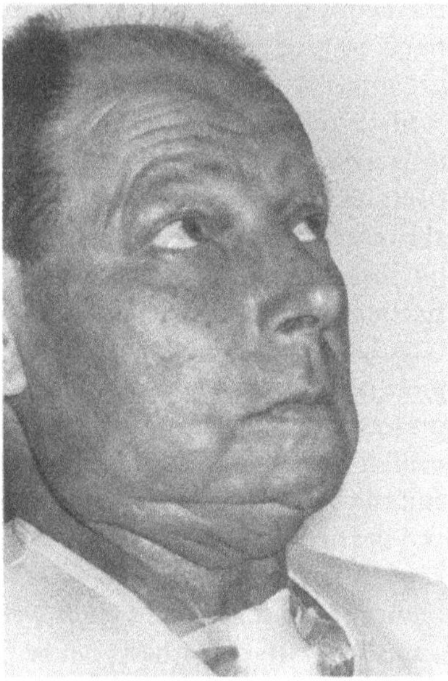

B

**Figure 8–9. A.** Replacement of the anterior mandibular arch with a composite pectoralis major myocutaneous flap containing rib: diagramatic.
**B.** Clinical photograph of a subject after replacement of anterior mandibular arch and cervical skin by a pectoralis major osteomycutaneous flap.

The successful survival of a free vascularised rib graft dependent on its periosteal blood supply has been reported by Ariyan [133]. The tremendous strides made in microvascular surgery over the past few years have found increasing application in the field of mandibular reconstruction. Ostrup and Fredrickson [134] in 1974 described the first free vascularised rib graft. Since then free vascularised osteocutaneous flaps based on dorsalis pedis and superficial circumflex artery have been successfully reported [135]. Following the work of Taylor [136], who demonstrated the superiority of a flap based on the deep circumflex iliac artery, a free vascularized ileal flap has been used increasingly with success [137,138]. Use of this flap is advantageous in that a 7- to 9-cm long vascular pedicle for anastomoses is provided and virtually half the size of the mandible can be carved out of the ileum with its adjoining muscle and skin. An immediate good vascularity of the graft overcomes the possibility of infection and necrosis. While these techniques are not free from complications and are being perfected, they shall certainly find increasing use in the future.

## 8. RECONSTRUCTION OF THE PALATE

Several methods of reconstruction of the palate by pedicle flaps were described in the past [139]. While some of these procedures succeed, they are necessarily multistaged procedures necessitating prolonged hospital stay. Guerrero-Santos [140] described tongue flaps for this purpose. The deltopectoral flap has been successfully used for palatal reconstruction after orbitomaxillary resections for cancer [141]. Delaying of the flap is advisable. A method of closing hard palate defects with flaps of nasal mucoperiosteum strengthened by fascialata and surgicel has been described by Björklund, Koch, and Pettersson [142]. Fascialata is placed into the nasal cavity. The defect in the hard palate is filled with surgicel and the substitutes are held in place by a dental plate. Surgicel stimulates fibrosis thus allowing mucosa to grow over. Closure of the anterior palate fistulas with buccal flaps and bone grafts have been reported by Lehman and his colleagues [143]. Defects of soft palate can be closed by the palatal island flap [144]. While smaller lesions may be closed by any of the above methods, larger defects are best managed by the use of prosthesis [145]. The ultimate choice of method depends on the general condition and motivation of the patient, the pathology, the degree and size of the defect, the condition of local tissues, and the experience of the surgeon concerned.

## 9. LARYNGEAL SUSPENSION

The loss of muscular attachment of the hyoid to the mandible produces an immediate lowering of the larynx in relation to the vertebral column. This is reflected in the increased possibility of aspiration, a major complication after surgery of the floor of the mouth when the elevator muscles are removed. Utilization of simple methods of laryngeal suspension reduces the risk of this complication [146,147]. The larynx is pulled upward and forward under the base of the tongue, thus decreasing pooling of saliva with overflow. Jabaley [148] described a technique of laryngeal suspension in cases with complete loss of hyomandibular complex.

## 10. POSTOPERATIVE CARE

Management of a clear airway through tracheotomy, care of nutrition of the patient, administration of suitable prophylactic antibiotics, and early ambulation are important steps in the postoperative care. Attention should be paid to the replacement of blood loss, and albumin levels should be controlled biweekly. Zinc levels have been shown to affect wound healing. The bacteriologist should be consulted from time to time before formulating an antibiotic therapy. In general no antibiotics are needed for clean and clean-contaminated wounds such as a neck dissection or a hemiglossectomy with neck dissection. For contaminated wounds and for procedures of very high magnitude requiring reconstruction and bone grafts, a broad-spectrum antibiotic administered two hours before and until 48 hours after is advisable. Early ambulation and physiotherapy help to prevent pulmonary complications. Bacterial swabs from the tracheal cannula should be done twice a week. Wound drains should be regularly checked and sent for bacteriological examination on removal. Half-hourly suction of the saliva by trained personnel prevents further aspiration and constant bathing of the wound in the immediate postoperative phase. Patients should be taught to do this by themselves as soon as they are ambulant. Oral hygiene must be strictly maintained and the wound areas regularly cleaned. No external dressings are usually necessary. Regular contact with the surgical and nursing team helps these patients maintain confidence during this critical phase.

## REFERENCES

1. Lockhart RD, Hamilton GF, Fyfe FW. Anatomy of the Human Body. London: Faber and Faber, 1959.
2. Edgerton MT. Rehabilitation of oral cavity by plastic surgery. In Proceedings of the Seventh National Cancer Conference. Philadelphia: J.B. Lippincott, p. 199, 1973.
3. Edgerton MT. Role of immediate reconstruction in treatment of head and neck cancer. In Symposium on Malignancies of the Head and Neck, Anderson R, Hoopes JE (eds). St. Louis: C.V. Mosby, pp. 169–177, 1975.
4. Harrison DFN. Problems of reconstruction following preoperative radiotherapy. Proc Roy Soc Med (67): 601–603, 1974.
5. Forrester JC. Wound healing and fibrosis. In Jamieson and Kay's Textbook of Surgical Physiology, Ledingham JMcA, MacKay C (eds). Edinburgh: Churchill Livingstone, p. 7, 1978.
6. Daniel RK, Taylor GI. Distant transfer of an island flap by microvascular anastomoses. Plast Reconstr Surg (52): 111–117, 1973.
7. McGregor I, Morgan G. Axial and random pattern flaps. Brit J Plast Surg (26): 202–213, 1973.
8. McCraw JB, Dibbel DG, Carraway JH. Clinical definition of independent myocutaneous vascular territories. Plast Reconstruc Surg (60): 341–352, 1977.
9. Jabaley ME, Orcutt TW, Clement RL. Applications of the Karapandzic principle of lip reconstruction after excision of lip cancer. Am J Surg (132): 529–532, 1976.
10. Davidson TM, Bartlow GA, Bone RC. Surgical excisions from and reconstructions of the oral lips. J Dermatol Surg Oncol (6): 134, 1980.
11. MacIntosh RB: Sliding block resection and reconstruction in cases of carcinoma of the lower lip. J Oral Surg (38): 417–423, 1980.
12. Johanson B, Aspelund E, Breine V, Holmström H. Surgical treatment of nontraumatic lower lip lesions with special reference to the step technique. Scan J Plast Reconstr Surg (8): 232–240, 1974.
13. Picoto, ADS, Oliviera ADS, Verde SF, Martins O. Management of squamous cell carcinoma of the lip. J Dermatol Surg Oncol (6): 562–566, 1980.
14. Estlander JA. Methode d'autoplastic de la joue ou d'une lèvre par un lambeau emprunté à l'autre lèvre. Rev Mens Med et Chir (1): 344, 1877.
15. Abbé R. A new plastic operation for the relief of deformity due to double hairlip. M Rec (53): 1898.
16. Stein SAW. Laebedannelse (cheiloplastik) udfört paa en ny methode. Hospitalsmeddelelser (Copenhagen) (1): 212, 1848.
17. Pagani WA, Capozzi O. Excision of a malignant neoplasm from a lower lip and reconstruction by a step technique of flaps. J Dermatol Surg Oncol 7 (2): 145–147, 1981.
18. Converse JM: The bridge flap for reconstruction of a full-thickness defect of the upper lip. Plast Reconstr Surg 57 (4): 442–44, 1976.

19. Karapandzic M. Reconstruction of lip defects by local arterial flaps. Brit J Plast Surg (27): 93–97, 1974.
20. Bernard C. Cancer de la lèvre inférieure opéré par un procédé nouveau. Bull. et mém Soc Chir Paris (3): 357, 1853.
21. Ginestet G. Reconstruction de toute la Lèvre inférieure par les lambeaux naso-génieus totaux. Revue d'odontologie et stomatologie (8): 28, 1946.
22. Freeman BS. Myoplastic modification of the Bernard cheiloplasty. Plast Reconstr Surg (21): 453–460, 1958.
23. Webster RC, Coffey RJ. Total and partial reconstruction of lower lip with innervated muscle bearing flaps. Plast Reconstr Surg (25): 360–371, 1960.
24. Fries RH. Advantages of a basic concept in lip reconstruction after tumour resection. J Max Fac Surg (1): 13–18, 1973.
25. Platz H, Werner F. Results of standardized lip repair after tumour resection. J Max Fac Surg (5): 108–114, 1977.
26. Meyer R, Shapiro DO. A technique for immediate reconstruction of the lower lip after ablation of tumour. Chir Plast (2): 1–16, 1973.
27. Jabaley ME. Reconstruction in patients with oral and pharyngeal cancer. In Current Problems in Surgery, Ravitch MM, Steichen FM (eds). Chicago: Year Book, 1977, pp. 1–65.
28. Clairment AA. Versatile karapandzic lip reconstruction. Arch Otolaryngol (103): 631–633, 1977.
29. Dieffenbach JF. Chirurgische Erfahrungen besonders über die Wiederherstellung zerstörter Theile des menschlichen Körpers nach neuen Methoden. T.C.F. Enslin, Berlin, 1829–1834.
30. Dieffenbach JF. Die operative chirurgie. FA Brockhaus. Leipzig, 1845–1848.
31. Bakamjian V. Use of tongue flaps in lower lip reconstruction. Brit J Plast Surg (17): 76–87, 1964.
32. McGregor IA. The tongue flap in lip surgery. Brit J Plast Surg (19): 253–263, 1966.
33. Jackson IT. Use of tongue flaps to resurface lip defects and close palate fistulae in children. Plast Reconstr Surg (49): 537–541, 1972.
34. Grabb WC, Myers MB. Skin Flaps. Boston: Little, Brown, 1975.
35. Pers M. Cheek flaps and partial rhinoplasty. Scand J Plast Surg (1): 37, 1967.
36. Pierce GW, O'Connor GB. A new method of reconstruction of the lip. Arch Surg (38): 317–334, 1934.
37. Meyer R, Failat ASA. New concepts in lower lip reconstruction. Head & Neck Surg (4): 240–245, 1982.
38. Gillies HD, Millard DR Jr. Principles and Art of Plastic Surgery. Boston: Little, Brown, 1957.
39. Brusati R. Reconstruction of the labial commissure by a sliding U-shaped cheek flap. J Max Fac Surg (7): 11–14, 1979.
40. Wang MKH, Converse JM, Macomber WB, Smith DW. Deformities of the lip and cheeks. In Reconstructive and Plastic Surgery, vol. II, Converse JM (ed). Philadelphia: W.B. Saunders, pp. 940–941, 1964.
41. Wilkinson TS. Tumours of the lip. In Symposium on Malignancies of the Head and Neck, Anderson R, Hoopes JE (eds). St. Louis: C.V. Mosby, p. 78, 1975.
42. Bakamjian V. A technique for primary reconstruction of the palate. Plast Reconstr Surg (31): 103–117, 1963.
43. O'Brien B. A muscle skin pedicle for total reconstruction of the lower lip. Plast Reconstr Surg (45): 395–399, 1970.
44. Owens N. A compound neck pedicle designed for the repair of massive facial defects. Plast Reconstr Surg (15): 369–398, 1955.
45. Schramm NL, Myers EN. Skin grafts in oral cavity reconstruction. Arch Otolaryngol (106): 528–532, 1980.
46. Conley J. Regional Flaps of the Head and Neck. Stuttgart: Georg Thieme, 1976.
47. Teh BT. Why do skin grafts fail? Plast Reconstr Surg (63): 323–332, 1979.
48. Bunji H. The Enzymes. New York: Academic Press, 1960.
49. Wilson GS, Miles AA. Principles of bacteriology, virology and immunity, London: Edward Arnold Co., 1975.
50. Conley JJ. The use of tongue flaps in head and neck surgery. Surgery (41): 745–751, 1957.

51. Gosserez M. Tongue the material of choice in the repair of labial substance losses. Ann Chir Plast (11): 159, 1966.
52. Chambers RG, Darrell A, Jacques MC, Mahiney MC. Tongue flaps for intraoral reconstruction. Am J Surg (118): 783–786, 1969.
53. Sessions DG, Dedo DD, Ogura JH. Tongue flap reconstruction in cancer of the oral cavity. Arch Otolaryngol (101): 166–169, 1975.
54. McGregor IA. The temporal flap in intraoral cancer. Its use in repairing the post-excisional defect. Br J Plast Surg (16): 318–335, 1963.
55. Edgerton MT, De Vito RT. Reconstructive surgery in treatment of oral pharyngeal and mandibular tumours. In Reconstructive Plastic Surgery, Converse JM (ed). Philadelphia: W.B. Saunders, pp. 981–983, 1964.
56. Davis GN, Hoopes JE. New route for passage of forehead flap to inside of mouth. Plast Reconstr Surg (47): 390, 1971.
57. McGregor IA, Reid WH. Simultaneous temporal and deltopectoral flaps for full thickness defects of the cheek. Plast Reconstr Surg (45): 326–331, 1970.
58. Shah JT. Folded forehead flap for reconstruction of full thickness defects of the cheek. Head & Neck Surg (2): 248–252, 1980.
59. Hancock DM. The repair of facial defects resulting from surgery for locally advanced buccal carcinoma. Plast Reconstr Surg (20): 117–132, 1957.
60. Prakash S, Ramakrishnan K, Ananthakrishnan N. Sternomastoid based island flap for lining after resection of oral carcinomas. Brit J Plast Surg (33): 115–118, 1980.
61. Chongehet V. Subcutaneous pedicle flaps for reconstruction of the lining of the lip and cheek. Brit J Surg (38): 38–41, 1977.
62. Becker DW. A cervicopectoral rotation flap for cheek coverage. Plast Reconstr Surg (61): 868–870, 1978.
63. Harashina T, Imai T, Wada M. The omental sandwich reconstruction for a full thickness cheek defect. Plast Reconstr Surg (64): 411–415, 1979.
64. Gabriel A. Unlined repairs of defects following oral cancer ablation. Br J Plast Surg (29): 165–169, 1976.
65. Stewart Watson J. The use of the latissimus dorsi island flap for intraoral reconstruction. Brit J Plast Surg. (35): 408–412, 1982.
66. McGregor IA. Quilted skin grafting in the mouth. Brit J Plast Surg (28): 100–102, 1975.
67. Mayer AW, Morfit HM. Reconstruction of the tongue after complications of treatment of lymph-haemagioma. Am J Surg (110): 603, 1965.
68. Washio H. Use of a pterygoid muscle sling to provide glossomimic function after total glossectomy. Plast Reconstr Surg (51): 497, 1973.
69. Matulic A, Barlovic M, Mikolji V, Viray M. Tongue reconstruction by means of the sternocleidomastoid muscle and a forehead flap. Brit J Plast Surg (31): 147–151, 1978.
70. Conley J, Sachs ME, Parke RB. The new tongue. Otolaryngol Head and Neck Surg (90): 58–68, 1982.
71. Feind CR, Cole RM. Cancer of the floor of the mouth and its lymphatic spread. Am J Surg (116): 482–486, 1968.
72. Druck NS, Lurton J. Repair of anterior floor of mouth defects. The island pedicle tongue flap. Laryngoscope (88): 1372–1377, 1978.
73. Shah JT, Cendon RA, Farr HW, Strong EW. Carcinoma of the oral cavity. Factors affecting treatment failure at the primary site and neck. Am J Surg (132): 504–507, 1976.
74. Farr HW, Goldfarb PM, Farr CM. Epidermoid carcinoma of the mouth and pharynx at Memorial Sloan-Kettering Cancer Centre 1965 to 1969. Am J Surg (140): 563–567, 1980.
75. Binnie WH. Epidemiology and etiology of oral cancer in Britain. Proc Roy Soc Med (69): 737–740, 1976.
76. Decker J, Goldstein JC. Risk factors in head and neck cancer. N Eng J Med (306): 1151–1154, 1982.
77. McCraw JB, Dibbell DG. Experimental definition of independent myocutaneous vascular territories. Plast Reconstr Surg (60): 341–352, 1977.
78. Hoopes JE. The forehead flap in intraoral reconstruction. In Symposium on Malignancies of the Head and Neck, Anderson J, Hoopes JE (eds). St. Louis: C.V. Mosby, 1975, pp. 193–195, 1975.

79. Bakamjian VY, Long M, Rigg B. Experience with the medially based deltopectoral flap in reconstructive surgery of the head and neck. Br J Plast Surg (24): 174–183, 1971.
80. Krizek TJ, Robson MC. Potential pitfalls in the use of the deltopectoral flap. Plast Reconstr Surg (59): 326–331, 1972.
81. Gingrass RP, Culf NK, Garrett WS Jr, Mladick RA. Complications with deltopectoral flap. Plast Reconstr Surg (49): 501–507, 1972.
82. Tiwari RM, Gorter H, Snow GB. Experience with the deltopectoral flap in reconstructive surgery of the head and neck. Head and Neck Surg (3): 379–383, 1981.
83. Edgerton MT, Desprez JD. Reconstruction of the oral cavity in the treatment of cancer. Plast Reconstr Surg (43): 247, 1969.
84. Zarem HA. Current concepts in reconstructive surgery in patients with cancer of the head and neck. Surg Clin North Am (51): 149, 1971.
85. Cohen IK, Theogaraj SD. Nasolabial flap reconstruction of the floor of the mouth after extirpation of oral cancer. Am J Surg (130): 479, 1975.
86. McCraw JB, Magee JWP, Kalwaic H. Uses of the trapezius and sternomastoid myocutaneous flaps in head and neck reconstruction. Plast Reconstr Surg (63): 49–57, 1979.
87. Ariyan S. One-stage reconstruction for defects of the mouth using a sternomastoid myocutaneous flap. Plast Reconstr Surg (63): 618–625, 1979.
88. Sasaki CT. The sternomastoid myocutaneous flap. Arch Otolaryngol (106): 74–76, 1980.
89. Larson DL, Goepfert H. Limitations of the sternocleidomastoid musculocutaneous flap in head and neck cancer reconstruction. Plast Reconstr Surg (70): 328–331, 1982.
90. Demargasso F, Piazza MV. Trapezius myocutaneous flap in reconstructive surgery for head and neck cancer: An original technique. Am J Surg (138): 533–536, 1979.
91. Shapiro MJ. Use of trapezius myocutaneous flaps in the reconstruction of head and neck defects. Arch Otolaryngol (107): 333–336, 1981.
92. Goodwin WJ, Rosenberg GJ. Venous drainage of the lateral trapezius muscleocutaneous island flap. Arch Otolaryngol (108): 411–413, 1982.
93. Tiwari RM, Snow GB. Role of myocutaneous flaps in reconstruction of the head and neck. J Laryngol and Otol (97): 441–458, 1983.
94. Ariyan S. The pectoralis major myocutaneous flap. A versatile flap for reconstruction in the head and neck. Plast Reconstr Surg (63): 73–81, 1979.
95. Baek S, Biller H, Krespu YP, Lawson W. The pectoralis major myocutaneous island flap for reconstruction of the head and neck. Head and Neck Surg. (1): 293–300, 1979.
96. Stell PM. Retraction of skin flaps. Clin Otolaryngol (7): 45–49, 1982.
97. Schuller DE. Limitations of the pectoralis major myocutaneous flap in head and neck cancer reconstruction. Arch Otolaryngol (106): 709–714, 1980.
98. Hodgkinson DJ. The pectoralis major myocutaneous flap for intraoral reconstruction—A word of warning. Brit J Plast Surg (35): 80–81, 1982.
99. Biller HF, Baek SM, Lawson W, Krespu YP, Blaugrund SM. Pectoralis major myocutaneous island flap in head and neck surgery. Analysis of complications. Arch Otolaryngol (107): 23–26, 1981.
100. Futrell HW, Johns ME, Edgerton MT, Cantrell RW, Fitz-Hugh GS. Platysma myocutaneous flap for intraoral reconstruction. Am J Surg (136): 504–507, 1978.
101. Cannon CR, Johns ME, Atkins JP, Keane WM, Cantrell RW. Reconstruction of the oral cavity using the platysma myocutaneous flap. Arch Otolaryngol (108): 491–494, 1982.
102. Mazzarella LA, Friedlander AH, Lebb DC. Floor of mouth reconstruction with free dorsalis pedis flap. Arch Otolaryngol (104): 38–41, 1978.
103. Panje WR, Krause CJ, Bardach J, Baker SR. Reconstruction of intraoral defects with the free groin flap. Arch Otolaryngol (103): 78–83, 1977.
104. Harii K, Ohmore K, Sekiguchi J. The free musculocutaneous flap. Plast Reconstr Surg (57): 294–303, 1976.
105. Soutar DS, Scheker LR, Tanner SB, McGregor IA. The radial forearm flap: A versatile method for intraoral reconstruction. Br J Plast Surg (36): 1–8, 1983.
106. Byars LT. Surgical management of mandible invaded by cancer. Surg Gynecol Obstet (98): 564–572, 1954.
107. Som ML, Nussbaum M. Marginal resection of the mandible with reconstruction by tongue flap for carcinoma of the floor of the mouth. Am J Surg (121): 679–683, 1971.

108. Flynn MB, Moore C. Marginal resection of the mandible in the management of squamous cancer of the floor of the mouth. Am J Surg (128): 490–493, 1974.
109. Conley JJ. The crippled oral cavity. Plast Reconstr Surg (30): 477, 1962.
110. Millard DR, Garst WP, Campbell RC, Stokley PH. Composite lower jaw reconstruction. Plast Reconstr Surg (46): 22–30, 1970.
111. Lindemann A. Bruhn's Ergebnisse aus dem Düsseldorfer Lazarett Behandlungen der Kieferschussverletzungen. Wiesbaden, p. 243, 1916.
112. Gordon S. The role of cancellous bone in plastic surgery. Surgery (20): 202, 1946.
113. Branemark PI, Lindstrom J, Hallen O, Breine U, Jeppson PH, Ohman A. Reconstruction of the defective mandible. Scand Plast Reconstr Surg (9): 116–128, 1975.
114. Salyer KE, Newsom HT, Homes R, Hahn G. Mandibular reconstruction. Am J Surg (134): 461–464, 1977.
115. Behringer WH, Schweiger JW. Mandibular replacement after resection for tumor. Laryngoscope (87): 1922–1931, 1977.
116. Adamo AK, Szal RL. Timing results and complications of mandibular reconstructive surgery. J Oral Surg (37): 755–763, 1979.
117. Benoist M. Experiences with 220 cases of mandibular recontruction. J Max Fac Surg (6): 40–49, 1978.
118. Kodsi MS, Culf NK, Hulnick SJ, Cramer LM. Reconstruction management of the mandible in treatment of head and neck cancer. In Symposium on Malignancies of the head and neck, Anderson R, Hoopes JE (eds). St. Louis: C.V. Mosby, pp. 196–210, 1975.
119. Snow GB, Kruisbrink JJ, van Slooten, EA. Reconstruction after mandibulectomy for cancer. Arch Otolaryngol (102): 207–210, 1976.
120. Lawson W, Baek SM, Loscalzo LT, Biller HF, Krespi YP. Experience with immediate and delayed mandibular reconstruction. Laryngoscope (92): 5–10, 1982.
121. Piggot TA, Logan AM: Mandibular reconstruction by "simple" bone graft. Brit J Plast Surg (36): 9–15, 1981.
122. Cuono CB, Ariyan S. Immediate reconstruction of a composite mandibular defect with a regional osteomusculocutaneous flap. Plast Reconstr Surg (65): 477–483, 1980.
123. Green MF, Gibson JR, Bryson JR, Thomson E. A one-stage correction of mandibular defects using a split sternum pectoralis major osteomusculocutaneous transfer. Brit J Plast Surg (34): 11–16, 1981.
124. Panje W, Cutting C. Trapezius osteomyocutaneous island flap for reconstruction of the anterior floor of mouth and mandible. Head and Neck Surgery (3): 66–71, 1980.
125. Barnes DR, Ossoff H, Pecaro B, Sisson G. Immediate reconstruction of mandibular defects with a composite sternocleidomastoid musculoclavicular graft. Arch Otolaryngol (107): 711–720, 1981.
126. Snyder C, Bateman JM, Davis CW, Warden GD. Mandibulo-facial restoration with live osteocutaneous flaps. Plast Reconstr Surg (45): 14–19, 1970.
127. Conley J. Use of composite flaps containing bone for major repairs in head and neck. Plast Reconstr Surg (49): 522–526, 1972.
128. Medgyeshi S. Observations of pedicled bone grafts in goats. Scand J Plast Surg (7): 110–115, 1975.
129. Brookes M. The Blood Supply of Bone, An Approach to Bone Biology. London: Butterworth, 1971.
130. Gothman L. The normal arterial pattern of the rabbits tibia. A microangiographic study. Acta Chir Scand (120): 211–220, 1960.
131. Rhinelander FW. The normal microcirculation of a diaphysial cortex and its response to fracture. J Bone Joint Surg Am (50): 784–800, 1968.
132. Cohen J, Harris WH. The three-dimensional anatomy of haversian systems. J Bone Joint Surg (40a): 419, 1958.
133. Ariyan S. The viability of rib grafts transplanted with the periosteal blood supply. Plast Reconstr Surg (65): 140–151, 1980.
134. Ostrup LT, Fredrickson JM. Distant transfer of a free living bone graft by microvascular anastomosis. Plast Reconstr Surg (54): 274–285, 1974.
135. Rosen IB, Bell MSG, Barron PT, Zuker RM, Manktelow RT. Use of microvascular flaps including free osteocutaneous flaps in reconstruction after composite resection for radiation recurrent oral cancer. Am J Surg (138): 544–549, 1978.

136. Taylor GL, Townsend P, Corlett R. Superiority of the deep circumflex iliac vessels as the supply for free groin flap. Plast Reconstr Surg (64): 745, 1979.
137. Franklin JD, Shack RB, Stone JD, Madden JJ, Lynch JB. Single-stage reconstruction of mandibular and soft tissue defects using a free osteocutaneous groin flap. Am J Surg (140): 492–498, 1980.
138. Salibian AH, Rappaport I, Furnas DW, Achauer BM. Microvascular reconstruction of the mandible. Am J Surg (140): 499–502, 1980.
139. Edgerton MT Jr, Zovickian A. Reconstruction of major defects of the palate. Plast Reconstr Surg (17): 105–128, 1956.
140. Guerrero-Santos J, Altamirano JT. The use of lingual flaps in repair of fistulas of the hard palate. Plast Reconstr Surg (38): 123–128, 1966.
141. Bakamjian VY, Poole M. Maxillofacial and palatal reconstructions with the deltopectoral flap. Brit J Plast Surg (39): 17–37, 1977.
142. Björklund A, Koch HJ, Pettersson KI. A new method for strengthening palatal closure defects of the hard palate. Acta Otolaryngol (82): 147–150, 1976.
143. Lehman JA, Curtin P, Mass DG. Closure of anterior palate fistulae. Cleft Palate J (15): 33–38, 1978.
144. Millard R Jr, Seider HA. The versatile palatal island flap. Its use in soft palate reconstruction and nasopharyngeal and choanal atresia. Br J Plast Surg (3): 300–305, 1977.
145. Conley J. Concepts in Head and Neck Surgery. Stuttgart: Georg Thieme Verlag, 1970.
146. Edgerton MT, McKee DM. Reconstruction with loss of hyomandibular complex in excision of large cancers. Arch Surg (78): 425–436, 1959.
147. Goode RL. Laryngeal suspension in head and neck surgery. Laryngoscope (86): 349–355, 1976.
148. Jabaley ME, Hoopes JE. A simple technique for laryngeal suspension after partial or complete resection of the hyomandibular complex. Am J Surg (118): 685–690, 1969.

# 9. PROSTHETIC REHABILITATION AND DENTAL CARE

S.E.W. ENGELS

## 1. INTRODUCTION

Dentists, prosthodontists, and dental hygienists may play an important role in the care of patients with an oral malignancy. Before any type of treatment is instituted, the patient should be seen by a dentist or prosthodontist who is acquainted with the specific problems related to the treatment of oral cancer. Additionally, establishing a good relationship at this stage is extremely helpful both for the patient and the dentist. The patient's own dentist should be contacted and correctly informed when dental treatment is required.

Caries and periodontal disease have to be taken care of adequately before therapy, whether surgical or radiological, is instituted. The type of dental restorations required depends partly on the dental mindedness of the patient and on the costs involved in such a treatment. Besides, time can be a limiting factor, especially in case of a fast-growing tumor. In any case, periapical inflammations should be eliminated either by endodontic treatment or by extraction. Root remnants and impacted teeth should be removed as well, especially when radiotherapy is anticipated in the course of treatment of an oral tumor in order to minimize the risk of osteoradionecrosis of the jaw bones. If extractions or surgical removal of teeth are necessary, a time interval of two weeks should be allowed in case of primary treatment by radiotherapy. In the

*I. van der Waal and G.B. Snow (eds), ORAL ONCOLOGY.* 

**Table 9–1.** The results of 58 consecutive patients in whom reconstruction was initially planned

| Results | No. of cases |
|---|---|
| Good oral functions, good to satisfactory cosmetic appearance. | 30 |
| No functional denture can be worn, but the appearance is acceptable. | 5 |
| The patient could not face further surgery after the initial resection. | 3 |
| Radiotherapy and/or persistent infection precluded grafting procedures. | 3 |
| Reconstruction abandoned because of locoregional recurrence and/or distant metastasis. | 11 |
| Postoperative death after resection. | 5 |
| Intercurrent death, N.E.D. | 1 |
| total | 58 |

From reference 5.

presence of an ulcerative oral malignancy, extraction or surgical removal of teeth is a debatable procedure because of the risk of contamination of the wound with tumor cells. This may lead to compromises, in most cases resulting in postponed dental treatment.

All patients, including those who wear dentures, should be instructed to maintain proper oral hygiene. For dentate patients who will receive radiotherapy, a dental hygienist is extremely helpful in maintaining a good oral hygiene. Another important measurement is the regular application of fluorides during and after radiotherapy.

In patients who will be treated by surgery in which the jaws are involved, preoperative casts of dental stone are made and a proper bite registration is performed for the construction of an immediate surgical resection splint. In case of surgical treatment, the extent of the procedure should be thoroughly discussed with the prosthodontist well in advance (see table 9–1).

## 2. RESECTION OF THE MAXILLA

In case of a superficial defect in the palate or the alveolar ridge, leaving the bone intact, a splint may be used to hold the dressing of the wound in its position. The dressing can be either a split skin or just a WHV gauze, as shown below:

Pig. Iodof. Co., Whitehead's Varnish:

| | |
|---|---|
| Benzoin, sumatra in coarse powder | 44 gr |
| Prepared storax | 33 gr |
| Balsam of Tolu | 22 gr |
| Jodoform | 44 gr |
| Solvent ether | to 1 fl. oz. |

When it is not possible to have a separate resection splint made, one may use the patient's denture, if he or she has one, for that purpose. However, it should be realized that dentures do not always fit properly and that such dentures, when used for fixation of some weeks' duration, may cause damage to the oral mucous membranes. In case of a very small bare surface of a few square centimeters, the wound may even be left uncovered. Granulation and secondary epithelialization will than take place in a matter of weeks.

Resection of the maxilla, however, will almost always result in a communication with the nasal cavity and/or the maxillary sinus. Although in some cases closure of such a defect with a pedicle flap is possible, most oncologic surgeons prefer to use a prosthetic appliance instead. This appliance will allow proper inspection of the field of surgery during follow-up.

A surgical resection splint is made of acrylic and will further be adapted to the defect with a thermoplastic material such as gutta-percha. For the retention of the gutta-percha to the splint, extensions of stainless steel wire 1.0 mm in diameter are partially embedded in the acrylic material of the splint. Another possibility consists of making multiple 2- to 3-mm perforations in the splints. In adapting the splint with gutta-percha, one should try to create an extension into the cheek(s), which will later on provide an undercut for retention of the final prosthetic appliance. The size of the adapted resection splint can be a problem if it is too large to remove from the mouth in one piece. In such instances a two-piece splint has to be made. It is also possible to pack the upper part of the maxillary defect with a WHV gauze. Prior to insertion of such a WHV gauze, any excess of medicament should be removed by squeezing the gauze thoroughly. It can usually be left in situ for several weeks without any adverse reactions.

The resection splint may also serve to accommodate a split skin graft (figures 9–1 to 9–5). This is an important function of the splint since it prevents the formation of a hematoma underneath the skin graft. Also, contraction of soft tissues is made impossible. When enough teeth are left in the maxilla, the resection splint can be attached to those teeth with clasps, or wires around the teeth, to allow easy removal. When no teeth are present, two 0.5 mm stainless steel circumzygomatic suspension wires are usually sufficient for fixation of the splint in position for at least some weeks. When the zygomatic arch has been removed, the wire may be passed through a hole drilled in the zygomatic process of the frontal bone.

The soft palate, if still intact, and the buccal mucosa can be attached with sutures to the borders of the resection splint. For that purpose holes can be drilled in the splint or special loops of stainless steel wire, embedded in the acrylic splint, can be applied. It is important to assure that the maxillary splint does not interfere with the normal movements of the mandible. Removal of the coronoid process together with a generous portion of the temporalis muscle eliminates a source of postoperative limitation of the mandibular movement [7]. Also recommended is the removal of the pterygoid plates and the

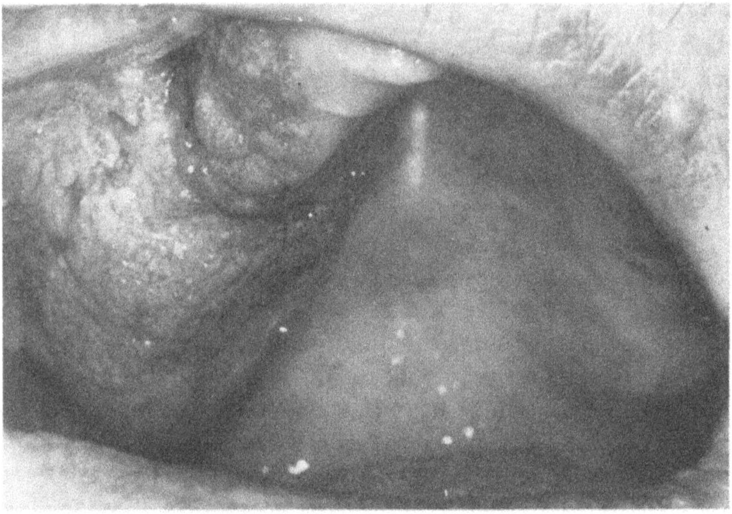

**Figure 9–1.** Squamous cell carcinoma of the right side of the maxilla in a 62-year-old man.

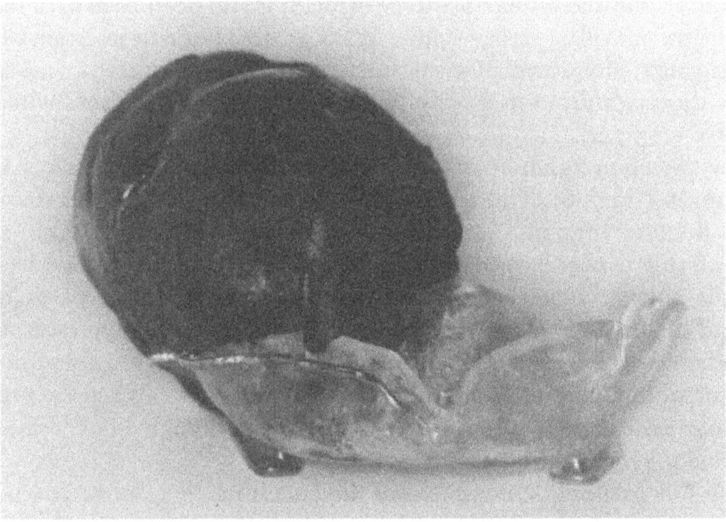

**Figure 9–2.** Splint for partial maxillectomy with bollards for the circumzygomatic wires and loops for fixation of the buccal mucosa. The splint is built up with gutta-percha and can now be covered with the skin graft.

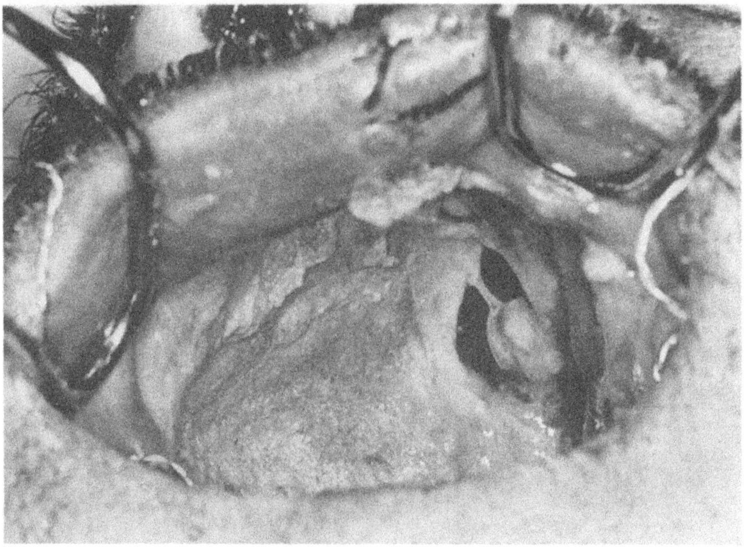

**Figure 9–3.** Surgical defect two weeks postoperatively, immediately upon removal of the surgical splint.

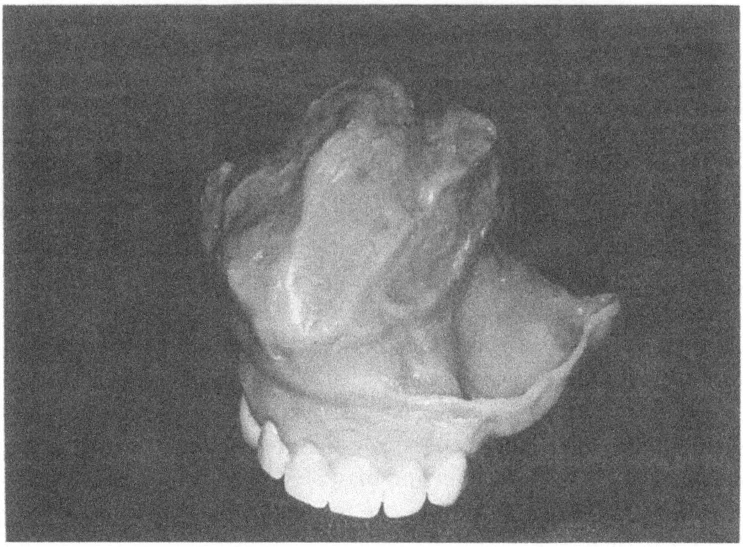

**Figure 9–4.** Semipermanent denture. In the final stage molar teeth will also be placed.

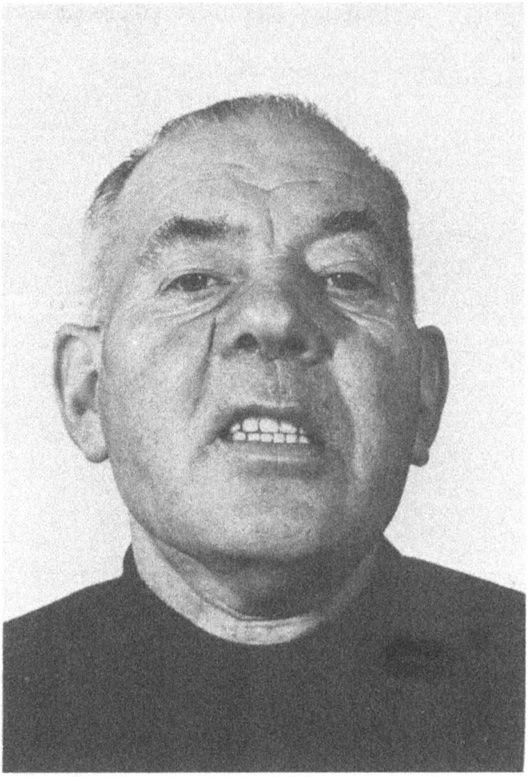

**Figure 9–5.** Postoperative picture three months after surgery with the dentures in place.

medial and lateral pterygoid muscles at their attachment since those structures are a source of postoperative limitation of movement as well. Apart from the patient's inability to close the mouth properly, overextension of the splint may exert pressure to the ramus of the mandible, which may cause local necrosis or even osteomyelitis. Ideally, the adaptation of the resection splint in the theatre should be done by the prosthodontist, who also will take care of the preparation of the final prosthetic appliance.

Removal of the resection splint can safely take place after 10 days. If possible, it should be done under general anesthesia since the removal of the splint at this stage can be quite difficult and may be very painful for the patient. The circumzygomatic suspension wires are untwisted but left in place for reuse. The splint can then be removed to allow proper inspection and cleaning of the surgical defect. If necessary, the splint is readapted with gutta-percha, and an impression of the splint is made in alginate. From this impression a temporary appliance is made in acrylic. Having such a temporary appliance of exactly the same shape is very helpful in the further management of the patient. At no time should the splint be left out of the mouth for more than 30 minutes since contraction of the skin graft occurs rapidly [7].

About one to two weeks after the first inspection of the wound, the resection splint can usually be replaced by the duplicated splint or by a temporary appliance, which in case of a large defect is made hollow in order to reduce the weight as much as possible. At this time it should be possible to remove the suspension wires. This can usually be done without any type of anesthesia. When the patient has undergone radiotherapy in the maxillary region, prophylactic administration of antibiotics is mandatory when removing the circumzygomatic wires, since in radiated areas chronic inflammation along the pathway of the wires may lead to a persistent inflammation and even necrosis of the skin.

Further description of the preparation of the final prosthetic treatment is beyond the scope of this book [1,2].

### 3. RESECTION OF THE MANDIBLE

In case of marginal resection of the mandible, usually no surgical splint is necessary, although one may consider the application of intermaxillary fixation for some weeks. However, when the thickness of the remaining mandibular bone is less than 1 cm, a secondary fracture is likely to occur in the course of time. Therefore, the rationale of a marginal resection is determined not only by considerations of an oncologic nature, but also by the clinical judgment of whether the remaining mandibular bone will be strong enough to withstand the chewing forces and whether it will be possible to prepare a lower denture.

When the continuity of the mandible has to be sacrificed, a resection splint is needed, irrespective of the type of reconstruction, being primary or secondary or not aimed for at all. In dentate patients the upper and lower teeth can be splinted in the usual way, taking care of the correct occlusion of the upper and lower teeth. In edentulous patients usually a monobloc type of device is constructed and kept in place by peralveolar or circumzygomatic and perimandibular wires around the remaining part(s) of the mandible. A monobloc has the advantage of optimal stabilization of the fragment(s) of the lower jaw. It has a disadvantage when a temporary opening of the mouth is needed for inspection. Immobilisation of the remaining part(s) of the mandible will facilitate proper wound healing of the soft tissues and will prevent a disfiguring deviation of the remaining mandibular bone.

When secondary reconstruction of the mandible is envisaged, the intermaxillary fixation is maintained (figures 9–6 to 9–11). Reconstruction of the mandible with an iliac bone graft (see chapter 8) is usually carried out three months after the resection of the tumor, when the local tissue reactions have sufficiently subsided. Intermaxillary fixation is left in place until there is sufficient clinical and radiological evidence of continuity of bone. This usually takes two to three months. In case of postoperative radiotherapy in a patient

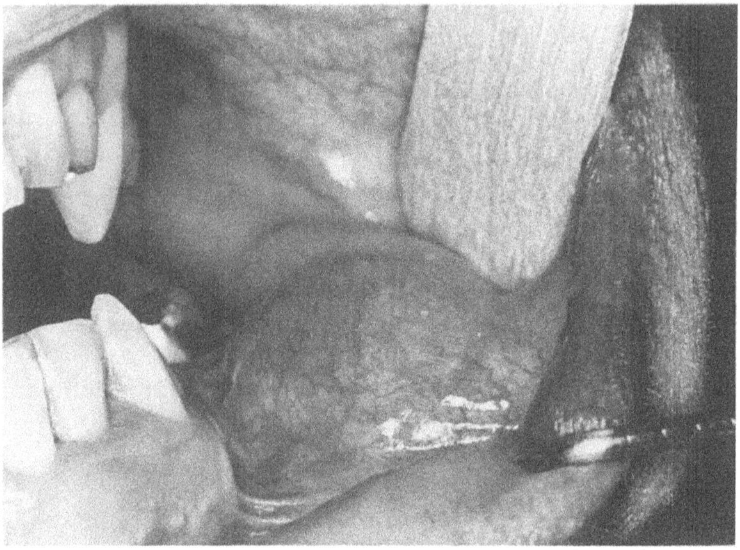

**Figure 9–6.** Juxtacortical osteogenic sarcoma of the left part of the mandible in a 40-year-old man.

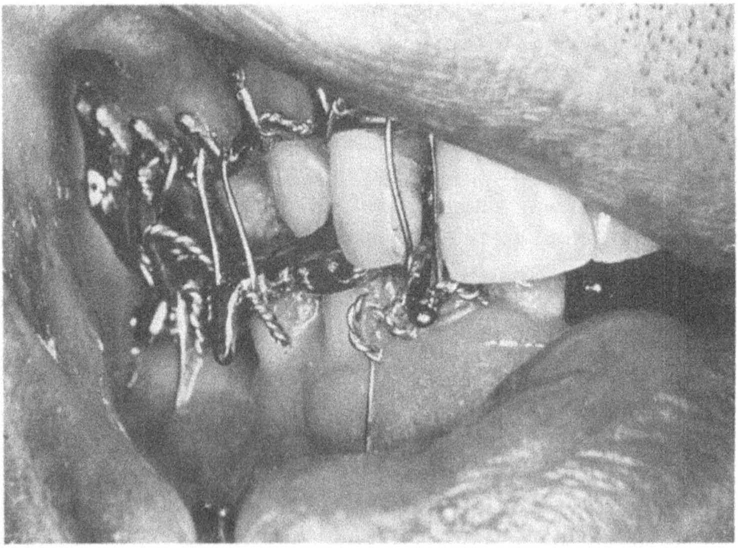

**Figure 9–7.** After a left hemimandibulectomy had been performed, the right side of the mandible was immobilized using intermaxillary fixation. Three months later a reconstruction was carried out.

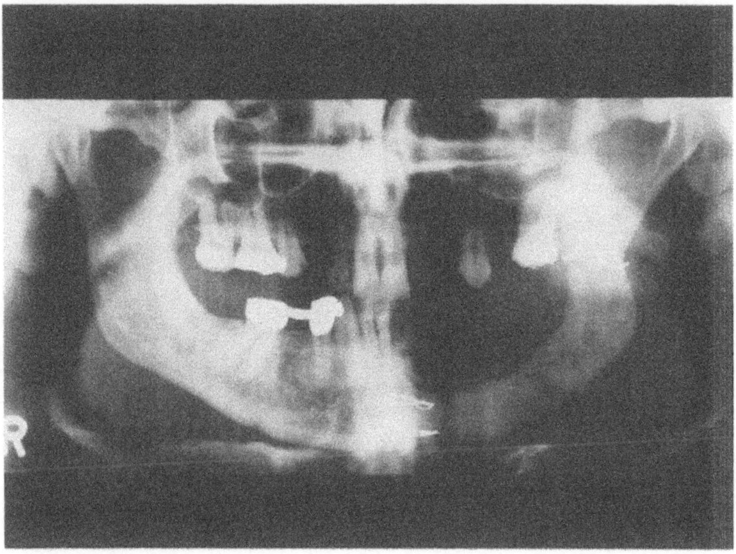


**Figure 9–8.** Same patient from figures 9–6 and 9–7 three months after reconstruction with bone from the iliac crest. At this stage a buccal-inlay procedure was required.

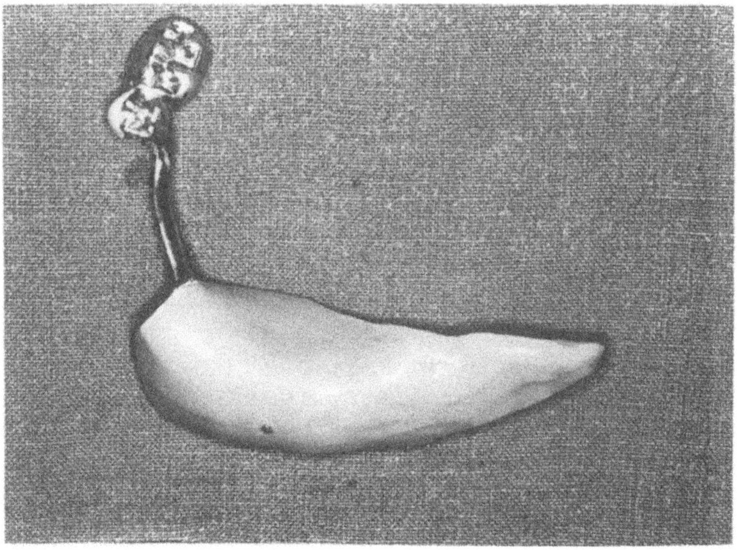

**Figure 9–9.** A temporary splint was made after completion of the preprosthetic procedure.

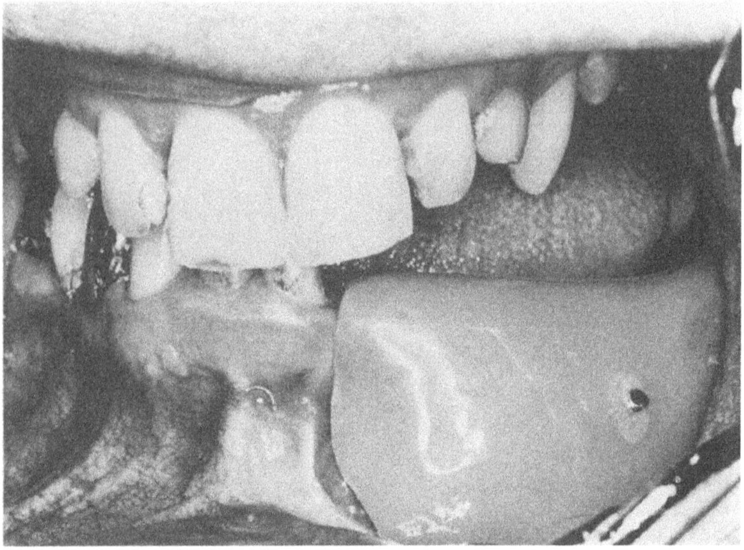

**Figure 9–10.** Appliance from figure 9–9 in place. In the final stage teeth will be adapted to this partial denture.

who needs a secondary reconstruction of the mandible, the intermaxillary fixation is maintained during the time of radiotherapy and until two to three months after reconstruction has taken place. When such a fixation is applied for a total period of five to six months, a vigorous oral hygiene program is required to prevent infection along the circumzygomatic and perimandibular wires.

Reconstruction of the bony part of the mandible also must always be followed by intraoral adaptation of the soft tissues around the bone graft in order to create sufficient room for a lower denture. Such a preprosthetic procedure can be performed as soon as there is evidence of a successful union of the bony graft, usually two to three months after reconstruction. However, it is advisable to allow a somewhat longer period between the bone grafting and the preprosthetic surgery. In most cases a vestibuloplasty is done, together with a reconstruction of a part of the floor of the mouth. The successful use of split thickness skin grafts over supraperiosteal dissections has been well documented in the literature.

When no reconstruction of the mandible is planned, the appliance can be removed after some weeks. In general, the patient will be able to have reasonable control of jaw movements, accept for some deviation of the chin. Dentate patients often manage to eat reasonably well with their remaining teeth. In edentulous patients it is usually very difficult or even impossible to

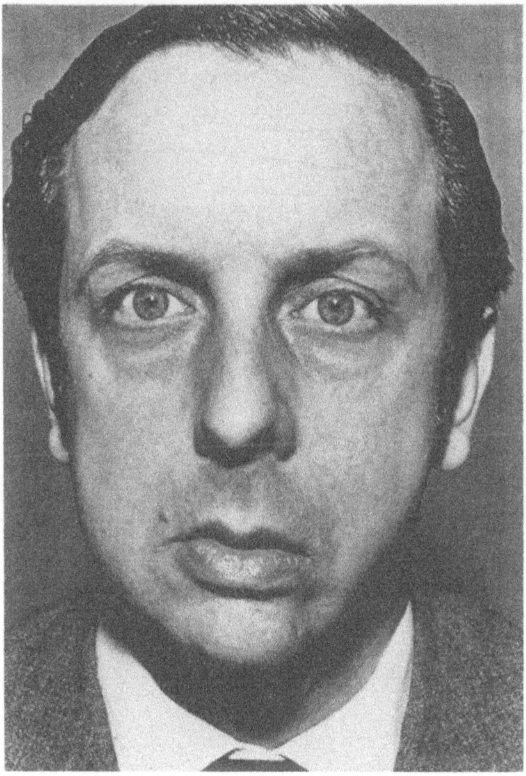

**Figure 9–11.** Extraoral view after completion of mandibular reconstruction.

make a lower denture in a partial resected mandible. Therefore, reconstruction of the mandible is aimed for in most cases.

#### 4. RESECTION OF THE TONGUE AND THE FLOOR OF THE MOUTH

Resections of the tongue and the floor of the mouth usually do not require the use of a surgical splint. Depending on the loss of tissue and the use of flaps, preprosthetic surgery—consisting of lowering of the floor of the mouth, mobilizing of the tongue, and deepening of the mandibular vestibule—may be required in edentulous patients to enable the accommodation of a lower denture. Such a surgical correction should not be done within three months after the surgical removal of the tumor to allow the tissues to heal properly. In patients who have received postoperative radiotherapy, even a longer period should be observed. The final result of a resection of part of the tongue or floor of the mouth is usually quite acceptable in dentate patients from a functional point of view. This is not always the case in edentulous patients, even when a

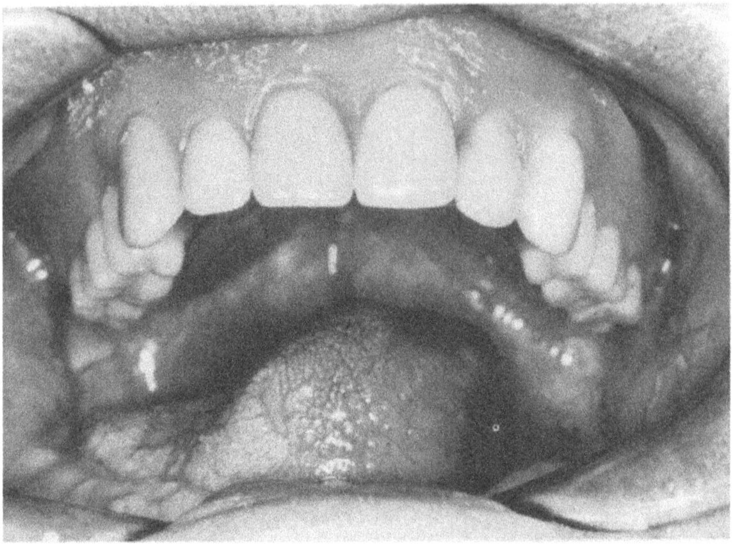

**Figure 9–12.** After tongue resection the volume of the tongue is insufficient to fill up the oral cavity.

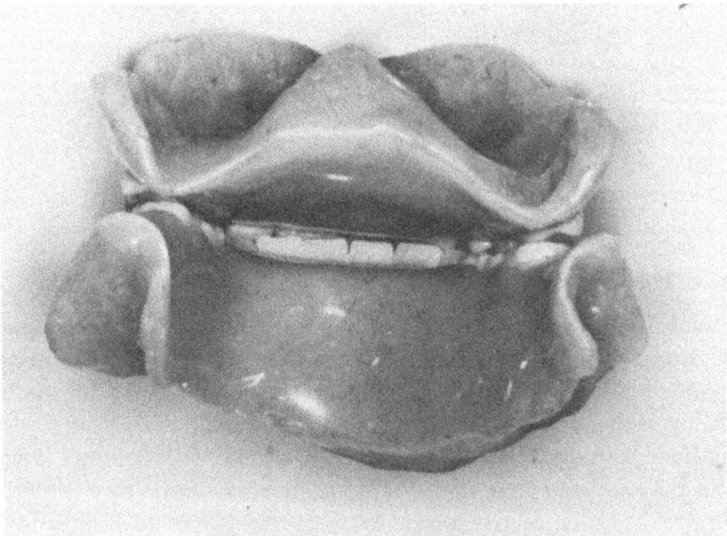

**Figure 9–13.** Adaptation of the upper denture because of diminished tongue volume and movement.

full set of dentures has been prepared. Some patients use their dentures just for esthetic reasons, being able to speak and to eat better without them. Improvement may be obtained by adapting the lingual surface of the upper denture to the movements of the tongue (figures 9–12 and 9–13). In the literature even the successful use of a tongue prosthesis after total glossectomy has been reported [6].

## 5. RESECTION OF FACIAL STRUCTURES

Since the contents of this book are focused upon tumors of the oral cavity, the possibilities of prosthetic reconstruction of structures such as the nose, the eyes, or the ears will not be discussed here.

## REFERENCES

1. Beumer J, Curtis ThA, Firtell DN. Maxillofacial Rehabilitation, Prosthodontic and Surgical Considerations. St. Louis: C.V. Mosby, 1979.
2. Chalian VA, Drane JB, Standish SM. Maxillofacial Prosthetics. Baltimore: Williams & Wilkins, 1971.
3. Conroy B, Bowforman J. Maxillofacial Prosthetics in Oral Surgery. London: Butterworth, 1980.
4. Rahon AO, Boucher LJ. Maxillofacial Prosthetics, Principles and Concepts. Philadelphia: W.B. Saunders, 1970.
5. van Slooten EA, Snow GB, Kruisbrink JJ. The place of reconstruction of the lower jaw in the treatment of oral cancer. In Tumoren im Kiefer-Gesichts-Bereich, Pape K (ed). Leipzig: Johann Ambrosius Barth, pp. 96–100, 1980.
6. de Souza LJ, Martins OJ. Swallowing and speech after radical total glossectomy with tongue prosthesis. Oral Surg (39): 356–360, 1975.
7. Towers JF. Some essentials for rehabilitation following maxillectomy. In Tumoren im Kiefer-Gesichts-Bereich, Pape K (ed). Leipzig: Johann Ambrosius Barth, 102–105, 1980.

# INDEX

GPSR Compliance
The European Union's (EU) General Product Safety Regulation (GPSR) is a set of rules that requires consumer products to be safe and our obligations to ensure this.

If you have any concerns about our products, you can contact us on

ProductSafety@springernature.com

In case Publisher is established outside the EU, the EU authorized representative is:

Springer Nature Customer Service Center GmbH
Europaplatz 3
69115 Heidelberg, Germany

www.ingramcontent.com/pod-product-compliance
Ingram Content Group UK Ltd.
Pitfield, Milton Keynes, MK11 3LW, UK
UKHW020238160926
475610UK00001B/40
* 9 7 8 1 4 6 1 2 9 7 9 6 3 *